IRON METABOLISM

Edited by **Sarika Arora**

Iron Metabolism
Edited by Sarika Arora

Published by InTech
Janeza Trdine 9, 51000 Rijeka, Croatia

Publishing Process Manager Masa Vidovic

Technical Editor Teodora Smiljanic

Cover Designer InTech Design Team

Additional hard copies can be obtained from orders@intechopen.com

Iron Metabolism, Edited by Sarika Arora
p. cm.
ISBN 978-953-51-0605-0

For EU product safety concerns:
IN TECH d.o.o., Prolaz Marije Krucifikse Kozulić 3, 51000 Rijeka, Croatia,
info@intechopen.com or visit our website at intechopen.com.

Meet the editor

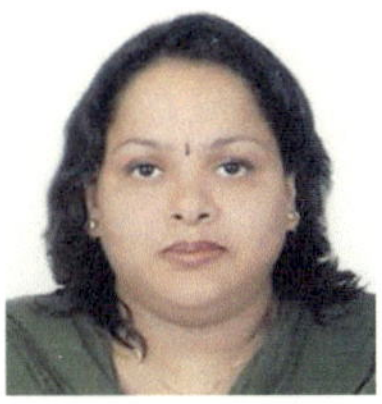

Dr Sarika Arora is currently working as an Associate Professor in the Department of Biochemistry, ESI Post-graduate Institute of Medical Sciences & Research, New Delhi, India. She has done her graduation and M.D. in Biochemistry from Lady Hardinge Medical College, New Delhi. She has also worked in Gobind Ballabh Pant Hospital and Lady Hardinge Medical College as Assistant Professor. She has more than ten years of teaching and research experience and more than forty publications in national and international journals. Her areas of expertise are mainly Iron metabolism, Insulin resistance, neuropeptides and studies on cardiovascular risk factors.

Contents

Preface

Iron is the most abundant element on earth representing nearly 90% of the mass in the earth's core, yet only trace elements are present in living cells. Most of the iron in the body is located within the porphyrin ring of heme, which is incorporated into proteins such as hemoglobin, myoglobin, cytochromes, catalases and peroxidases. Although iron appears in a variety of oxidation states, in particular as hexavalent ferrate, the ferrous and ferric forms are of most importance. The transition from ferrous to ferric iron and vice versa occurs readily, meaning that Fe(II) acts as a reducing agent and Fe(III) as an oxidant. Iron is closely involved with the metabolism of oxygen in a variety of biochemical processes. Iron, as either heme or in its "nonheme" form, plays an important role in cell growth and metabolism because of its involvement in key reactions of DNA synthesis and energy production.

However, low solubility of iron in body fluids and the ability to form toxic hydroxyl radicals in presence of oxygen make iron uptake, use and storage a serious challenge. Iron metabolism in complex organisms involves two levels of regulation. The lower level is cellular and comprises the mechanisms of cellular uptake and storage as well as the intracellular use of iron in enzymes. In this regard, two principles effectively control iron uptake, the use of cell surface receptors for iron-containing proteins or direct iron import by metal transporters. This aspect has been studied in detail during the last three decades with a special focus on the mechanisms and regulation of receptor-mediated cellular iron uptake and storage. In contrast, the knowledge about the upper level of iron metabolism, the systemic level, was inadequate up to the end of the last century. This involves various unsolved questions pertaining to the regulation of intestinal iron uptake, various signalling pathways involved in the iron demand of individual cells and how these signals are transmitted to the iron stores and the intestine. The discovery of new metal transporters, receptors and peptides and as well as the discovery of new cross-interactions between known proteins are now leading to a breakthrough in the understanding of systemic iron metabolism. The objective of this book is to review and summarize recent developments in our understanding of iron transport and storage in living systems and how iron metabolism may be affected in anemias associated with chronic diseases and hemodialysis patients. It begins with a focus on normal systemic iron metabolism in humans focusing on the role of various iron containing proteins and the mechanisms involved in iron absorption and utilization. It then progresses to a detailed review on Cellular Iron metabolism with a special focus on the IRP/IRE regulatory network. One of the major roles of iron is in erythropoiesis which has been appropriately covered in one of the chapters. Though the emphasis is on human iron metabolism in physiological and pathological states, further knowledge is derived from the chapter on iron metabolism in pathogenic trypanosomes. These parasites have developed distinct strategies to scavenge efficiently iron from the surrounding medium and support their metabolic needs, which differ between trypanosomatid species and life stages.

This book provides knowledge about iron metabolism and related diseases in 6 coordinated Chapters which can also be read as stand-alone. The new and essential path breaking insights into iron metabolism have been addressed in this book. Together with the efforts of experienced and committed authors who spent their time and fundamentally contributed to the success of this book, I hope that a number of readers will enjoy the review Chapters and find a lot of information to develop new ideas in this rapidly ongoing field of investigation.

Dr Sarika Arora
Department of Biochemistry
ESI Postgraduate Institute of Medical Sciences & Research
Basaidarapur, New Delhi
India

Section 1

Systemic Iron Metabolism in Physiological States

1

Iron Metabolism in Humans: An Overview

Sarika Arora and Raj Kumar Kapoor
Department of Biochemistry, ESI Postgraduate Institute of Medical Sciences, Basaidarapur, New Delhi, India

1. Introduction

Iron is the most abundant element on earth, yet only trace elements are present in living cells. The four major reasons leading to limited availability of iron in living cells despite environmental abundance would be:

1. When iron was available some 10 billion years ago, it was available as Fe (II), but Fe (II) is not a very strong Lewis acid. Thus, it does not bind strongly to most small molecules or activate them strongly toward reaction.
2. Today iron is not readily available from sea or water solutions due to oxidation and hydrolysis.
3. Iron in ferrous state is not easily retained by proteins since it does not bind very strongly to them.
4. Free Fe (II) is mutagenic, especially in the presence of dioxygen.

To overcome, the above problems with availability of iron, specific ligands have evolved for its transport and storage because of its limited solubility at near neutral pH under aerobic conditions [1].

Iron is involved in many enzymatic reactions of a cell; hence it is believed that the presence of iron was obligatory for the evolution of aerobic life on earth. Furthermore, the propensity of iron to catalyze the oxygen radicals in aerobic and facultative anaerobic species indicates that the intracellular concentration and chemical form of the element must be kept under tight control.

2. Overview of iron metabolism

2.1 Oxidation states

The common oxidation states are either ferrous (Fe^{2+}) or ferric (Fe^{3+}); higher oxidation levels occur as short-lived intermediates in certain redox processes. Iron has affinity for electronegative atoms such as oxygen, nitrogen and sulfur, which provide the electrons that form the bond with iron, hence these atoms are found at the heart of the iron-binding centers of macromolecules. When favorably oriented on the macromolecules, these anions can bind iron with high affinity. During formation of complexes, no bonding electrons are derived from iron. The non bonding electrons in the outer shell of iron (the incompletely filled *3d* orbitals) can exist in two states. When bonding interactions with iron are weak, the outer non-bonding electrons will avoid pairing and distribute throughout the *3d* orbitals. When bonding electrons interact strongly with iron, there will be pairing of the outer non-bonding electrons, favoring lower energy *3d* orbitals. These two different distributions for each oxidation state of iron can be determined by electron spin resonance measurements. Dispersion of *3d* electrons to all orbitals leads to the high-spin state, whereas restriction of *3d* electrons to lower energy orbitals, because of electron pairing, leads to a low-spin state.

3. Distribution and function

The total body iron in an adult male is 3000 to 4000 mg. In contrast, the average adult woman has only 2000-3000 mg of iron in her body. This difference may be attributed to much smaller iron reserves in women, lower concentration of hemoglobin and a smaller vascular volume than men.

Iron is distributed in six compartments in the body.

i. Hemoglobin

Iron is a key functional component of this oxygen transporting molecule. About 65% to 70% total body iron is found in heme group of hemoglobin. A heme group consists of iron (Fe^{2+}) ion held in a heterocyclic ring, known as aporphyrin. This porphyrin ring consists of four pyrrole molecules cyclically linked together (by methene bridges) with the iron ion bound in the center [Figure 1] [2]. The nitrogen atoms of the pyrrole molecules form coordinate covalent bonds with four of the iron's six available positions which all lie in one plane. The iron is bound strongly (covalently) to the globular protein via the imidazole ring of the F8 histidine residue (also known as the proximal histidine) below the porphyrin ring. A sixth position can reversibly bind oxygen by a coordinate covalent bond, completing the

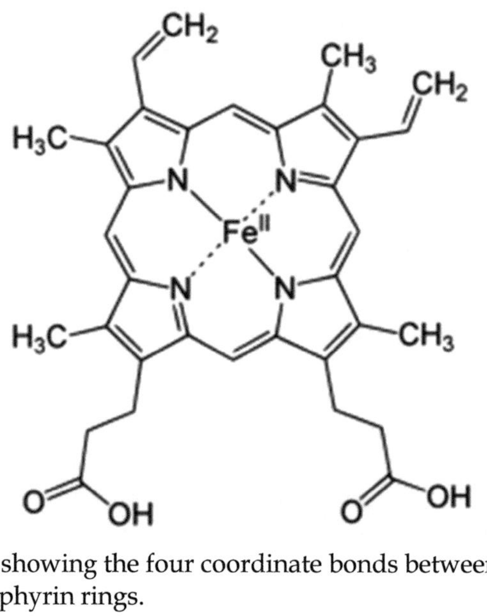

Fig. 1. Structure of heme showing the four coordinate bonds between ferrous ion and four nitrogen bases of the porphyrin rings.

octahedral group of six ligands [Figure 2]. This site is empty in the nonoxygenated forms of hemoglobin and myoglobin. Oxygen binds in an "end-on bent" geometry where one oxygen atom binds Fe and the other protrudes at an angle. When oxygen is not bound, a very weakly bonded water molecule fills the site, forming a distorted octahedron.

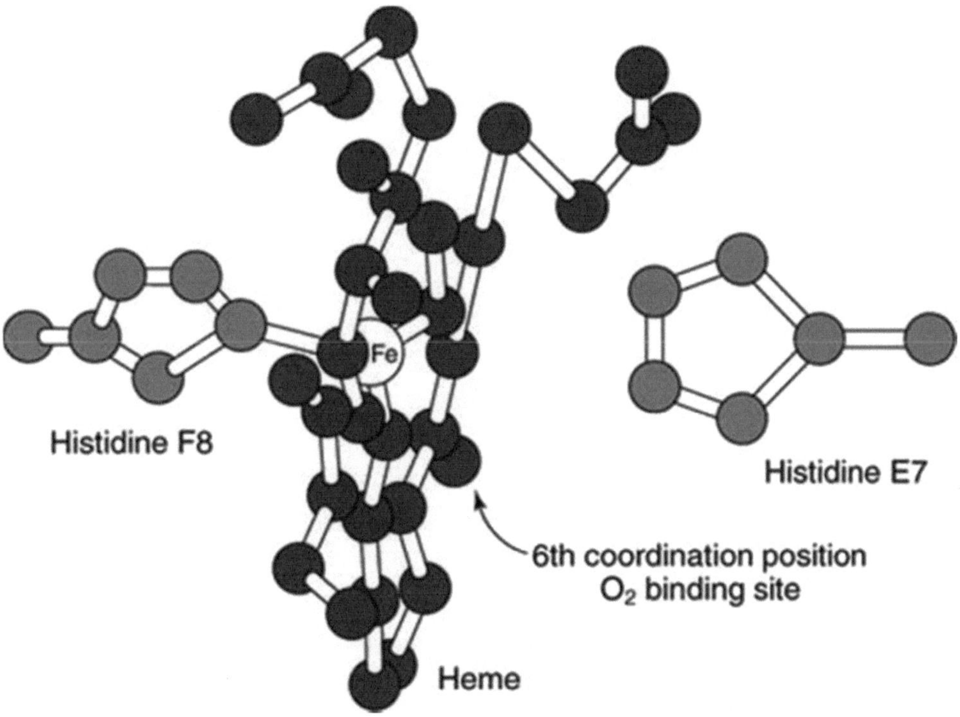

Fig. 2. Structure of heme showing the square planar tetrapyrrole along with the proximal and the distal histidine.

Even though carbon dioxide is also carried by hemoglobin, it does not compete with oxygen for the iron-binding positions, but is actually bound to the protein chains of the structure. The iron ion may be either in the Fe^{2+} or in the Fe^{3+} state, but ferrihemoglobin also called methemoglobin (Fe^{3+}) cannot bind oxygen [3]. In binding, oxygen temporarily and reversibly oxidizes (Fe^{2+}) to (Fe^{3+}) while oxygen temporarily turns into superoxide, thus iron must exist in the +2 oxidation state to bind oxygen. If superoxide ion associated to Fe^{3+} is protonated the hemoglobin iron will remain oxidized and incapable to bind oxygen. In such cases, the enzyme methemoglobin reductase will be able to eventually reactivate methemoglobin by reducing the iron center.

ii. Storage Iron- Ferritin and Hemosiderin

Ferritin is the major protein involved in the storage of iron. The protein consists of an outer polypeptide shell (also termed apoferritin) composed of 24 symmetrically placed protein chains (subunits), the average outside diameter is approximately 12.0 nm in hydrated state. The inner core (approximately 6.0 nm) contains an electron-dense and chemically inert inorganic ferric "iron-core" made of ferric oxyhydroxyhydroxide phosphate [$(FeOOH)_8(FeO\text{-}OPO_3H_2)$]. [Figure 3]. The ferritins are extremely large proteins (450kDa)

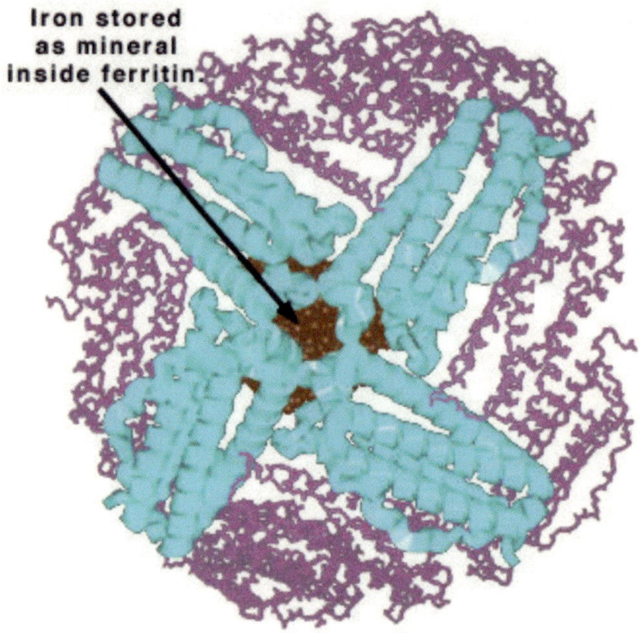

Fig. 3. Structure of ferritin showing the outer polypeptide shell with inner iron-core containing iron stored as mineral –ferric oxyhydroxyhydroxide phosphate $[(FeOOH)_8 (FeO\text{-}OPO_3H_2)]$.

which can store upto 4500 iron atoms as hydrous ferric oxide. The ratio of iron to polypeptide is not constant, since the protein has the ability to gain and release iron according to physiological needs. Channels from the surface permit the accumulation and release of iron. All iron-containing organisms including bacteria, plants, vertebrates and invertebrates have ferritin [4,5].

Ferritin from humans, horses, pigs and rats and mice consists of two different types of subunits- H subunit (*heavy; 178 amino acids*) and L (*Light, 171 amino acids*) that provide various isoprotein forms. H subunits predominate in nucleated blood cells and heart. L - subunits in liver and spleen. H-rich ferritins take up iron faster than L-rich *in –vitro* and may function more in iron detoxification than in storage [6]. Synthesis of the subunits is regulated mainly by the concentration of free intracellular iron. The bulk of the iron storage occurs in hepatocytes, reticuloendothelial cells and skeletal muscle. When iron is in excess, the storage capacity of newly synthesized apoferritin may be exceeded. This leads to iron deposition adjacent to ferritin spheres. This amorphous deposition of iron is called **hemosiderin** and the clinical condition is termed as hemosiderosis.

Multiple genes encode the ferritin proteins, at least in animals, which are expressed in a cell-specific manner. All cells synthesize ferritin at some point in the cell cycle, though the amount may vary depending on the role of the cell in iron storage, i.e housekeeping for intracellular use or specialized for use by other cells.

Expression of ferroportin (FPN) results in export of cytosolic iron and ferritin degradation. FPN-mediated iron loss from ferritin occurs in the cytosol and precedes ferritin degradation by the proteasome. Depletion of ferritin iron induces the monoubiquitination of ferritin subunits. Ubiquitination is not required for iron release but is required for disassembly of ferritin nanocages, which is followed by degradation of ferritin by the proteasome [7].

iii. Myoglobin

Myoglobin is an iron- and oxygen-binding protein found in the muscle tissue of vertebrates in general and in almost all mammals. It is a single-chain globular protein of 153 or 154 amino acids [8,9], containing a heme prosthetic group in the center around which the remaining apoprotein folds. It has eight alpha helices and a hydrophobic core. It has a molecular weight of 17,699 daltons (with heme), and is the primary oxygen-carrying pigment of muscle tissues [9]. Unlike the blood-borne hemoglobin, to which it is structurally related [10], this protein does not exhibit cooperative binding of oxygen, since positive cooperativity is a property of multimeric /oligomeric proteins only. Instead, the binding of oxygen by myoglobin is unaffected by the oxygen pressure in the surrounding tissue. Myoglobin is often cited as having an "instant binding tenacity" to oxygen given its hyperbolic oxygen dissociation curve [Figure 4].

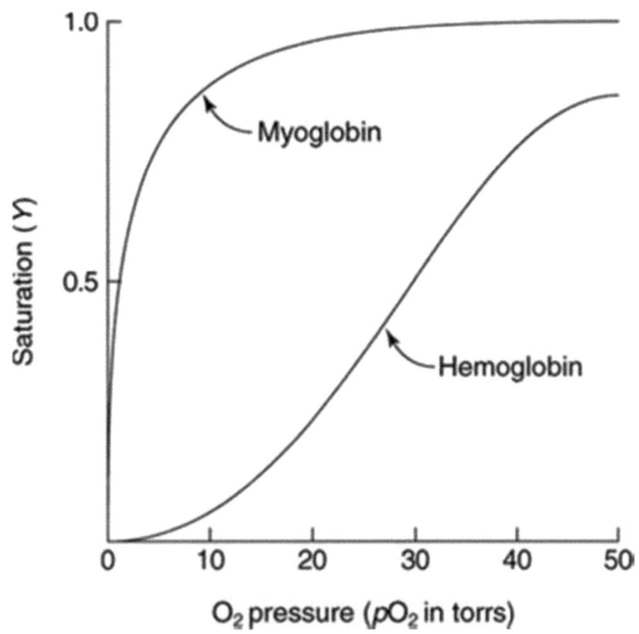

Fig. 4. Iron dissociation curve of hemoglobin and myoglobin.

iv. Transport Iron- Transferrin

Transferrin is a protein involved in the transport of iron. The transferrins are glycoproteins with molecular weight of approximately 80, 000 Da, consisting of a single polypeptide chain of 680 to 700 amino acids and no subunits. The transferrins consist of two non cooperative iron- binding lobes of approximately equal size. Each lobe is an ellipsoid of approximate dimensions 55 x35 x 35A° and contains a metal binding site buried below the surface of the protein in a hydrophilic environment [Figure 5]. The two binding sites are separated by 42 A° [11]. There is approximately 40% identity in the amino acid sequence between the two

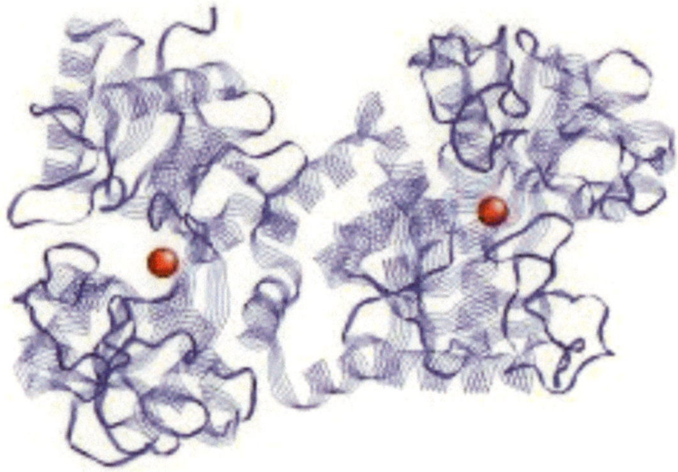

Fig. 5. Bilobar structure of Human transferrin

lobes [12, 13]. The protein is a product of gene duplication derived from a putative ancestral gene coding for a protein binding only one atom of iron.

The transferrins are highly cross-linked proteins, the number of disulfide bridges varying between proteins and between domains within each protein. There are six disulfide bonds conserved in each of the two-domains of all the transferrins, plus additional ones for the individual proteins. Human serum transferrin is the most cross- linked, having 8 and 11 disulfide bridges in the N- and C- terminal metal-binding lobes. The transferrins, with the exception of lactoferrin, are acidic proteins, having an isoelectric point (pI) value around 5.6 to 5.8.

Several metals bind to transferrin; the highest affinity is for Fe^{3+}; Fe^{2+} ion is not bound. Various spectroscopic and chemical modification studies have implicated histidine, tyrosine, water (or hydroxide) and (bi) carbonate as ligands to the Fe^{3+} in the metal-protein complex.

The transferrins are unique among proteins in their requirement of coordinate binding of an anion (bicarbonate) for iron binding [14,15]. Several studies suggest that the bicarbonate is directly coordinated to the iron, presumably forming a bridge between the metal and a cationic group on the protein. In the normal physiological state, approximately one-ninth of all the transferrin molecules are saturated with iron at both sides; four-ninths of transferrin molecules have iron at either site; and four-ninth of transferrin molecules are free of iron.

Transferrin delivers iron to cells by binding to specific cell surface receptors (TfR) that mediate the internalization of the protein. The TfR is a transmembrane protein consisting of two subunits of 90,000 Da each, joined by a disulfide bond. Each subunit contains one transmembrane segment and about 670 residues that are extracellular and bind a transferrin molecule, favoring the diferric form. Internalization of the receptor- transferrin complex is dependent on receptor phosphorylation by a Ca^{2+}- Calmodulin- protein kinase C complex. Release of the iron atoms occurs within the acidic milieu of the lysososme after which the receptor- apotransferrin complex returns to the cell surface where the apotransferrin is released to be reutilized in the plasma [Figure 6]. Inside the cell, iron is used for heme synthesis within the mitochondria, or is stored as ferritin.

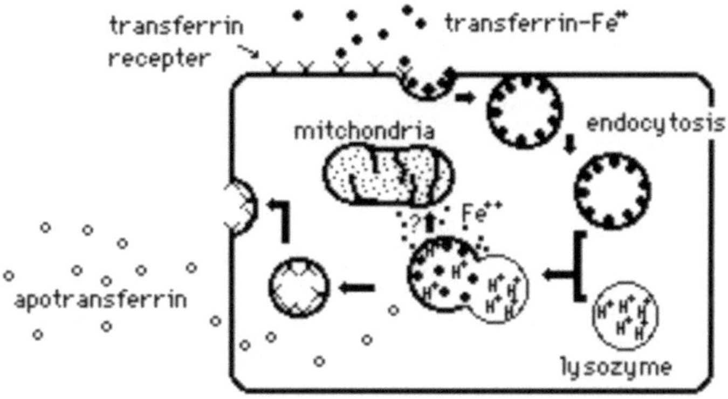

Fig. 6. Cellular uptake of iron by transferrin receptor

v. Labile iron Pool

The uptake and storage of iron is carried out by different proteins, hence a pool of accessible iron ions, called labile iron pool (LIP) exists, that constitutes crossroads of the metabolic pathways of iron containing compounds [16]. The LIP is localized primarily but not exclusively, within the cytoplasm of the cells. It is bound to low-affinity ligands [17] and is accessible to permeant chelators and contains the cells' metabolically and catalytically reactive iron. LIP is maintained by a balanced movement of iron from extra- and intracellular sources [18].

The trace amounts of "free" iron can catalyse production of a highly toxic hydroxyl radical via Fenton/Haber-Weiss reaction cycle. The critical factor appears to be the availability and abundance of cellular labile iron pool (LIP) that constitutes a crossroad of metabolic pathways of iron-containing compounds and is midway between the cellular need of iron, its uptake and storage. To avoid an excess of harmful "free" iron, the LIP is kept at the lowest sufficient level by transcriptional and posttranscriptional control of the expression of principal proteins involved in iron homeostasis [19].

vi. Other heme proteins and flavoproteins

Certain enzymes also contain heme as part of their prosthetic group (e.g. catalase, peroxidases, tryptophan pyrrolase, guanylate cyclase, Nitric oxide synthase and mitochondrial cytochromes).

Iron readily forms clusters linked to the polypeptide chain by thiol groups of cysteine residues or to non-proteins by inorganic sulphide and cysteine thiols leading to generation of iron- sulphur clusters. Examples of iron-sulphur proteins are the ferredoxins, hydrogenases, nitrogenases, NADH dehydrogenases and aconitases. Structure of most of these proteins dictates their function.

4. Physiological turnover of iron in the body

Daily requirements for iron vary depending on the person's age, sex and physiological status. Although iron is not excreted in the conventional sense, about 1 mg is lost daily through the normal shedding of skin epithelial cells and cells that line the gastrointestinal and urinary tracts. Small numbers of erythrocytes are lost in urine and feces as well. Humans and other vertebrates strictly conserve iron by recycling it from senescent erythrocytes and from other sources. The loss of iron in a typical adult male is so small that it can be met by absorbing approximately 1 mg of iron per day [20] [Figure 7]. In comparison, the daily iron requirement for erythropoiesis is about 20 mg. Such conservation of iron is essential because many human diets contain just enough iron to replace the small losses. However, the blood lost in each menstrual cycle drains 20 to 40 mg of iron, so women in their reproductive years need to absorb approximately 2 mg of iron per day. However, when dietary iron is more abundant, absorption is appropriately attenuated.

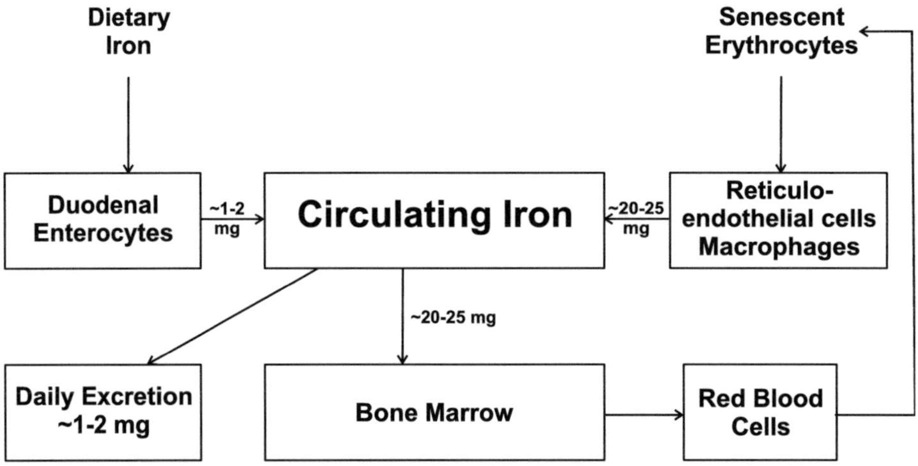

Fig. 7. Diagram showing the physiological turnover of iron in the body

5. Mechanisms regulating Iron absorption

The iron stores in the body are regulated by intestinal absorption. Intestinal absorption of iron is itself a regulated process and the efficacy of absorption increases or decreases depending on the body requirements of iron.

The dietary iron, which exists mostly in the ferric form, is converted to the more soluble ferrous form, which is readily absorbed. The ferric form is reduced to ferrous by the action of acids in stomach, reducing agents such as ascorbic acid, cysteine and –SH groups of proteins. Entry of Fe^{3+} into the mucosal cells may be aided by an enzyme on the brush-border of the enterocyte (the enzyme possesses ferric reductase activity also). The ferrous ion is then transported in the cell by a divalent metal transporter (DMT1) [Figure 8].

In the intestinal cell, the iron may be (a) stored by incorporation into ferritin in those individuals who have adequate plasma iron concentration. A ferroxidase converts the absorbed ferrous iron to the ferric form, which then combines with apoferritin to form ferritin, or (b) transported to a transport protein at the basolateral cell membrane and released into the circulation. However, the basolateral-transport protein has not yet been identified, It is believed to work in combination with hephaestin, a copper-containing protein, which oxidizes Fe^{2+} back to Fe^{3+} .

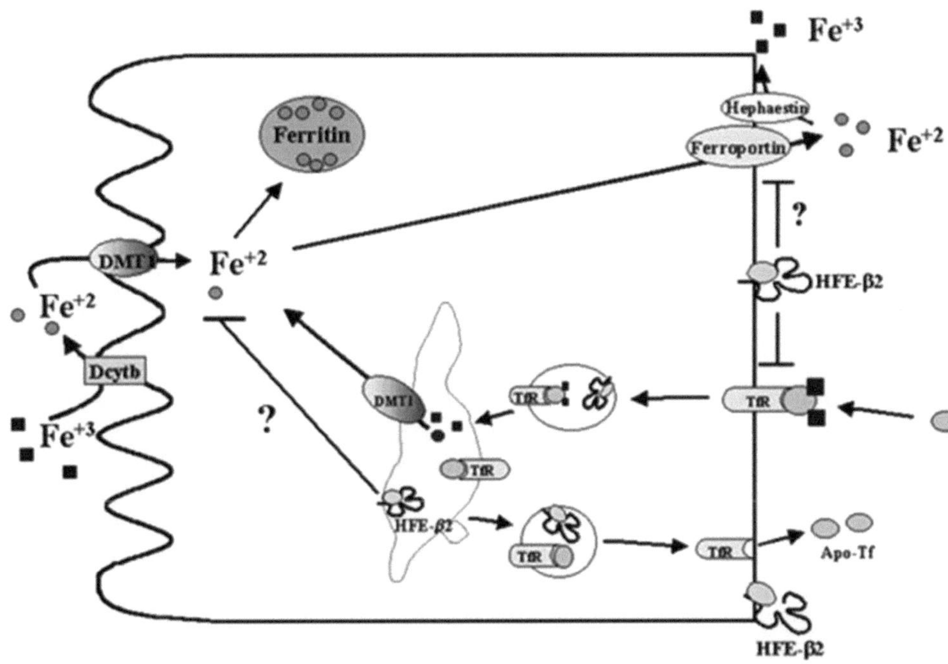

Fig. 8. Mechanism of intestinal Iron absorption

The intestinal cells internalize more iron than the amount that will eventually enter the circulation. The surplus, incorporated into ferritin for storage, is subsequently mobilized, if necessary. The ferritin stores are gradually built up, but most are lost when the mucosal cells are shed.

Thus during the dietary iron absorption, iron needs to traverse both the apical and basolateral membranes of absorptive epithelial cells in the duodenum to reach the blood, where it is incorporated into transferrin. The transport of non-heme iron across the apical membrane occurs via the divalent metal transporter 1 (DMT1), the only known intestinal iron importer. Dietary non-heme iron exists mainly in ferric form (Fe^{+3}) and must be reduced prior to transport. Duodenal cytochrome B (DcytB) is one of the major reductases localized in the apical membrane of intestinal enterocytes [21]. A heme protein, Dcytb, is upregulated by conditions that stimulate iron absorption, including iron deficiency, chronic anaemia and hypoxia. The mechanism by which its expression is upregulated in these conditions is unclear, as there are no obvious IREs in the mRNA of Dcytb. Nevertheless, the localization of Dcytb on the brush border of duodenal enterocytes closely mirrors that of DMT1, supporting the concept that Dcytb supplies ferrous iron to DMT1.

In addition, iron is also absorbed as heme. The transporter responsible for heme uptake at the apical membrane has not yet been conclusively identified. Cytosolic iron in intestinal enterocytes can be either stored in ferritin or exported into plasma by the basolateral iron exporter ferroportin (FPN). FPN is most likely the only cellular iron exporter in the duodenal mucosa as well as in macrophages, hepatocytes and the syncytial trophoblasts of the placenta. The export of iron by FPN depends on two multicopper oxidases, ceruloplasmin (Cp) in the circulation and hephaestin on the basolateral membrane of enterocytes, which convert Fe^{+2} to Fe^{+3} for incorporation of iron into transferrin (Tf).

Intestinal iron absorption is dependent on the body iron needs and is a tightly controlled process. Recent studies indicate that this process is accomplished by modulating the expression levels of DMT1, DcytB and FPN by multiple pathways.

Iron regulatory proteins (IRPs) are essential for intestinal iron absorption. DMT1 mRNA has an iron responsive element (IRE) at the 3'UTR and is stabilized upon IRP binding. In contrast, FPN mRNA has IRE at the 5'UTR and IRP binding inhibits translation. Specific intestinal depletion of both IRP1 and IRP2 in mice markedly decreases the DMT1 and increases FPN, resulting in the death of the intestinal epithelial cells [22]. The mice die of malnutrition within two weeks of birth, underscoring the importance of these proteins. These results demonstrate the critical role of IRPs in the control of DMT1 and FPN expression. A novel isoform of FPN lacking an IRE was recently identified in enterocytes [23]. This FPN isoform is hypothesized to allow intestinal cells to export iron into the body under low iron conditions. DMT1 also expresses multiple isoforms with and without 3'IRE. The IRP/IRE regulatory network is described in detail in the subsequent chapters.

Secondly, the hypoxia-inducible factor (HIF)-mediated signaling plays a critical role in regulating iron absorption. Two studies [24,25] show that acute iron deficiency induces HIF signaling via HIF-2α in the duodenum, which upregulates DcytB and DMT1 expression and increases iron absorption. A conditional knockdown of intestinal HIF-2α in mice abolishes this response. In addition to DMT1 and FPN, both HIF signaling and IRP1 activation are associated with the regulation of iron absorption [26, 27]. HIF-2α mRNA contains an IRE within its 5'-UTR [26]. Under conditions of cellular hypoxia, HIF-2α is derepressed through the inhibition of IRP-1–dependent translational repression [27].

Thirdly, FPN protein is negatively regulated by hepcidin, a critical and one of the most important iron regulatory hormones, predominantly secreted by liver hepatocytes. Thus, intestinal iron absorption is coordinately regulated by several signaling pathways and is sensitive to hypoxia by HIF-2α, enterocyte iron levels by IRP/IRE and bodily iron levels by hepcidin.

Although iron uptake into the body is tightly controlled, iron loss does not appear to be regulated. Under normal conditions iron is excreted through blood loss, sweat, and the sloughing of epithelial cells. These losses amount to approximately 1 to 2 mg of iron per day. Under certain pathological states, Tf, and therefore iron, can be lost when the kidney fails to reabsorb proteins from the urinary filtrate. These proteinurea syndromes result from the lack of functional cubulin, megalin, or ClC-5 [28]. Cubulin and megalin are protein scavenging receptors, whose function in the proximal renal tubule is the reuptake of nutrients from the urinary filtrate. ClC-5, a voltage-gated chloride channel, is required for the acidification of endocytic vesicles and the release of iron from Tf.

6. Mechanisms of cellular iron transport and uptake

(This section is only briefly described here. The topic is discussed in detail in subsequent chapter by Dr Sanchez etal).

The abundance and availability of transferrin receptor for cellular iron uptake is regulated by cellular iron status. Cellular iron content determines the composition of a cytosolic protein termed iron regulatory protein 1 (IRP1). Under iron-replete conditions, IRP1 contains a 4Fe–4S cluster that is unable to bind to iron-responsive elements (IRE) in the mRNAs of TfR1 and ferritin. When cellular iron content is low, the iron–sulphur cluster is disassembled, liberating an apo-IRP that binds to specific stem–loop structures in the 3′ or 5′ untranslated regions (UTRs) of the mRNAs encoding these proteins. In the case of TfR1, the IREs are located in the 3′ UTR, and binding of IRP1 increases the stability of the message and enhances the synthesis of TfR1.

Conversely, binding of IRP1 to the IREs in the 5′ UTR of ferritin mRNA mediates translation repression. Thus, under iron replete conditions, there is more rapid turnover of TfR1 mRNA, leading to diminished translation and cell-surface expression of TfR1, reduced uptake of transferrin-bound iron and an expanded capacity for iron storage through increased synthesis of ferritin. Hepatic transferrin receptor (TfR2) expression is not downregulated by iron overload [29]. Given that the liver is a major site for iron storage, the high level of expression of TfR2 and its lack of responsiveness to iron status might be viewed as a protective mechanism, selectively diverting iron to hepatocytes under conditions in which circulating levels of transferrin bound iron are high and peripheral iron stores are replete.

In normal individuals, nearly all cellular acquisition of iron from blood occurs via transferrin receptor-mediated uptake, since most of the iron in circulation is bound to transferrin. In circumstances in which the binding capacity of transferrin becomes saturated, as in case of iron loading disorders, iron forms low-molecular-weight complexes, the most abundant being iron citrate. It has been known for years that hepatic clearance of this non-transferrin-bound iron (NTBI) is rapid and highly efficient. Furthermore, studies in isolated perfused rat livers and cultured hepatocytes indicated that hepatic uptake of NTBI involves a membrane carrier protein whose iron transport function is subject to competition by other divalent metal ions. Based on these characteristics, it appears that the recently discovered divalent metal transporter 1 (DMT1; also known as DCT1 and Nramp-2) is the major transporter accounting for hepatic uptake of NTBI. Using a cDNA library prepared from iron-deficient rat intestine, the DMT1 transcript was identified by its ability to increase iron uptake in *Xenopus* oocytes [30]. DMT1 has subsequently been shown to transport various divalent metal ions in a manner that is coupled to the transport of protons. Although DMT1 mRNA is broadly expressed in mammalian tissues including liver, its highest level of expression is found in the proximal intestine, consistent with its role in the absorption of dietary non-heme iron. Two isoforms of DMT1 have been described. The form of DMT1 that predominates in the intestine has an IRE in its 3′ UTR, indicating that the stability of this transcript is regulated by cellular iron status in a manner similar to that of TfR1. Reciprocal changes in duodenal DMT1 expression *vis-àvis* iron status have been demonstrated in iron-deficient rats and in humans with iron deficiency and iron overload [31].

Collectively, these data provide evidence for a negative feedback loop in which iron status regulates intestinal DMT1 expression, which in turn controls iron uptake.

7. Mechanism of iron mobilization and export from storage sites

Liver is the main site of iron storage under physiological conditions, hence various mechanisms regulate the mobilization and export of stored iron from liver to extrahepatic tissues. Under normal physiological circumstances, Kupffer cells play a prominent role in inter organ iron trafficking. One of the primary sites of erythrocyte turnover, Kupffer cells, along with the reticuloendothelial cells of the spleen and bone marrow, ingest senescent or damaged red blood cells, catabolize the haemoglobin and release the iron. Collectively, the quantity of iron that is recycled from erythrocytes through the macrophage compartment on a daily basis is several fold greater than that taken up through the intestine. Hence, the contribution of Kupffer cells to total body iron economy is both qualitatively and quantitatively important. It is therefore not surprising that Kupffer cells are the major type of liver cell that express a recently described iron exporter, FPN (also known as Ireg1 and MTP1) [32-34]. Consistent with its role in iron absorption, FPN is expressed at high levels along the basolateral membrane in mature enterocytes of the duodenal villi. In the intestine, FPN expression is upregulated by iron deficiency and anaemia. In addition, FPN transcripts are also detected in liver, spleen, kidney and placenta. In murine liver, hepatocytes as well as Kupffer cells show immunoreactivity for FPN, albeit less intense. The quantitative PCR study on isolated cells from rat livers discussed above reported similar levels of FPN transcripts in hepatocytes, Kupffer cells and stellate cells, and lower levels in sinusoidal endothelial cells [35]; however, FPN protein has not been demonstrated in the last two cell types. Interestingly, the subcellular localization of FPN appears to differ between hepatocytes and Kupffer cells, being localized to the plasma membrane along the sinusoidal border in the former and cytoplasmic in the latter [34]. It has been proposed that the intracellular localization of FPN in Kupffer cells (which is also observed in RAW267.4 cells, a murine macrophage cell line) indicates that FPN does not directly export iron across the plasma membrane in these cells but, rather, that it may participate in intracellular trafficking of iron, perhaps through the secretory pathway. Further studies are needed to determine whether FPN is involved in multiple pathways of iron export.

Like cellular uptake of iron, efflux of iron from cells requires ferroxidase activity. It has been known for some time that ceruloplasmin, a copper-containing plasma ferroxidase synthesized by hepatocytes, plays an important role in iron homeostasis. Aceruloplasminaemia results in a form of iron overload that is recapitulated in mice with a targeted disruption of the ceruloplasmin gene [36]. Interestingly, although the ceruloplasmin knockout mice accumulate iron in both hepatocytes and Kupffer cells, intestinal iron absorption is unaffected by ceruloplasmin deficiency. This observation could probably be explained by the recent demonstration of ceruloplasmin homologue, termed hephaestin in the intestinal villi. Despite their similarities, the function of hephaestin is distinct from that of ceruloplasmin,as mutations in hephaestin lead to iron deficiency rather than iron overload.

In this context, it is interesting to contrast hepatocytes, which have low levels of FPN protein and lack detectable hephaestin transcripts, with Kupffer cells, which have higher levels of FPN and express hephaestin transcripts, at levels that are considerably lower than the intestine [35]. Taken together, these observations suggest that the ferroxidase activity of ceruloplasmin can indeed substitute for hephaestin in FPN-expressing cells in the liver (but not in the intestine). Another possibility is that hepatocytes and Kupffer cells may employ additional means to promote iron export, such as upregulation of hephaestin in response to iron loading and/or the expression of alternative exporters or ferroxidases.

A major advance in the understanding of iron metabolism was the discovery of the iron regulatory hormone hepcidin nearly 10 years ago. Hepcidin was originally identified as an antimicrobial peptide isolated from human urine [37]. The liver is the predominant source of hepcidin, where the 84-amino-acid prepropeptide is synthesized and cleaved to yield 20- and 25-amino-acid peptides that are released into the circulation and filtered by the kidney. Consistent with release into the blood from hepatocytes, hepcidin immunoreactivity is observed along the sinusoidal borders of hepatocyte membranes, with accentuated staining of periportal (zone 1) hepatocytes which decreases towards the central vein and sinusoids [38].

Hepcidin acts as a systemic iron-regulatory hormone as it controls iron transport from iron-exporting tissues into plasma [39]. [Figure 9] Studies have demonstrated that hepcidin knockout mice develop a form of iron overload reminiscent of hereditary haemochromatosis [40], while mice with over expression of hepcidin have severe iron-deficiency anaemia [41]. Hepcidin inhibits the intestinal absorption [37,41], macrophage release [42,43] and placental passage [41] of iron. A pharmacodynamic study of the effects of a radiolabelled hepcidin injection in mice, showed that a single 50 µg dose resulted in 80% drop in serum iron within 1 h which did not return to normal until 96 hours [44]. This time course is consistent with the blockage of recycled iron from macrophages and previous reports of the rapid hepcidin response to IL-6 administration [45]. The rapid disappearance of plasma iron was followed by a delayed recovery, possibly due to the slow resynthesis of membrane FPN. Tissue concentrations revealed that hepcidin preferentially accumulates in the proximal duodenum and spleen, reflecting the high expression of FPN in these areas.

Hepatocytes evaluate body iron status and release or downregulate hepcidin according to the iron status of the body [Figure 9]. An oral load of 65 mg of iron in healthy volunteers caused > 5-fold increase in hepcidin within 1 day [45]. Hepcidin mRNA moves with the

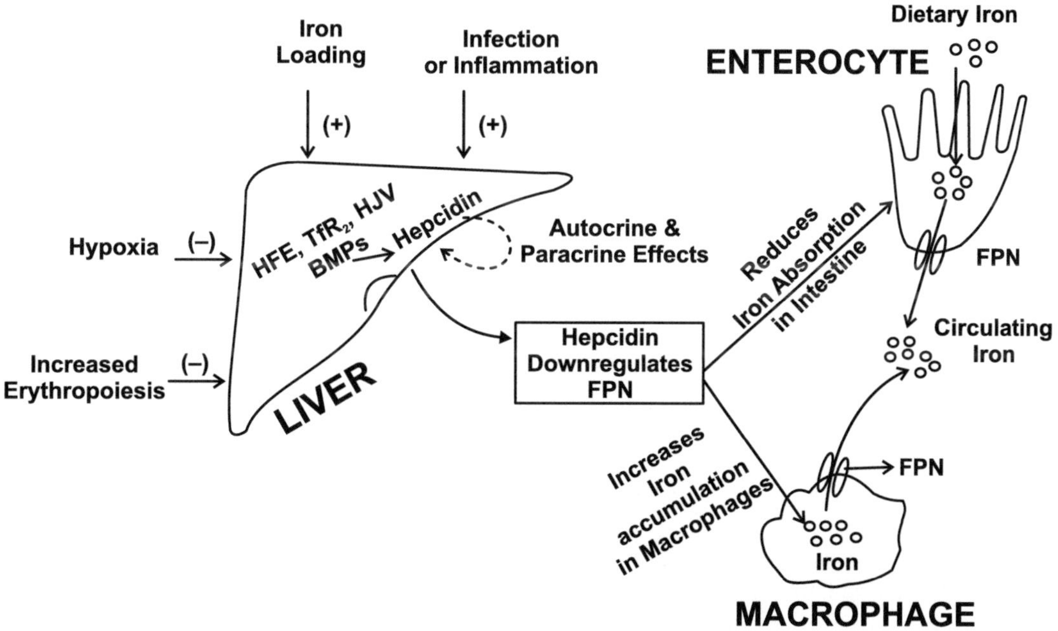

Fig. 9. Schematic Diagram showing the regulation of circulating iron levels by Hepcidin

body's iron levels, increasing as they increase and decreasing as they decrease [46]. Hepcidin regulates iron uptake constantly on a daily basis, to maintain sufficient iron stores for erythropoiesis [47], as well as its feedback mechanism to prevent iron overload. Hepcidin negatively regulates the uptake of iron by Tf, the major iron transport protein in the blood. Since Tf is the major source of iron for hemoglobin synthesis by red blood cell precursors, increased hepcidin limits erythropoiesis and is a major contributor to the anemia of chronic disease [48]. In humans, patients with large hepatic adenomas found to overexpress hepcidin, had a severe iron refractory microcytic anaemia, which was corrected by removal of the adenoma [49].

Recent studies have provided insight into the mechanisms by which hepcidin modulates iron absorption. Within a week of being placed on a low-iron diet, rats show a twofold increase in intestinal iron absorption that is temporally associated with a significant drop in hepatic hepcidin expression, and increases in duodenal mRNAs for Dcytb, DMT1 and FPN [50]. Although the increase in FPN mRNA under these circumstances is of relatively small magnitude, the increase in FPN protein is more substantial. A similar pattern is seen in the intestine of hepcidin knockout mice, providing additional evidence that hepcidin suppresses the expression of these iron transporters. While the role of hepcidin in the regulation of Dcytb and DMT1 has not been characterized, several reports have established that FPN is a major target of hepcidin's action. As suggested by the observations discussed above, hepcidin appears to regulate FPN expression by two distinct mechanisms. The first is at the level of FPN transcripts, which are decreased following stimulation of endogenous hepcidin production or administration of recombinant hepcidin [51]. The second involves binding of hepcidin to FPN at the cell membrane, causing internalization and degradation of FPN, thus diminishing iron transfer [39, 52,53]. These mechanisms are clearly not mutually exclusive and, either or both may probably contribute to the decrease in intestinal iron absorption in response to hepcidin. However, it is unclear at present whether FPN expression in liver cells is regulated in the same manner. In mice treated with iron, intestinal FPN expression is low, consistent with the known effects of hepcidin. In the liver, however, FPN is increased, particularly in Kupffer cells [34]. This may result from enhanced translation due to the presence of the IRE in the 5′ UTR of FPN mRNA. If so, this effect must predominate over the hepcidin-induced increase in FPN turnover. Alternatively, the distinctive intracellular pattern of FPN in Kupffer cells implies that FPN may not physically interact with hepcidin in macrophages, again raising the possibility of differential regulation of FPN in liver vs. intestine.

Hepcidin inhibits the release of iron by macrophages and lessens the iron uptake in the gut by diminishing the effective number of iron exporters on the membrane of enterocytes or macrophages. In FPN mutations it has been observed that iron accumulates mainly in macrophages and is often combined with anemia [54].

The development of iron overload in hepcidin knockout mice [40] and humans with mutations in the hepcidin gene [55] is clearly explicable by the effects of hepcidin on intestinal iron absorption. Since the discovery of hepcidin, several authors have reported that hepcidin expression fails to increase in response to increased iron stores in other disease states characterized by iron loading. For example, hepcidin expression is inappropriately low in iron-loaded subjects with hereditary haemochromatosis [56] and haemojuvelin (HJV) mutations [57]. Similar findings are reported in a variety of iron-loading anaemias [58]. Under physiological conditions, hepatic hepcidin expression is regulated by a cohort of proteins that are expressed in hepatocytes, including the hereditary hemochromatosis (HH) protein called HFE, transferrin receptor 2 (TfR2), hemojuvelin (HJV), bone morphogenetic protein 6 (BMP6), matriptase-2 and Tf. Hepcidin expression can also be robustly regulated by erythroid factors, hypoxia, and inflammation, regardless of body iron levels. The inappropriately low levels of hepcidin production in HFE-associated Hereditary Hemochromatosis (HH) suggest that HFE is upstream of hepcidin in the molecular regulation of hepcidin production [59]. Similarly, the HJV gene, which is mutated in Juvenile Hemochromatosis [JH] , is associated with low hepcidin levels [60], suggesting regulation proximal to hepcidin. Type 3 haemochromatosis is due to homozygous mutations in TfR2, a membrane glycoprotein that mediates cellular iron uptake from transferrin. TfR2 mutant mice have low levels of hepcidin mRNA expression, even after massive intraperitoneal iron loading also suggestive of iron modulation proximal to hepcidin [61]

It is possible that hepcidin is the common pathway modulating iron absorption via HFE, TfR2 and HJV, mutations of which all result in an iron overload phenotype. Mutations in these proteins, or their genetic ablation, result in diminished hepcidin expression, indicating that they positively regulate hepcidin production. Signaling through the BMP pathway has been shown to be a central axis for hepcidin regulation. BMPs (such as BMP2, 4, 6, or 9) are secreted soluble factors that interact with cell-surface BMP receptors, initiating an intracellular signaling cascade that activates hepcidin transcription [62].

In vivo, BMP6 seems especially important for iron homeostasis; because Bmp6-null mice display reduced hepcidin expression and iron overload [63]. Efficient BMP signaling through BMP receptor requires HJV, a 50-kDa protein with a glycosylphosphatidylinositol (GPI) anchor that tethers the protein to the extracellular surface of the plasma membrane. This membrane-bound hemojuvelin (m-HJV) is capable of binding BMPs, facilitating their association with the BMP receptor [64]. As such, m-HJV is often referred to as a BMP co-receptor. The potent contribution of m-HJV to BMP-mediated hepcidin activation is illustrated by mutations in HJV that abrogate cell surface expression. Individuals with such mutations develop juvenile hemochromatosis, characterized by exceedingly low serum hepcidin concentrations (<5 ng/mL) [65] and severe hepatic iron overload.

Several studies have proved that there is local production of hepcidin by macrophages [74], cardiomyocytes [66] and fat cells [67], suggesting that hepcidin is involved in different regulatory mechanisms to control iron imbalance. Apart from this, few studies have proposed that hepcidin might also directly inhibit erythroid-progenitor proliferation and survival [68]. At the same time hepcidin synthesis is increased by iron loading and decreased by anemia and hypoxia [69]. Anemia and hypoxia are associated with a dramatic decrease in liver hepcidin gene expression, which may account for the increase in iron release from reticuloendothelial cells and increase in iron absorption frequently observed in these situations [47].

HFE is highly expressed in the liver as well as the intestine and is involved in regulation of iron metabolism. Originally identified on the basis of a high frequency of HFE mutations in patients with genetic haemochromatosis, wild-type HFE protein forms a complex at the plasma membrane with TfR1 and β2-microglobulin [Figure 8]. Studies in transfected cells indicate that the stoichiometry of these components influences the rate of recycling of TfR1, thus modulating iron uptake [70]. Nonetheless, the precise mechanism whereby HFE mutations lead to iron loading remains speculative. While immunohistochemistry for HFE demonstrates a distinctive pattern of intracellular perinuclear staining in the epithelial cells of the small intestine [71], immunoreactivity for HFE in liver has been variously ascribed to bile ducts, sinusoidal lining cells, Kupffer cells and endothelial cells. Furthermore, these studies are at variance with results of PCR and Western blot analysis of isolated liver cells demonstrating that hepatocytes are the major source of HFE in rat liver, with a minor contribution from Kupffer cells [35]. Additional studies are needed to resolve this discrepancy and provide further insight into the function of HFE.

While the function of HJV is unknown, it has been proposed that HJV is 'upstream' of hepcidin in the pathways controlling iron metabolism, as both patients with iron overload resulting from HJV mutations and HJV knockout mice fail to respond to their iron burden with an appropriate increase in hepcidin. On treatment with parenteral iron in mice, hepatic expression of HJV is not altered despite an increase in hepcidin mRNA indicating that a direct interaction between these two proteins is unlikely. Thus, currently available studies demonstrate lack of responsiveness of HJV to iron as well as divergent regulation of HJV and hepcidin in normal animals treated with iron.

8. Conclusion

Iron is an essential element in the body but its effect in the body is like a two-edged sword. At one end it is essential for maintaining most of the body functions and at the other end it becomes potentially toxic if in excess. Thus, elaborate physiological mechanisms have evolved for regulation of uptake and disposition of iron. The earlier concept of regulation of iron levels by absorption could not explain several clinical conditions like hemochromatosis and severe anemias associated with chronic diseases and malignancies. However, a newer insight into the understanding of iron metabolism has been provided in the past few years, mainly as a result of the discovery of hepcidin, a key regulator of whole-body iron homeostasis.

9. References

[1] Brown EB, Aisen P, Fielding J, Crichton RC. Proteins of Iron Metabolism, Grune & Stratton, New York 1977.
[2] Hemoglobin." School of Chemistry - Bristol University - UK. N.p., n.d. Web. 12 Oct. 2009. http://www.chm.bris.ac.uk/motm/hemoglobin/hemoglobjm.htm.
[3] Linberg R, Conover CD, Shum KL, Shorr RG.. "Hemoglobin based oxygen carriers: how much methemoglobin is too much?" Artif Cells Blood Substit Immobil Biotechnol 1998; 26 (2): 133–48.
[4] Theil EC. Ferritin: structure, gene regulation in animals, plants, and micro-organisms. Ann. Rev. Biochem. 1987; 56: 289-315.
[5] Theil EC, Aisen P. The storage and transport of iron in animal cells, in *Iron Transport in Microbes, Plants and Animals,* van der Helm D, Neilands J and Winkelmann G Eds, VCH Publishers, Weinheim, Federal Republic of Germany, 1987: 421.
[6] Levi S, Luzzago A, Cesareni G, Cozzi A, Franceschinelli F, Albertini A, Arosio P. Mechanism of ferritin iron uptake: activity of the H-chain and deletion mapping of the ferro-oxidase site. J Biol Chem 1988; 263: 18086-92.

[7] De Domenico I, Vaughn MB, Li L, Bagley D, Musci G, Ward DM, etal. Ferroportin-mediated mobilization of ferritin iron precedes ferritin degradation by the proteasome. The EMBO Journal 2006; 25: 5396 - 04.

[8] Hendgen-Cotta U, Kelm M, Rassaf T. A highlight of myoglobin diversity: the nitrite reductase activity during myocardial ischemia-reperfusion. Nitric oxide : biology and chemistry / official journal of the Nitric Oxide Society 2009; 22: 75–82.

[9] Ordway GA, Garry DJ. Myoglobin: an essential hemoprotein in striated muscle. J Experimen Biol 2004; 207 : 3441–6.

[10] Lodish H, Berk A, Zipursky LS, Matsudaira P, Baltimore D, Darnell J. Evolutionary tree showing the globin protein family members myoglobin and hemoglobin. Molecular Cell Biology (4th ed.). W. H. Freeman 2000; 3136-3.

[11] Anderson BF, Baker HM, Norris GE, Rice DW, Baker EN. Structure of human lactoferrin: crystallographic analysis and refinement at 2.8 A° resolution. J Mol Biol 1989; 209: 711-34.

[12] MacGillivray RTA, Mendez E, Sinha SK, Sutton MR, Lineback Zins J, Brew K. The complete amino acid sequence of human serum transferrin. Proc. Natl Acad Sci USA 1982; 79: 2504-8.

[13] Metz- Boutique MH, Jolles J, Mazurier J, Schoentgen F, Legrand D, Spik G, Montreuil J, Jolles P. Human lactotransferrin: amino acid sequence and structural comparisons with other transferrins. Eur J Biochem 1984; 145: 659- 76.

[14] Baldwin DA, Egan TJ. An inorganic perspective of human serum transferrin. S Afr J Sci 1987; 83:22.

[15] Chasteen ND. Identification of the probable locus of iron and anion binding in the transferrins. Trends Biochem Sci 1983; 8: 272-5.

[16] Kruszewski M, Iwanenko T. Labile iron pool correlates with iron content in the nucleus and the formation of oxidative DNA damage in mouse lymphoma L5178Y cell lines. Acta Biochimica Polonica 2003; 50: 211-215.

[17] Prus E, Fibach E. Flow cytometry measurements of the labile iron pool in human hematopoietic cells. Cytometry2008; 73A: 22-27.

[18] Epsztejn S, Kakhlon O, Glickstein H, Breuer W, Cabantchik ZI. Fluorescence analysis of the labile iron pool of mammalian cells. Analyt Biochem 1997; 248: 31-40.

[19] Kruszewski M. Labile iron pool: the main determinant of cellular response to oxidative stress. Mutat Res 2003; 531: 81-92.

[20] Andrews NC. Disorders of iron metabolism. N Engl J Med. 1999; 341: 1986-95.

[21] McKie AT, Barrow D, Latunde-Dada GO, Rolfs A, Sager G, Mudaly E, et al. An iron regulated ferric reductase associated with the absorption of dietary iron. Science 2001; 291: 1755–8.

[22] Galy B, Ferring-Appel D, Kaden S, Grone HJ, Hentze MW. Iron regulatory proteins are essential for intestinal function and control key iron absorption molecules in the duodenum. Cell Metab. 2008;7: 79–85.

[23] Zhang DL, Hughes RM, Ollivierre-Wilson H, Ghosh MC, Rouault TA. A ferroportin transcript that lacks an iron-responsive element enables duodenal and erythroid precursor cells to evade translational repression. Cell Metab. 2009; 9: 461–73.

[24] ShahYM, MatsubaraT, Ito S, Yim SH, Gonzalez FJ. Intestinal hypoxia-inducible transcription factors are essential for iron absorption following iron deficiency. Cell Metab. 2009; 9: 152–64.

[25] Mastrogiannaki M, Matak P, Keith B, Simon MC, Vaulont S, Peyssonnaux C. HIF-2alpha, but not HIF-1alpha, promotes iron absorption in mice. J Clin Invest. 2009; 119: 1159–66.

[26] Sanchez M, Galy B, Muckenthaler MU, Hentze MW. Iron-regulatory proteins limit hypoxia-inducible factor-2alpha expression in iron deficiency. Nat Struct Mol Biol. 2007; 14: 420–6.

[27] Zimmer M, Ebert BL, Neil C, Brenner K, Papaioannou I, Melas A, et al. Small-molecule inhibitors of HIF-2a translation link its 5'UTR iron-responsive element to oxygen sensing. Mol Cell. 2008; 32: 838–48.

[28] Devuyst O, Jouret F, Auzanneau C, Courtoy PJ. Chloride channels and endocytosis: new insights from Dent's disease and ClC-5 knockout mice. Nephron Physiol. 2005; 99: 69–73.

[29] Fleming RE, Migas MC, Holden CC, Waheed A, Britton RS, Tomatsu S, et al. Transferrin receptor 2: continued expression in mouse liver in the face of iron overload and in hereditary hemochromatosis. Proc Natl Acad Sci USA 2000; 97: 2214–9.

[30] Gunshin H, Mackenzie B, Berger U, Gunshin Y, Romero MF, Boron WF, et al. Cloning and characterization of a mammalian proton-coupled metal-ion transporter. Nature 1997; 388: 482–8.

[31] Zoller H, Koch RO, Theurl I, Obrist P, Pietrangelo A, Montosi G, et al. Expression of duodenal iron transporters divalent-metal iron transporter 1 and ferroportin 1 in iron deficiency and iron overload. Gastroenterology 2001; 120: 1412–19.

[32] Donovan A, Brownlie A, Zhou Y, Shepard J, Pratt SJ, Moynihan J, et al. Positional cloning of zebrafish *ferroportin*1 identifies a conserved vertebrate iron exporter. Nature 2000; 403: 776–81.

[33] McKie AT, Marciani P, Rolfs A, Brennan K, Wehr K, Barrow D, et al. A novel duodenal iron regulated transporter, IREG1, implicated in the basolateral transfer of iron to the circulation. Mol Cell 2000; 5: 299–309.

[34] Abboud S, Haile DJ. A novel mammalian iron-regulated protein involved in intracellular iron metabolism. J Biol Chem 2000; 275: 19906–12.

[35] Zhang AS, Xiong S, Tsukamoto H, Enns CA. Localization of iron metabolism-related mRNAs in rat liver indicate that HFE is expressed predominantly in hepatocytes. Blood 2004; 103: 1509–14.

[36] Harris ZL, Durley AP, Man TK, Gitlin JD. Targeted gene disruption reveals an essential role for ceruloplasmin in cellular iron efflux. Proc Natl Acad Sci USA 1999; 96: 10812-7.

[37] Park CH, Valore EV, Waring AJ, Ganz T. Hepcidin, a urinary antimicrobial peptide synthesized in the liver. J Biol Chem 2001; 276: 7806–10.

[38] Kulaksiz H, Gehrke SG, Janetzko A, Rost D, Bruckner T, Kallinowski B, et al. Pro-hepcidin: expression and cell specific localisation in the liver and its regulation in hereditary haemochromatosis, chronic renal insufficiency, and renal anaemia. Gut 2004; 53: 735–43.

[39] Ganz T. Hepcidin and its role in regulating systemic iron metabolism. Hematol Am Soc Hematol Educ Program 2006; 507: 29–35.

[40] Nicolas G, Bennoun M, Devaux I, BeaumontC, Grandchamp B, Kahn A, et al. Lack of hepcidin gene expression and severe tissue iron overload in upstream stimulatory factor 2 (USF2) knockout mice. Proc Natl Acad Sci USA 2001; 98: 8780–5.
[41] Nicolas G, Bennoun M, Porteu A, Mativet S, Beaumont C, Grandchamp B, et al. Severe iron deficiency anemia in transgenic mice expressing liver hepcidin. Proc Natl Acad Sci USA 2002; 99: 4596–601.
[42] Fleming RE, Sly WS. Hepcidin: a putative iron regulatory hormone relative to hereditary hemochromatosis and the anemia of chronic disease. Proc Natl Acad Sci U S A 2001; 98: 8160–2.
[43] Singh PK, Parsek MR, Greenberg EP, Welsh MJ. A component of innate immunity prevents bacterial biofilm development. Nature 2002; 417: 552–5.
[44] Rivera S, Nemeth E, Gabayan V, Lopez MA, Farshidi D, Ganz T. Synthetic hepcidin causes rapid dose-dependent hypoferremia and is concentrated in ferroportin-containing organs. Blood 2005; 106: 2196–9.
[45] Nemeth E, Rivera S, Gabayan V, Keller C, Taudorf S, Pederson BK, et al. IL-6 mediates hypoferremia of inflammation by inducing the synthesis of the iron regulatory hormone hepcidin. J Clin Invest 2004; 113: 1271–6.
[46] Pigeon C, Ilyin G, Courselaud B, Leroyer P, Turlin B, Brissot P, et al. A new mouse liver specific gene, encoding a protein homologous to human antimicrobial peptide hepcidin, is overexpressed during iron overload. J Biol Chem 2001; 276: 7811–9.
[47] Finch C. Regulators of iron balance in humans. Blood 1994; 84: 1697–702.
[48] Zhang AS, Enns CA. Molecular mechanisms of normal iron homeostasis. Hematology 2009; 2009: 207-214.
[49] Weinstein DA, Roy CN, Fleming MD, Loda MF, Wolfsdorf JI, Andrews NC. Inappropriate expression of hepcidin is associated with iron refractory anemia: implications for the anemia of chronic disease. Blood 2002; 100: 3776–81.
[50] Frazer DM, Wilkins SJ, Becker EM, Vulpe CD, Mc Kie AT, Trinder D, et al. Hepcidin expression inversely correlates with the expression of duodenal iron transporters and iron absorption in rats. Gastroenterology 2002; 123: 835–44.
[51] Yeh KY, Yeh M, Glass J. Hepcidin regulation of ferroportin 1 expression in the liver and intestine of the rat. Am J Physiol 2004; 286: G385–G94.
[52] Nemeth E, Tuttle MS, Powelson J, Vaughn MB, Donovan A, Ward DM, et al. Hepcidin regulates cellular iron efflux by binding to ferroportin and inducing its internalization. Science 2004; 306: 2090–3.
[53] De Domenico I, Mc Vey Ward D, Kaplan J. Regulation of iron acquisition and storage: consequences for iron-linked disorders. Nat Rev Mol Cell Biol 2008; 9: 72–81.
[54] Njajou OT, de Jong G, Berghuis B, Vaessen N, Snijders PJ, Goossens JP, et al. Dominant hemochromatosis due to N144H mutation of SLC11A3: clinical and biological characteristics. Blood Cells Mol Dis 2002; 29:439–43.
[55] Roetto A, Papanikolaou G, Politou M, Alberti F, Girelli D, Christakis J, et al. Mutant antimicrobial peptide hepcidin is associated with severe juvenile hemochromatosis. Nature Genet 2003; 33: 21–22.
[56] Bridle KR, Frazer DM, Wilkins SJ, Dixon JL, Purdie DM, CrawfoDHG, et al. Disrupted hepcidin regulation in *HFE*-associated haemochromatosis and the liver as a regulator of body iron homeostasis. Lancet 2003; 361: 669–73.

[57] Papanikolaou G, Samuels ME, Ludwig EH, MacDonald ML, Franchini PL, Dube MP, et al. Mutations in *HFE*2 cause iron overload in chromosome 1q-linked juvenile hemochromatosis. Nature Genet 2004; 36: 77–82.

[58] Papanikolaou G, Tzilianos M, Christakis JI, Bogdanos D, Tsimirika K, MacFarlane J, et al. Hepcidin in iron overload disorders. Blood 2005; 105: 4103–5.

[59] Ahmad KA, Ahmann JR, Migas MC, Waheed A, Britton RS, Bacon BR, etal. Decreased liver hepcidin expression in the Hfe knockout mouse. Blood Cells, Molecules and Diseases 2002; 29: 361–6.

[60] Ganz T. Hepcidin - a regulator of intestinal iron absorption and iron recycling by macrophages. Best Practice and Research. Clinical Haematology 2005; 18: 171–82.

[61] Kawabata H, Fleming RE, Gui D, Moon SY, Saitoh T, O'kelly J, etal. Expression of hepcidin is down-regulated in Tfr2 mutant mice manifesting a phenotype of hereditary hemochromatosis. Blood 2005; 105: 376–81.

[62] Truksa J, Peng H, Lee P, Beutler E. Bone morphogenetic proteins 2, 4, and 9 stimulate murine hepcidin 1 expression independently of Hfe, transferrin receptor 2 (Tfr2), and IL-6. Proc Natl Acad Sci USA. 2006; 103: 10289–93.

[63] Andriopoulos B, Corradini E, Xia Y, Faasse SA, Chen S, Grgurevic L, et al. BMP-6 is a key endogenous regulator of hepcidin expression and iron metabolism. Nat Genet. 2009; 41: 482-7.

[64] Babitt JL, Huang FW, Wrighting DM, Xia Y, Sidis Y, Campagna JA, et al. Bone morphogenetic protein signaling by hemojuvelin regulates hepcidin expression. Nat Genet. 2006; 38: 531–9.

[65] Ganz T, Olbina G, Girelli D, Nemeth E, Westerman M. Immunoassay for human serum hepcidin. Blood. 2008;112: 4292–4297.

[66] Merle U, Fein E, Gehrke SG, Stremmel W, Kulaksiz H. The iron regulatory peptide hepcidin is expressed in the heart and regulated by hypoxia and inflammation. Endocrinology 2007; 148: 2663–8.

[67] Bekri S, Gaul P, Anty R, et al. Increased adipose tissue expression of hepcidin in severe obesity is independent from diabetes and NASII. Gastroenterologia 2006; 131: 788–96.

[68] Dallalio G, Law E, Means Jr RT. Hepcidin inhibits in vitro erythroid colony formation at reduced erythropoietin concentrations. Blood 2006;107:2702–4.

[69] Nicolas G, Chauvet C, Viatte L, Danan JL, Bigard S, Devaux I, et al. The gene encoding the iron regulatory peptide hepcidin is regulated by anemia, hypoxia, and inflammation. J Clin Invest 2002; 110: 1037–44.

[70] Waheed A, Grubb JH, Zhou XY, Tomatsu S, Fleming RE, Costaldi ME. Regulation of transferrin mediated iron uptake by HFE, the protein defective in hereditary hemochromatosis. Proc Natl Acad Sci USA 2002; 99: 3117–22.

[71] Parkkila S, Waheed A, Britton RS, Feder JN, Tsuchihashi Z, Schatzman RC, et al. Immunohistochemistry of HLA-H, the protein defective in patients with hereditary hemochromatosis, reveals unique pattern of expression in gastrointestinal tract. Proc Natl Acad Sci USA 1997;94: 2534–9.

Section 2

Cellular Iron Metabolism

2

Cellular Iron Metabolism – The IRP/IRE Regulatory Network

Ricky S. Joshi, Erica Morán and Mayka Sánchez
Institute of Predictive and Personalized Medicine of Cancer (IMPPC), Badalona, Barcelona, Spain

1. Introduction

General Overview of iron homeostasis

Iron is the most abundant transition metal in cellular systems and is an essential micronutrient required for many cellular processes including DNA synthesis, oxidative cell metabolism, haemoglobin synthesis and cell respiration. Despite iron being an absolute requirement for almost all organisms, caution should be taken with an inappropriate disequilibrium in iron levels because excess iron is toxic and a lack of it leads to anaemia.

As a transition metal, iron can exist in various oxidation states (from -2 to +6). Usually, iron exists and switches between two different ionic states (Fe^{+2} and Fe^{+3}). Iron in the reduced state is known as ferrous iron and has a net positive charge of two (Fe^{+2}). In the oxidized state it is known as ferric iron and has a net positive charge of three (Fe^{+3}). This electron switch property of iron as a metal element allows it to be used as a cofactor by many enzymes involved in oxidation-reduction reactions and also confers its toxicity. Iron toxicity relates to the intracellular labile iron pool (LIP), a pool of transitory, chelatable (i.e. free) and redox-active iron that can catalyze the formation of oxygen-derived free radicals via the Fenton reaction. Iron-catalyzed oxidative stress causes lipid peroxidation, protein modifications, DNA damage (promoting mutagenesis) and depletion of antioxidant defences.

Iron containing proteins can be classified into 3 groups (for an extensive revision see (Crichton, 2009)):

Haemoproteins, in which iron is bound to four ring nitrogen atoms of a porphyrin molecule called haem and one or two axial ligands from the protein. Examples of haemoproteins are the oxygen transport protein haemoglobin, the muscle oxygen storage protein myoglobin, peroxidases, catalases and electron transport proteins such as the cytochromes a, b and c.

Iron-sulphur proteins are proteins that contain iron atoms bound to sulphur forming a cluster linked to the polypeptide chain by thiol groups of cysteine residues or to non-protein structures by inorganic sulphide and cysteine thiols. Examples of iron-sulphur proteins are the ferredoxins, hydrogenases, nitrogenases, NADH dehydrogenases and aconitases.

Non-haem non iron-sulphur proteins, these proteins can be of three types:

Mononuclear non-haem iron enzymes such as catechol or Rieske dioxygenases, alpha-keto acid dependent enzymes, pterin-dependent hydrolases, lipoxygenases and bacterial superoxide dismutases

Dinuclear non-haem iron enzymes, also known as diiron proteins, like the H-ferritin chain, haemerythrins, ribonucleotide redictase R2 subunit, stearoyl-CoA desaturases and bacterial monoxygenases

Proteins involved in ferric iron transport, for instance the transferrin family that includes serotransferrin, lactotransferrin, ovotransferrin and melanotransferrin and are found in physiological fluids of many vertebrates.

As previously mentioned, many proteins involved in very different cellular pathways contain iron. Therefore, cells require iron to function properly. However, mammals have no physiological excretion mechanisms to release an excess of iron and consequently, iron homeostasis must be tightly controlled on both the systemic and cellular levels to provide just the right amounts of iron at all times. If an adequate balance of iron is not achieved, it will cause a clinical disorder. Iron is therefore crucial for health. Iron deficiency leads to anaemia —a major world-wide public health problem— and iron overload is toxic and increases the oxidative stress of body tissues leading to inflammation, cell death, system organ dysfunction, and cancer (Hentze et al., 2010).

Systemic iron homeostasis is regulated by the hepcidin/ferroportin system in vertebrates (Ganz & Nemeth, 2011). Hepcidin is a liver-specific hormone secreted in response to iron loading and inflammation and is the master regulator of systemic iron homeostasis. Increased hepcidin levels result in anaemia while decreased expression is a causative feature in most primary iron overload diseases. Transcription of hepcidin in hepatocytes is regulated by a variety of stimuli including cytokines (TNF-α, IL-6), erythropoiesis, iron stores and hypoxia (De Domenico et al., 2007). At the molecular level, the binding of hepcidin to the iron exporter ferroportin (FPN) induces its internalization and degradation; and thus prevents iron entry into plasma (Nemeth et al., 2004).

Cellular iron homeostasis is mainly controlled by a system composed of RNA binding proteins and RNA binding elements that constitutes a post-transcriptional gene expression regulation system known as the Iron Regulatory Protein (IRP) / Iron-Responsive Element (IRE) regulatory network (Hentze et al., 2010; Muckenthaler et al., 2008; Recalcati et al., 2010). This chapter will focus on the IRP/IRE regulatory network, addressing in depth, its role in the regulation of cellular iron homeostasis, its alterations in diseases and new research lines to be explored in the future.

2. Cellular iron homeostasis

Cellular iron maintenance involves the coordination of iron uptake, utilization, and storage to ensure appropriate levels of iron inside the cell. Although transcriptional regulation of iron metabolism has been reported in the literature; cellular iron homeostasis is mainly controlled at the post-transcriptional level (Muckenthaler et al., 2008). In general, post-transcriptional regulation ensures a faster and easier way of controlling protein expression levels in mammalians by changing the rate of specific mRNA synthesis using repressor or stabilizer proteins. Particularly in iron metabolism, this system involves the so-called IRP/IRE regulatory network.

2.1 The IRP/IRE regulatory network

The Iron Regulatory Protein (IRP) / Iron-Responsive Element (IRE) regulatory network is a post-transcriptional gene expression regulation system that controls cellular iron homeostasis. This network comprises two RNA binding proteins called Iron Regulatory Proteins (IRP1 and IRP2) and *cis*-regulatory RNA elements, named Iron-Responsive Elements, or IRE, that are present in mRNAs encoding for important proteins of iron homeostasis.

IRP/IRE interactions regulate the expression of the mRNAs encoding proteins for iron acquisition (transferrin receptor 1, TFR1; divalent metal transporter 1, Slc11a2), iron storage (H-ferritin, Fth1; L-ferritin, Ftl), iron utilization (erythroid 5-aminolevulinic acid synthase, Alas2), energy (mitochondrial aconitase, Aco2; *Drosophila* succinate dehydrogenase, Sdh), and iron export (ferroportin, Fpn-Slc40a1) (Figure 1) (Muckenthaler et al., 2008). Less well known is the role of the IRP/IRE regulatory network in the control of other pathways (for details see section 2.1.3.5).

The IRE binding activities of IRP1 and IRP2 are regulated by intracellular iron levels and other stimuli (including nitric oxide, oxidative stress, and hypoxia) through distinct mechanisms (for details see sections 2.1.2.1 and 2.1.2.2). IRP/IRE binding activity is high in iron-deficient cells and low in iron-replete cells. When iron levels inside the cells are increased the IRPs are unable to bind the IREs, because IRP1 in these conditions assemble an iron-sulphur cluster (Fe-S cluster) and it is transformed into a cytosolic aconitase; while IRP2 is degraded by a mechanism that involves the proteosome (see section 2.1.2.1). Therefore, only in iron-starved cells, the IRPs became an IRE binding protein (Figure 1).

Depending on the location of the IRE in the untranslated regions (UTR), IRP binding regulates gene expression differentially. Both IRPs inhibit translation initiation when bound to IREs at the 5'UTR by preventing the recruitment of the small ribosomal subunit to the mRNA (Muckenthaler et al., 1998). Although the cap binding complex eIF4F can assemble when IRP1 is bound to a cap-proximal IRE, the small ribosomal subunit cannot be established in the presence of IRP1, which interferes with the bridging interactions that need to be established between eIF4F and the small ribosomal subunit. The IRPs association with the 3'IREs of the TRF1 mRNA decreases its turnover by preventing an endonucleolytic cleavage and its mRNA degradation (Binder et al., 1994). This mechanism of IRP mRNA stabilization has not been fully probed for other 3' IRE-containing mRNAs such as DMT1 and CDC14A, which only have a single 3'IRE and may require additional factors for their regulation. Overall, the regulation of the IRE-binding activities of IRP1 and IRP2 assures the appropriate expression of IRP target mRNAs and cellular iron balance.

The IRP/IRE regulatory system was initially described as a simple post-transcriptional regulatory gene expression circuit controlling the production of the ferritins and Transferrin Receptor 1. The identification of other mRNAs associated with this system has added considerable complexity and has extended the role of the IRPs to interconnect different cellular pathways, which should be regulated by iron metabolism in a coordinated way.

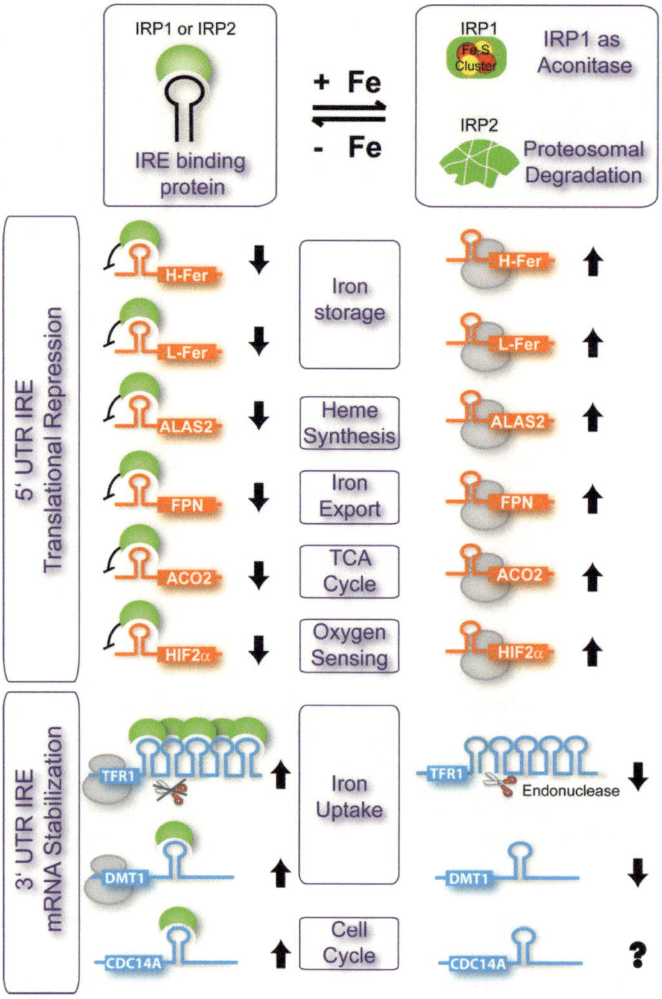

Fig. 1. The iron-regulatory protein/iron-responsive element (IRP/IRE) regulatory system. IRP1 and IRP2 bind to IREs in iron-deficient conditions (-Fe). This binding mediates translation repression in those mRNAs with an IRE at the 5′ UTR, decreasing their protein levels. If the IRE is in the 3′ UTR the IRP binding enhances mRNA stabilization by preventing an endonucleotic cleavage in TFR1 mRNA. The exact mechanism of IRP regulation in DMT1 and CDC14A mRNA is not yet well known. H-Fer: H-ferritin, L-Fer: L-ferritin, ALAS2: erythroid-specific delta-aminolevulinate synthase, FPN: Ferroportin, ACO2: mitochondrial aconitase 2, HIF2α: Hypoxia inducible factor 2 alpha, TFR1: Transferrin Receptor 1, DMT1: divalent metal transporter 1, CDC14A: Cell Division Cycle 14, *S. Cerevisiae*, homolog A.

2.1.1 Iron-Responsive Elements (IRE)

Iron-responsive elements or IREs are conserved *cis*-regulatory mRNA motifs of 25-30 nucleotides located in the untranslated regions (UTR) of mRNAs that encode proteins involved in iron metabolism.

The mRNAs of H-ferritin (FTH1), L-ferritin (FTL), erythroid-specific delta-aminolevulinate synthase (ALAS2), ferroportin (FPN), mitochondrial aconitase 2 (ACO2), and others (see section 2.1.3.5) contain one single IRE in their 5´UTRs (Figure 1 and 2). The mRNA encoding for Transferrin Receptor 1 (TFR1) is so far the only known mRNA with multiple (five) IREs, all of them located in its 3´UTR. The mRNA encoding for DMT1 protein (gene SLC11A2) also contains a single IRE in its 3´UTR (Figure 1 and 2). In addition, a single 3′ IRE has been reported in other not so well documented mRNAs (see section 2.1.3.5).

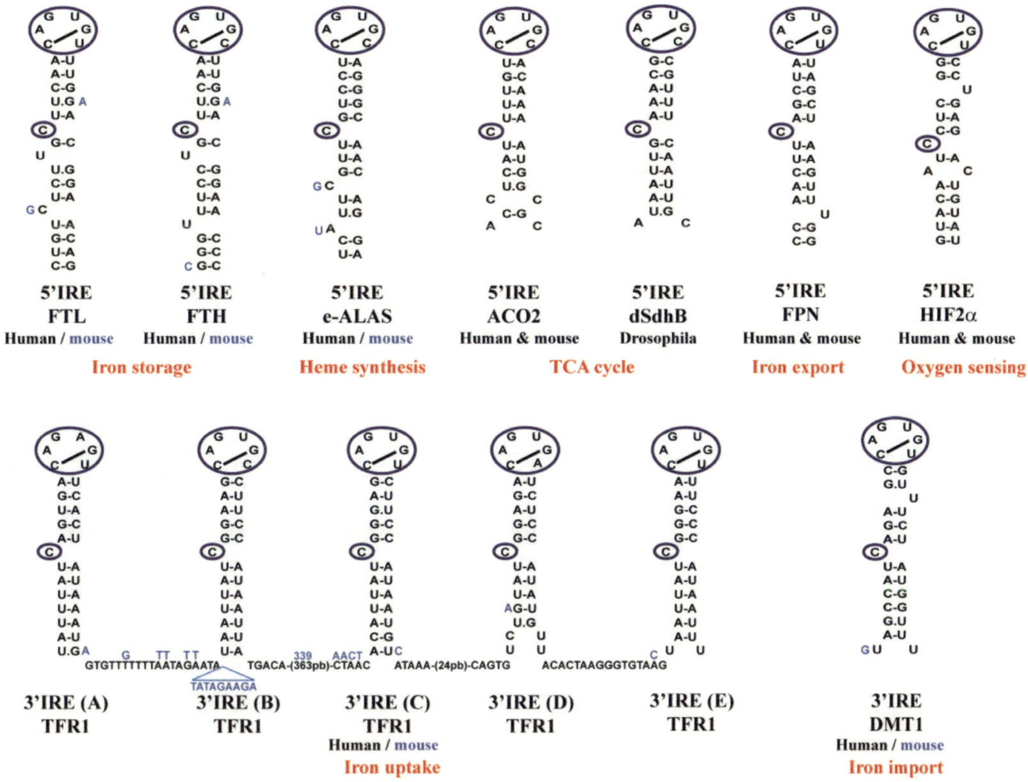

Fig. 2. Functional Iron-Responsive Elements (IREs) and the role of their encoded protein. Note all motifs contain the characteristic C-bulge (C8) present in the stem motif and a 6-nucleotide -CAGAGU/C- apical loop both circled in blue. 5′ IREs are shown at the top of the figure and 3′ IREs at the bottom. The 5 IREs from TFR1 mRNAs are depicted and named as IRE-A to IRE-E. Nucleotides shown in blue represent changes in mouse with respect to the human sequence. The function of the encoded protein is shown in red. FTL: L-Ferritin, FTH:H- Ferritin, e-ALAS2: erythroid-specific delta-aminolevulinate synthase, ACO2: mitochondrial aconitase 2, dSdhB: Drosophila succinate dehydrogenase B, FPN: Ferroportin, HIF2α: Hypoxia inducible factor 2 alpha, TFR1: Transferrin Receptor 1, DMT1: divalent metal transporter 1.

The canonical IRE hairpin-loop is composed of a six-nucleotide apical loop (5′-CAGWGH-3′; whereby W stands for A or U and H for A, C or U) on a stem of five paired nucleotides, a small asymmetrical bulge with an unpaired cytosine on the 5′strand of the stem, and an additional lower stem of variable length (see Figure 2 for IREs examples). The IRE stem forms base pairs of moderate stability, and folds into an α-helix (Figure 3B) distorted by the presence of a small 5′ bulge (an unpaired C8 nucleotide) in the middle of the IRE. IRE base pairs can be Watson-Crick bonding or wobble pairs (U.G or G.U). The IRE (CAGWGH) terminal loop forms a pseudotriloop (AGW) isolated by a conserved base pair (C14:G18) and followed by an unpaired nucleotide (N19, Figure 3A). The base pair C14:G18 and the unpaired nucleotide do not make contact with the protein, which suggests that the bridge C14:G18 serves only a structural role for IRP1 recognition (Walden et al., 2006). The pseudotriloop and the C8 nucleotide make multiple contacts with IRP1 (for more details see section 2.1.2.1). It is most likely that all these important structural details, revealed in the 2.8 angstrom resolution crystal structure of the IRP1:H-ferritin IRE complex reported by Walden and collaborators, also apply to IRP2:IRE structures (Walden et al., 2006).

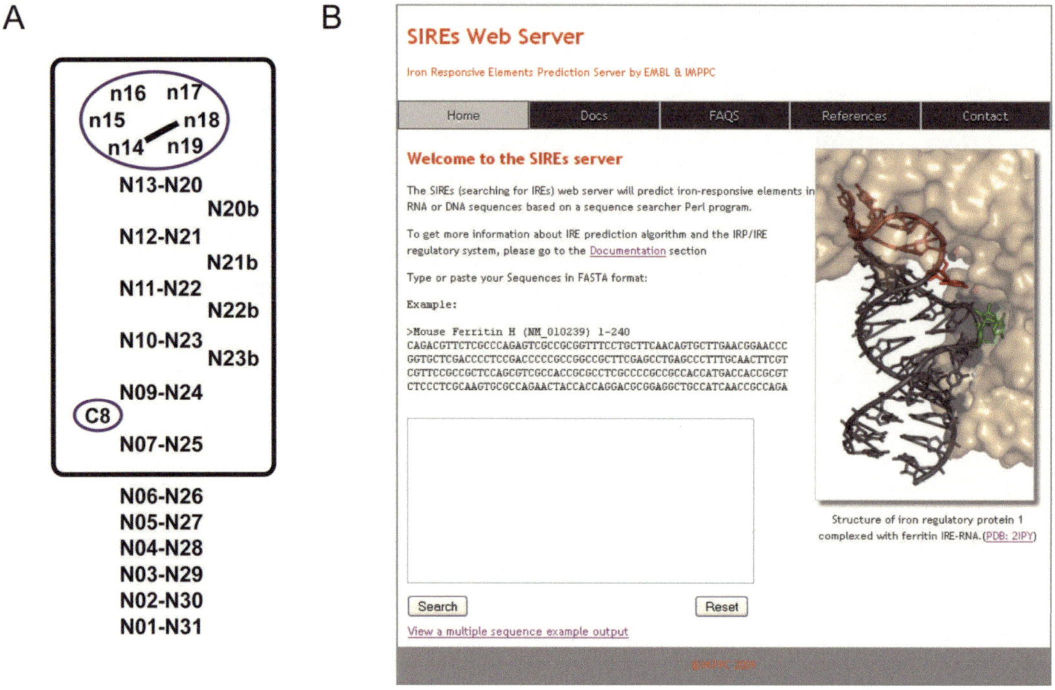

Fig. 3. SIREs, Searching for Iron-Responsive Elements, the bioinformatic program for the prediction of IREs. A. Schematic representation of an IRE motif, rectangular region indicates the IRE core region predicted by SIREs software. C-bulge (C8) and 6 nucleotide apical loop are shown within a blue circle. The presence of possible 3′ bulge nucleotides are represented as N20b, N21b, N22b and N23b. B. SIREs freely available web-server home page at http://ccbg.imppc.org/sires/index.html.

The differential regulation of the IRPs on the different 5′ and 3′ IREs is discussed in the section above. Mutations in the Iron-Responsive Elements disrupt the IRP/IRE regulatory system and cause iron-related disorders in humans (for details see sections 3).

2.1.1.1 Bioinfomatic predictions of iron-responsive elements

One of the biggest challenges facing researchers in the study of IREs is the availability of fast, reliable approaches to recognising possible IREs in known RNA sequences. Existing software tools to predict this type of *cis*-regulatory element (RNA Analyzer, UTRScan and RNAMotif) (Bengert & Dandekar, 2003; Macke et al., 2001; Mignone et al., 2005) are not sufficiently accurate to find atypical IREs due to their strict constraints for pattern matching searches. Therefore, these programs fail to identify mRNAs that have an atypical IRE with an unpaired 3′ bulged nucleotide in the upper stem, such as the HIF2α IRE (see Figure 2). In addition, previous SELEX (systematic evolution of ligands by exponential enrichment) experiments have reported that the six-nucleotide apical loop of an IRE can differ from the canonical CAG(U/A)GN sequence and still bind efficiently to IRPs *in vitro* (Butt et al., 1996; Henderson et al., 1996). Furthermore, current IRE prediction programs do not allow for the presence of a mismatch pair of nucleotides in the upper stem, although the IRE reported in the Gox mRNA contains one such mismatch (Kohler et al., 1999) (see Figure 5).

To overcome these limitations, the laboratory of Dr. Mayka Sanchez has created new software for the prediction of IREs which is implemented as a user-friendly web server tool. The SIREs (Search for iron-responsive elements) web server uses a simple data input interface and provides structural analysis, predicts RNA folds, folding energy data and an overall quality flag based on properties of well characterized IREs. The SIREs algorithm is implemented on a Perl script that screens for a 19 or 20 nucleotide sequence motif corresponding to the core sequence of an IRE (positions n07–n25) that includes the hexa-apical hairpin loop (n14–n19), the upper stem, the cytosine bulge (C8) and the lower base pair (n07–n25) (see Figure 3A). This core IRE region is sufficient to identify known IREs assigning them an equal RNA binding hierarchy as recently reported between IRP1 and 5′ IREs (Goforth et al., 2010). The SIREs results are displayed in a tabular format and as a schematic visual representation that highlights important features of the IRE. The major advantage of the SIREs program is that it is able to detect canonical and non-canonical IREs because it integrates and allows the combination of several experimentally reported IRE structures without losing stringency in its predictions. Therefore, with this new bioinformatic software one can screen an input sequence for the existence of IRE structures and will receive a scored output (as a high, medium or low) of the predicted IRE for prioritization of further studies (see Figure 3B for the home page of the SIREs website).

Overall, the SIREs web server represents a significant improvement on currently available programs to predict IREs, providing the scientific community with an easy-to-use bioinformatics platform to identify putative IRE motifs that can then be subjected to further experimental testing *in vitro* and *in vivo*. The SIREs web server is freely available on the web at: http://ccbg.imppc.org/sires/index.html (Figure 3) and was published by Campillos and collaborators (Campillos et al., 2010).

2.1.2 Iron regulatory proteins: IRP1 and IRP2

Iron regulatory proteins 1 and 2 (IRP1 and IRP2) are proteins sensitive to cytosolic iron concentrations that post-transcriptionally regulate the expression of iron metabolism genes to optimize cellular iron availability. IRP1 is encoded by the gene ACO1 found in chromosome 9p21.1 and IRP2 by the gene IREB2 found in chromosome 15q25.1. In iron-deficient cells, IRPs bind to iron-responsive elements (IREs) found in the mRNAs of ferritin, transferrin receptor and other iron metabolism transcripts, enhancing iron uptake and decreasing iron sequestration. IRP1 registers cytosolic iron status mainly through an iron-sulphur cluster switch mechanism, alternating between an active cytosolic aconitase form with an iron-sulphur cluster ligated to its active site and an apo-protein form that binds IREs. Although IRP2 is 60 to 70% identical to IRP1 (one of the major difference is an extra 73 amino acid insertion present in IRP2), both proteins are differentially regulated. IRP2 does not have an aconitase function and its activity is regulated primarily by iron-dependent degradation through a ubiquitin-proteasomal system in iron-replete cells (see next section).

Constitutive deletion of both IRPs is embryonic lethal, demonstrating that the IRP/IRE regulatory system is essential for life (Galy et al., 2008; Smith et al., 2006). The groups of Matthias W. Hentze (EMBL) and Tracey Rouault (NIH) have reported knock-out targeted deletion strategies for IRP1 and/or IRP2 in whole animals or tissue specific. Their publications show that adult mice that constitutively lack IRP1 develop no overt abnormalities under standard laboratory conditions; however, IRP2 KO mice developed microcytic anaemia, elevated red cell protoporphyrin IX levels, high serum ferritin, and adult-onset neurodegeneration. When mice are missing both copies of IRP2 and one copy of IRP1 they develop a more severe anaemia and neurodegeneration compared with mice with deletion of IRP2 alone (Smith et al., 2006). At the cellular level, Galy and collaborators reported that mitochondrial iron supply and function also require IRPs for cellular ATP, haem and iron-sulphur cluster production (Galy et al., 2010).

Both IRPs are expressed in all tissues, however IRP1 is particularly abundant in kidney and brown fat, and IRP2 expression is higher in brain, intestine, and cells of the reticuloendothelial system (reviewed in (Cairo & Pietrangelo, 2000)).

2.1.2.1 Structure and regulation of IRPs by iron

IRP1 is a dual-functional protein with a key role in the control of iron metabolism as an IRE-binding protein and with an additional function as a cytoplasmic isoform of the aconitase enzyme (Figure 4). Aconitases are a group of iron-sulphur enzymes that require a 4Fe-4S cluster (iron-sulphur cluster, ISC) for their function. The ISC is essential to catalyse the conversion of citrate to isocitrate via the intermediate cis-aconitate during the citric acid cycle. Three iron atoms are attached to cysteine residues of the active site, whereas a fourth iron remains free and mediates catalytic chemistry (reviewed in (Eisenstein, 2000)). IRP1, as cytosolic aconitase (c-aconitase), catalyses the citrate to isocitrate conversion in the cytosol and shares 30% amino acid sequence homology with mitochondrial aconitase (m-aconitase), which catalyzes the same reaction in the mitochondrial matrix. In contrast with m-aconitase, IRP1 only retains its ISC and enzymatic function in iron-replete cells, and thus only functions as a cytosolic aconitase when cells have high levels of iron. Under iron scarcity, the ISC dissemble from holo-IRP1 and the protein is converted into IRP1 apo-protein, acquiring IRE-binding ability. Hence, IRP1 is reversibly regulated by this unusual ISC switch (Wallander et al., 2006).

The IRP1 protein is composed of four globular domains. In its c-aconitase form, domains 1–3 are compact and join domain 4 through a polypeptide linker and the ISC is central at the interface of the four domains. The ISC structure and surrounding environment are fairly well conserved between c- and m-aconitases. Nevertheless, the overall structure of holo-

IRP1 (a 889 amino acid protein), shows differences to m-aconitase, which is smaller (780 amino acids). The short IRP1 fragments that do not superimpose with m-aconitase are exposed on the surface of the protein. As a result, the shapes and surface topologies of holo-IRP1 and m-aconitase diverge substantially, which may explain the fact that IRP1 is the only aconitase that can acquire IRE binding activity.

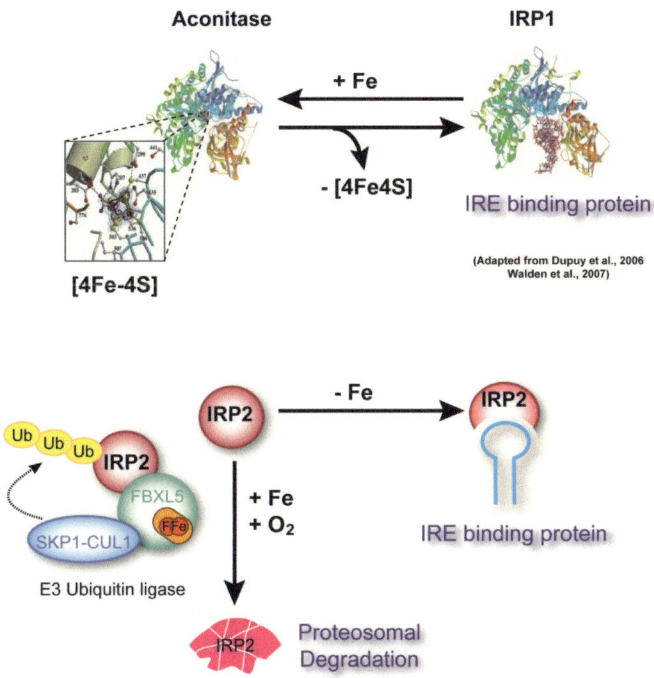

Fig. 4. Iron regulation of Iron-Regulatory Proteins IRP1 and IRP2. Under iron depleted conditions (-Fe) IRP1 and IRP2 bind to IREs. IRP1 is a bi-functional protein acting as an aconitase when it assembles an iron-sulphur cluster (4Fe-4S) or as an IRE binding protein. IRP2 undergoes proteosomal degradation via ubiquitinization (Ub) when iron (Fe) and oxygen (O_2) levels are high. FBXL5: F-Box and leucine rich repeat protein 5, SKP1: S-Phase kinase-associated protein 1, CUL1: Cullin 1.

IRP1 apo-protein shows an open conformation compared with that of cytosolic aconitase, allowing its interactions with IREs and controlling the gene expression of key proteins of iron metabolism. IRP1: H-ferritin IRE crystal structural complex has been resolved at a resolution of 2.8Å and the details of its reorganization upon loss of its ISC has been described by Walden and collaborators (Walden et al., 2006). IRP1 conformational changes after loss of its ISC reveals a rotation of domain 4 and an extensive rearrangement of domain 3, creating a hydrophilic cavity that allows access to the IRE (Figure 4). The RNA-protein interaction requires two important segments at the interface of domain 2 (residues 436-442) and domain 3 (residues 534-544). Thr438 and Asn439 make direct contact with the IRE. The terminal residues of the IRE motif, A15, G16 and U17 (see figure 3A), interact with Ser371, Lys379 and Arg269 respectively within a cavity between domains 2 and 3. A second binding site is present around the unpaired-C-bulge residue (C8 bulge, Figure 3A) located between the upper and lower stem, which occupies a pocket within domain 4, involving residues between Arg713 and Arg780. The IRE–IRP1 complex is also stabilized by additional ionic interactions. The evolutionary origin and selective advantage of the IRP1 dramatic conformational plasticity and dual functionality remains to be determined.

A second IRE-binding protein first named IRFB and lately renamed as IRP2 was isolated and characterized in rodents in 1993 (Henderson et al., 1993). This manuscript also reports that IRP1 IRE binding activity is predominant in liver, intestine, and kidney, while IRP2 revealed highest binding activity in intestine and brain. Human IRP2 has a molecular mass of 105 kD, slightly larger than human IRP1 (87kD) due to an extra 73 amino acid insertion. Human IRP2 shares 57% homology with human IRP1. Despite this homology, IRP2 is unable to assemble an iron-sulphur cluster and thus has no aconitase activity. IRP1 and IRP2's role in controlling mRNA translation and stabilization in IRE-containing mRNAs is similar, that is both proteins carry out a translational repression in 5′ IREs and mRNA stabilization in 3′ IREs. However unlike IRP1, IRP2 is rapidly targeted for degradation in iron-replete cells (Recalcati et al., 2010). It seems that the mechanism by which IRP2 undergoes iron-dependent degradation may involve different aspects. The 73 cysteine rich amino acid domain of IRP2 may be responsible for this degradation due to its ability to facilitate iron-dependent oxidation, ubiquitination, and proteasomal degradation (Wang & Pantopoulos, 2011). Recently, two groups have independently identified the protein FBXL5 as part of the ubiquitin ligase complex that promotes iron-dependent polyubiquitination and degradation of IRP2 (Salahudeen et al., 2009; Vashisht et al., 2009) (see Figure 4). As the stability of FBXL5 itself is controlled by iron and/or oxygen levels through an iron-binding hemerythrin-like domain located in the N-terminus, FBXL5 accumulates when iron is plentiful and is degraded upon iron depletion. By this mechanism the presence of FBXL5 in iron rich conditions works as a key sensor in the regulation of IRP2 degradation. No crystal structure of IRP2 is available as of yet, and forthcoming experiments will allow us to elucidate the role (if any) of the extra amino acid residues in IRP2 IRE binding specificity and/or their role in protein degradation. Ultimately, the crystallization of IRP2, especially in a complex with IRE, will be necessary to precisely map the RNA–protein interactions and further shed light on its mechanistic properties (Wang & Pantopoulos, 2011).

2.1.2.2 Regulation of IRPs by other stimuli than iron

Iron was the first identified regulator of the IRP/IRE network however various other stimuli, drugs and pathological agents have been reported to affect IRP activity.

Hypoxia

IRP1 and IRP2 are regulated by oxygen levels (reviewed in (Rouault, 2006)) which control their binding activity. Hypoxia has been shown to decrease the binding to IREs in IRP1 by favouring the assembly of the ISC and causing IRP1 to acquire aconitase activity, but increasing IRP2 activity (Meyron-Holtz et al., 2004). Other studies also reported an opposite regulatory effect of hypoxia on IRP1 and IRP2 IRE binding activities, though not all studies agree on the direction of this divergent modulation. As described in section 2.1.2.1 IRP2 degradation is controlled by FBXL5 in an iron- and oxygen-dependent manner, which suggests one possible explanation for the differential regulation of the two IRPs by hypoxia. At low oxygen concentrations, which favour the assembly of an ISC of IRP1 and stabilise IRP2, the latter regulates iron homeostasis but, at high oxygen concentrations, FBXL5 is stabilised, interacts with IRP2 and induces its degradation, whereas the apoform of IRP1 can bind and regulate the mRNAs encoding proteins of iron metabolism. These mechanisms may therefore allow cells to regulate iron metabolism effectively over a broad range of oxygen availability.

Hypoxia has also been shown to reduce IRP1 binding to HIF-2α mRNA via a newly identified 5′ IRE (see section 2.1.3.5), while slightly increasing binding to IRP2 (Zimmer et al., 2008). Interestingly, these authors describe a major effect of IRP1 on de-repression of HIF-2α translation in hypoxic conditions, and they suggest that IRP1 acts as a direct or indirect sensor of hypoxia, which is somehow contradictory to the previous reported predominant role of IRP2 at physiologically low oxygen levels (3%-5%). This work was done in the context of renal cells in which IRP1 is particularly abundant, and this may explain the main regulatory role of IRP1 in HIF translation during hypoxia.

Oxidative stress

Both IRP1 and IRP2 are sensitive to ROS (Reactive Oxygen Species) and RNS (Reactive Nitrogen Species) (reviewed in (Cairo & Pietrangelo, 2000)). As explained earlier, the redox regulation of IRP1 is mediated by its iron-sulphur cluster (ISC) switch. Exposure of cells to H_2O_2 leads to the removal of ISC and conversion of IRP1 into a null protein lacking both RNA binding and aconitase activities. This conversion can be reversed by myeloperoxidase-derived hypochlorite (Mutze et al., 2003).

Early studies of exogenous H_2O_2 exposure to cell lines were shown to increase IRP1 expression (Cairo & Pietrangelo, 2000) though this was later shown to be a consequence of signalling pathway effects rather than direct oxidative stress on IRP1 (Caltagirone et al., 2001). Successive studies in various cell models have reported a number of agents (superoxide, phorone, quinone) (reviewed in (Recalcati et al., 2010)) with the ability to increase cellular H_2O_2 and O_2- and reversibly inactivate IRP1. This opens up the question of whether IRP1 inactivation (and subsequent TFR1 down-regulation, ferritins up-regulation and therefore decreasing LIP) is a homeostatic response to subdue ROS formation.

ROS studies on IRP2 have revealed seemingly contradictory results to date. Iwai and collaborators suggested that ROS triggers down-regulation of IRP2 by alterations to "sensitive" amino acid residues leading to ubiquitin-dependent proteasomal degradation (Iwai et al., 1998). However, a more recent study reported that treatment of murine macrophage cells with exogenous H_2O_2 protects IRP2 against iron and increases its IRE-binding activity (Hausmann et al., 2011). Moreover, they also showed that IRP2 is stabilized during menadione-induced oxidative stress suggesting that the degradation of IRP2 in iron-replete cells is not only oxygen-dependent but also sensitive to redox perturbations. Overall, further in-depth analysis of the exact role of oxidative stress is needed to properly evaluate its specific role in iron homeostasis.

Nitric Oxide

Nitric Oxide (NO) is a vital signalling and effector molecule that can rapidly switch IRP1 from its holo- to the apo-form (Drapier, 1997). NO is produced by NO synthases and once released, attacks the ISC of IRP1 promoting its gradual disassembly and complete removal suggesting this NO-mediated switch could represent a homoeostatic response to iron starvation. NO has also been implicated in promoting iron efflux from cells (Drapier, 1997).

The effect of NO on IRP2 has also been studied, although with contradictory results. Wang and collaborators claimed that IRP2 was activated under NO exposure (Wang et al., 2005), whereas Kim and collaborators demonstrated that IRP2 degradation was NO-dependent (S. Kim et al., 2004). Mulero and collaborators showed that IRP2 had a lack of regulation by NO (Mulero & Brock, 1999). Furthermore, it has been reported that endogenous and exogenous NO increases (S. Kim & Ponka, 2002) or decreases (Pantopoulos & Hentze, 1995) ferritin levels and further discrepant results of TfR1 regulation by NO has been described (Pantopoulos & Hentze, 1995). As a result, the role of the IRP/IRE system in NO-mediated regulation of cellular iron metabolism still remains unknown.

Other antioxidants, such as ascorbate, α-tocopherol and N-acetylcysteine have also been shown to disturb the IRE/IRP regulation system by promoting the proteasomal turnover of IRP2 (Wang et al., 2004).

Other stimuli that affect IRP regulation: Hormones and viruses

A number of hormones and viruses have been documented as interacting with IRPs and regulating iron metabolism. In an extensive report, *in vitro* and *in vivo* studies of the thyroid hormone showed that it functionally regulates the IRE binding activity of the IRPs to ferritin mRNA (Leedman et al., 1996). Estrogens modulate the RNA binding of IRP1 in adipose tissue and consequently the expression of ferritin and TfR1 (Mattace Raso et al., 2009).

Given the importance of iron in viral infections and replication (Drakesmith & Prentice, 2008) several studies have outlined the impact of viruses on iron homeostasis. In the case of Herpes Virus-1 infection of Madin-Darby bovine kidney cells, IRP RNA binding activity was reported to be reduced (Maffettone et al., 2008). However, this effect may be due to different factors, as shown in studies on the hepatitis B virus X protein that produced an increase in ROS and thus IRP1 down modulation (Gu et al., 2008). Similarly, in a cell culture model of hepatitis C virus replication, the down-regulation of TfR1, increased FPN levels and reduced LIP were associated with concomitant induction of IRE-binding activity and IRP2 expression (Fillebeen et al., 2007).

Other stimuli that affect IRP regulation: Xenobiotics

Many studies of xenobiotic effects on the IRP/IRE regulatory system have been performed with Doxorubicin (DOX). DOX is an anti-cancer anthracycline that causes a severe form of chronic cardiomyopathy. The alcohol metabolite of DOX (DOXol) breaks iron away from the iron-sulphur cluster of cytoplasmic aconitase and the O_2 free radicals and H_2O_2 derived from the redox activation of DOX convert IRP1 to a null protein (Brazzolotto et al., 2003). In another study it was shown that this null protein does not actually rely on the action of DOXol but on anthracycline-iron complexes attacking both aconitase and IRP1 (Kwok & Richardson, 2002). IRP2 protein does not contain an ISC and is not affected by DOXol, but is degraded by the action of the ROS that is produced (Minotti et al., 2001). The ability of DOX to regulate the RNA binding activity of IRP1 and IRP2 may also be due to its anti-tumoral and cardiotoxic activities. The possibility of combining DOX with other anti-neoplastic drugs is currently being tested for clinical applications.

Other stimuli that affect IRP regulation: Cell growth

Iron homeostasis and cell growth are interrelated because iron is essential for cell proliferation and is especially required in neoplastic cells as they proliferate faster and thus require elevated iron supplies. This is demonstrated by a higher expression of TfR1 and higher transferrin iron uptake in cancer cells. In addition, iron is required for the function of many proteins involved in cell cycle and DNA synthesis (e.g. Ribonucleotide Reductase). Moreover, iron appears to play a critical role in the expression and regulation of a number of molecules that control cell cycle progression e.g. p53, GADD45 and WAF1/p21 (Gao et al., 1999). In fact, without iron, cells are unable to proceed from G1 to the S phase of the cell cycle due to post-transcriptional regulation caused by iron depletion in cyclin D1 expression (a protein that plays a critical role in G1 progression) (Nurtjahja-Tjendraputra et al., 2007).

The cell cycle further manipulates the IRP/IRE regulatory system as IRP2 is phosphorylated at Ser 157, independently of iron levels, by Cdk1/cyclin B1 during the G2/M phase of the cell cycle, and in turn dephosphorylated by CDC14A after mitosis. This reduces IRP2 RNA binding activity in the G2/M phase of the cell cycle, increasing ferritin synthesis and impairing TfR1 mRNA stability (Wallander et al., 2008). Therefore, it seems that this reversible phosphorylation of IRP2 facilitates cell cycle progression. It has been shown that IRP activity is high in a classical model of non-neoplastic cell growth such as liver regeneration (Cairo & Pietrangelo, 1994). Cell proliferation induces IRP2 activity possibly because of the combined effect of high iron consumption in growing cells and IRP2's preferential sensitivity to iron deprivation (Recalcati et al., 1999). However, the fact that IRP2 transcription is specifically stimulated by a c-myc oncogene (Wu et al., 1999) suggests that the induction of IRP2 activity (with consequent ferritin repression and TfR1 up-regulation) may be specifically aimed at ensuring sufficient iron for the metabolic requirement of proliferating cells.

In 2006, Sanchez and collaborators reported a novel IRE located in the 3' UTR of the cell division cycle 14A (CDC14A) mRNA that efficiently binds both IRP1 and IRP2 (Sanchez et al., 2006) (see also section 2.1.3.5). Differential splicing of CDC14A produces IRE- and non-IRE-containing mRNA isoforms. Interestingly, only the expression of the IRE-containing mRNA isoforms is selectively increased by cellular iron deficiency. This uncovered a previously unrecognized regulatory link between iron metabolism and the cell cycle.

2.1.3.1 The IRP/IRE regulatory network in iron uptake

The main cellular iron uptake pathway is mediated by Transferrin Receptor 1 (TFR1, gene located on chromosome 3q29), which internalises iron-bound transferrin (TF) via a receptor-mediated endocytosis mechanism (Ponka et al., 1998). Iron-loaded transferrin binds with high affinity to TFR1 on the surface of cells, and the complex undergoes endocytosis via clathrin-coated pits. Once inside the endosome, a proton pump lowers the pH to 5.5, resulting in the release of Fe^{3+} from transferrin. Subsequently, the affinity of transferrin to TFR1 falls about 500-fold, resulting in its de-attachment of the TFR1-TF complex. In the final step of the cycle, non-iron bound transferrin is secreted into the bloodstream to recapture more Fe^{3+} and the transferrin receptor 1 protein is again relocated in the cell surface for another round of endocytosis.

TFR1 is expressed in many cells and plays a relevant function in erythroid iron acquisition for haem synthesis and haemoglobinization. Its expression parallels the maturation of erythroid progenitors and is involved in the development of erythrocytes and the nervous system (Levy et al., 1999).

Knockout mice homozygous for a null mutation in the transferrin receptor 1 (Tfr1) gene die after 12.5 days from severe anaemia and neurological abnormalities during embryonic development (Levy et al., 1999). These mice have a more severe phenotype than homozygous hypotransferrinaemic (*hpx/hpx*) mice that carry a mutation in the transferrin gene and have a severe reduction of transferrin expression. Haploinsufficiency for Tfr1 (Trfr+/-) results in impaired erythroid development with microcytic, hypochromic erythrocytes and abnormal iron homeostasis with mild tissue iron depletion in liver and spleen. In this regard, Trfr+/- mice differ from *hpx/hpx* and +/*hpx* mice, which have increased intestinal iron absorption leading to tissue iron overload.

TFR1 expression is controlled by iron and oxygen status amongst other factors (Cairo & Pietrangelo, 2000). At the transcriptional level, TFR1 is regulated by the hypoxia-inducible factor HIF1 in response to low oxygen levels and iron starvation (Bianchi et al., 1999). In addition, the TFR1 promoter region contains potential binding sites for transcription factors such as c-myc (O'Donnell et al., 2006). Nevertheless, in most cells TFR1 expression is mainly controlled post-transcriptionally by cellular iron levels through binding of IRP1 and IRP2 to five IREs located in the 3' UTR of the TFR1 mRNA (see Figure 2). TFR1 mRNA is stabilized by the binding of IRPs under iron-starved conditions by a mechanism that involves the protection of the mRNA degradation by a cleavage of a putative, as yet unidentified, endonuclease (Figure 1). This mechanism will ensure an increased expression of TFR1 in the cell surface to stimulate the acquisition of iron from plasma transferrin, and it will be blocked in iron-replete cells. However, the IRP/IRE regulation of TFR1 mRNA is overridden in specialized cells such as the erythroid progenitor cells, where TFR1 mRNA stability is uncoupled from iron supply and IRP regulation to ensure efficient massive iron uptake needed in these cells for haem synthesis and haemoglobinisation. In these cells TFR1 expression is regulated transcriptionally by a promoter erythroid active element (Lok & Ponka, 2000).

The SLC11A2 gene, located on chromosome 12q13, encodes a member of the solute carrier 11 protein family named Divalent Metal Transporter 1 (DMT1) or natural resistance-associated macrophage protein 2 (Nramp2). DMT1 is a glycoprotein that consists of twelve transmembrane domains and transports reduced ferrous iron (Fe+2) and other divalent metals (manganese, cobalt, nickel, cadmium, lead, copper, and zinc) to the inside of duodenal enterocytes, where it is highly expressed at the apical (luminal) site (Mackenzie & Garrick, 2005).

Inorganic iron absorption via DMT1 is an important iron uptake pathway, as observed in homozygous *mk/mk* mice that have microcytic, hypochromic anaemia due to severe defects in intestinal iron absorption and erythroid iron utilization. By positional cloning, Fleming and collaborators discovered in 1997 that a missense mutation in the gene Nramp2 was responsible for the mk mouse phenotype (Fleming et al., 1997). One year later the same group also reported that a similar phenotype present in Belgrade (b) rats was due to the same missense mutation, a glycine-to-arginine missense mutation (G185R), in the Nramp2 gene (Fleming et al., 1998). Functional studies of the protein encoded by the mutated b allele of rat Nramp2 demonstrated that the mutation disrupted iron transport. Therefore, the phenotypic characteristics of *mk* mouse and Belgrade rats indicate that Nramp2 is not only essential for normal intestinal iron absorption but also for transport of iron out of the transferrin cycle endosome.

DMT1 is a conserved transporter in vertebrates and the phenotype called chardonnay (*cdy*) in zebrafish mutants with hypochromic, microcytic anaemia is due to a nonsense mutation in DMT1. The truncated DMT1 protein expressed in cdy mutants is not functional (Donovan et al., 2002). In humans, mutations in this gene are associated with hypochromic microcytic anaemia with iron overload. This is a very rare disease so far described in only five subjects (OMIM 206100).

The SLC11A2 gene encodes four transcripts that are the result of alternative splicing at the 5′ or 3′ end, yielding DMT-1A-IRE, DMT-1B-IRE, DMT-1A-nonIRE, and DMT-1B-nonIRE isoforms. The different isoforms of DMT1 are differentially expressed in tissues, increasing somewhat the complexity of the study of this gene (Hubert & Hentze, 2002). One of the two 3′ splicing forms (the IRE isoform) contains an IRE structure in its 3′ UTR (see Figure 2) and is up-regulated by iron deficiency via the IRPs (Mackenzie & Garrick, 2005); however, the regulation of DMT1 is very complex and both transcriptional and post-transcriptional regulations may be involved in its gene expression regulation. The ablation of both IRPs in intestinal epithelial cells reduces the levels of IRE-containing DMT1 mRNA and DMT1-dependent intestinal iron uptake (Galy et al., 2008), but transcriptional regulation may be important, as is also suggested by recent studies showing that HIF2α–dependent DMT1 transcription plays a role in intestinal iron uptake (Mastrogiannaki et al., 2009).

2.1.3.2 The IRP/IRE regulatory network in iron storage

In addition to iron recycling and absorption, the storage and potential release of (excess) iron are critical determinants of circulating iron levels. Under physiological conditions, approximately 20% (0.5 to 1g) of the body's total iron content is stocked in the storage compartment, and only 1 to 2mg of iron is lost each day. The iron stores become depleted when iron absorption does not meet the body's needs or in cases of excessive iron loss (e.g. bleeding, pregnancy); conversely, tissue iron overload occurs when intestinal iron absorption surpasses iron utilization and loss (Andrews, 2010). Iron storage should be therefore tightly controlled to avoid an iron imbalance that will lead to a disease stage.

Ferritins are the major iron storage protein, and are found in the cytoplasm, mitochondria, and nucleus of the cells (Arosio et al., 2009). In vertebrates, cytoplasmic ferritin is expressed in almost all tissues and plays an important role in the control of intracellular iron distribution. Ferritin consists of a 24-subunit heteromultimer of light (L) and heavy (H) chains (174 and 182 amino acids respectively) that form a spherical shell around a cavity where iron (as ferric oxide) is stored. Each subunit has a distinct role in iron metabolism: L-ferritin facilitates iron-core formation and H-ferritin subunit generates ferroxidase activity (converting Fe^{+2} to Fe^{+3}) to incorporate iron into the protein shell. Plant and bacteria ferritins have only a single type of subunit which probably fulfils both functions. L- and H-ferritin subunits are synthesized by two different genes located on chromosomes 19q13.2 and 11q13, respectively. Although both genes are ubiquitously expressed, post-transcriptional regulation mediates tissue-specific changes in the H/L mRNA ratio.

The best characterized system regulating ferritin expression is the post-transcriptional, iron-dependent machinery based on the interaction between the IRPs and IREs localized in the 5′ untranslated region of H- and L-ferritin mRNA (Muckenthaler et al., 2008) (see Figure 1 and 2). Iron deficient cells need to rapidly mobilize the iron storage pool and in these conditions there is no need for the production of ferritins. This is achieved through the formation of

IRP/IRE complexes in the 5'UTR of ferritins that inhibits translation in iron-starved cells. Mechanistically, this translational block is due to the IRP interference in the recruitment of the small ribosomal subunit to the mRNA by preventing the interactions between the cap binding complex eIF4F and the small ribosomal subunit (Muckenthaler et al., 1998). The rate of *de novo* synthesis and abundance of ferritin can change over a 50-fold range in response to variations in iron availability mainly via the IRP/IRE regulatory system and thus the transcripts of the H- and L-ferritin chains are the prototypes of IRP-mediated translational control.

In vivo disruption of the H-ferritin gene by homologous recombination (Fth-/- mice) is early embryonic lethal (Ferreira et al., 2000). Fth -/- embryos die between 3.5 and 9.5 days of development, suggesting that there is no functional redundancy between the two ferritin subunits and that, in the absence of H subunits, L-ferritin homopolymers are not able to maintain iron in a bioavailable and nontoxic form. Fth +/- mice are healthy, fertile, and do not differ significantly from their control littermates. To overcome this embryonic lethality of Fth -/- mice, the group of Dr. Lukas Kuhn has recently created an intestine-specific H-ferritin knock-out mouse model (Vanoaica et al., 2010), which shows that not only is hepcidin required for an accurate control of iron absorption, but H-ferritin is also critical for limiting iron efflux from intestinal cells. These mice with an intestinal H-ferritin gene deletion show increased body iron stores and transferrin saturation that resembles Hereditary Hemochromatosis (HH).

In humans defects in the L-ferritin gene are associated with a neurodegenerative disease (NBIA3, neurodegeneration with brain iron accumulation 3, OMIM #606159), genetic hyperferritinemia without iron overload (Kannengiesser et al., 2009) and hyperferritinemia-cataract syndrome (HHCS). A mutation in the H-ferritin gene causes the autosomal dominant Iron overload syndrome. The hyperferritinemia-cataract syndrome (HHCS, OMIM #600886) and the autosomal dominant Iron overload syndrome (OMIM +134770) are due to specific mutations in the IRE motif of H- and L-ferritin, respectively and are extensively discussed in sections 3.1 and 3.2.

2.1.3.3 The IRP/IRE regulatory network in iron release

The transmembrane protein Ferroportin (FPN) is encoded by the SLC40A1 gene (chromosome 2q32.2) and this protein is the only known cellular iron exporter (Donovan et al., 2005). FPN is ubiquitously expressed, but is more abundant on the basolateral membrane of enterocytes in the duodenum and in reticuloendothelial cells. Ferroportin plays an important role in iron absorption (i.e. iron transport from enterocytes into the plasma) and iron reuse (i.e. iron released out of macrophages and coming from erythrophagocytosis of senescent or damaged red blood cells) (Hentze et al., 2010).

FPN is post-translationally regulated by hepcidin, which plays a central role in controlling systemic iron levels. On hepcidin binding, FPN is internalized and degraded (Ganz & Nemeth, 2011), thus inhibiting iron efflux from enterocytes, macrophages, and other cells.

FPN is also regulated at the post-transcriptional level by the IRP/IRE regulatory system (Figure 1). FPN mRNA bears a functional IRE motif in its 5'UTR (see Figure 2) that allows it to respond to iron manipulations in hepatic, intestinal, and monocytic cells (Lymboussaki et al., 2003). Similarly to ferritin IRP control, in iron deprivation the IRP binding to the ferroportin 5′ IRE will inhibit its translation. The simultaneous ablation of IRP1 and IRP2 in mice markedly increases intestinal FPN expression, despite the increase in hepatic hepcidin expression, indicating that IRPs are as critical as hepcidin for physiological FPN expression in the intestine (Galy et al., 2008). The IRP-dependent translational control of FPN expression has been found in response to nitric oxide (NO) (X. B. Liu et al., 2002) and erythrophagocytosis (Delaby et al., 2008). Duodenal epithelial and erythroid precursor cells utilize an alternative upstream promoter to express a FPN1 transcript, FPN1B, which lacks the IRE and therefore this FPN isoform will escape the IRP repression in iron-deficient conditions (Zhang et al., 2009).

SLC40A1 gene mutations are associated with an autosomal inherited genetic iron disorders described as ferroportin disease. Indeed, ferroportin disease is phenotypically heterogeneous with two sub-types. Classical ferroportin disease is the usual form and is characterized by hyperferritinemia, normal or low transferrin saturation, and iron overload in macrophages. This form is generally asymptomatic with no tissue damage and is due to ferroportin mutations that lead to a loss of function. The non-classical ferroportin form is rarer and resembles Hereditary Hemochromatosis with hepatocellular iron deposits and high transferrin saturation. In this form, ferroportin mutations are responsible for a gain of function with full iron export capability but resistance to down-regulation by hepcidin, which leads to a phenotype similar to hepcidin deficiency-related HH (i.e. types 1, 2, and 3). In fact, the non-classical ferroportin form is also known as Hereditary Hemochromatosis type 4. Most of the described mutations in ferroportin are located in the coding region or in exon-intron boundaries, only one patient with iron-overload Hereditary Hemochromatosis type 4 has been described with a point mutation close to the FPN IRE. This mutation could alter the IRE structure and the IRP regulation of FPN, but this was not studied further (Liu et al., 2005). In addition, radiation-induced polycythaemia (Pcm) mice were shown to have a ferroportin promoter microdeletion that also eliminates the iron-responsive element (IRE) in the 5' untranslated region (Mok et al., 2004) (see section 3.3).

2.1.3.4 The IRP/IRE regulatory network in iron utilization and energy metabolism

The erythroid iron utilization is also controlled by the IRP/IRE system through the interaction with ALAS2 mRNA. ALAS2 (erythroid-specific 5-aminolevulinic acid synthase) mRNA encodes for the first and rate-limiting enzyme in the haem biosynthesis pathway. This mRNA contains a 5′ UTR IRE (see Figure 1) identified using an *in silico* approach, and it is translationally repressed by the binding of the IRPs in iron-deficient conditions preventing the accumulation of toxic intermediates of the haem biosynthesis pathways such as protoporphyrin IX (Dandekar et al., 1991). The regulation of the Alas2 mRNA by the IRPs is affected in the zebrafish mutant *shiraz*, which presents severe hypochromic anaemia and early embryonic lethality due to defects in the Grx5 gene (Wingert et al., 2005). Grx5 protein is required for iron-sulphur cluster assembly and its abrogation shifts IRP1 conformation to an IRE-binding protein that leads to Alas2 repression and cytosolic iron depletion that also activates IRP2, which will further contribute to the repression of Alas2. A patient with iron overload and mild sideroblastic anaemia was described as bearing a homozygous mutation that interferes with intron 1 splicing and drastically reduces GLRX5 mRNA levels (Camaschella et al., 2007). Surprisingly, in this patient the anaemia was worsened by blood transfusions but partially reversed by iron chelation, presumably because iron chelation will redistribute iron to the cytosol, which might decrease IRP2 excess, improving haem synthesis and anaemia. These intricate mechanisms reveal the control of the IRP/IRE regulatory system in haem biosynthesis during erythroid differentiation, as well as the coordination of the regulation of haemoglobin with the iron-sulphur cluster assembly machinery.

The IRP/IRE system also controls energy metabolism by the regulation of two iron-sulphur containing enzymes of the tricarboxylic acid cycle (TCA cycle), the mitochondrial aconitase Aco2 and the Drosophila succinate dehydrogenase B, SdhB. These two mRNAs contain a single 5′ UTR IRE that were identified using the same IRE bio-computational searching approach as previously mentioned (Gray et al., 1996) (see Figure 1). The translational regulation of these mRNAs by the IRPs may co-ordinate their expression with iron availability since these are iron-containing enzymes, and altogether influence energy metabolism.

There is evidence that the translational repression exerted by the IRPs varies depending on the targeted mRNA. For instance, IRP regulation of ferritin transcripts is stronger than IRP Aco2 repression (Schalinske et al., 1998), this is in part due to differences in binding affinities of the IRPs for each particular transcript (Goforth et al., 2010).

2.1.3.5 The IRP/IRE regulatory network in other pathways

Apart from the IREs found in transferrin receptor 1, DMT1, H- and L-ferritins, ferroportin, Alas2, Aco2 and DSdhB already discussed, it seems that the IRP/IRE regulatory network is wider than previously thought and may regulate pathways not directly related to iron homeostasis (Sanchez et al., 2011).

Several groups have reported new IRE-containing mRNAs using different approaches

By computational searches, an IRE was described in the 3′ UTR of the human MRCKα, also known as CDC42 binding protein kinase alpha (CDC42BPA) (Cmejla et al., 2006) (see Figure 5). This kinase is the effector of a small Rho GTPase Cdc42 and promotes cytoskeletal reorganization. The authors claim that the mRNA of MRCKα is regulated by iron in a similar but less intense way to TFR1 mRNA and they proposed a novel molecular link between iron metabolism and the cellular cytoskeleton.

Members of our group have found a conserved and functional 3′ UTR IRE in a splicing mRNA isoform coding for CDC14A, a highly evolutionarily conserved cell-cycle phosphatase (Sanchez et al., 2006) (see Figure 5). The CDC14A mRNA and other mRNAs were bioinformatically predicted to bear a conserved IRE and subsequently spotted on a home-made iron-specific microarray. The CDC14A and HIF2α mRNAs (see below) were isolated by IRP immunoprecipitation, using total RNA derived from human cell lines, and identified using this same iron-specific microarray. The mRNA levels of the human CDC14A IRE isoform were shown to be specifically increased upon iron deprivation and it is possible that the regulation of CDC14A by the IRPs participates in the cell-cycle arrest observed during iron scarcity in cells. This finding opens up new interesting links between iron metabolism and cell cycle regulation.

The approach described above also revealed an atypical IRE in the 5′ UTR of HIF2α mRNA, which encodes for a key transcription factor induced by lack of oxygen (hypoxia) or iron (Sanchez et al., 2007). The IREs of HIF2α and DMT1 mRNAs have an additional bulge on the

3′ strand of the upper stem (see Figure 2). Under normoxic conditions, IRPs bind to the 5′ IRE of HIF2α mRNA and repress its translation, whereas hypoxia de-represses HIF2α mRNA translation by impairing IRP binding activity and prevents HIF2α degradation by inhibiting prolyl hydroxylase activity. This mechanism was proposed to modulate the levels of erythropoietin, a major target of HIF2α, adjusting the rate of red blood cell production to iron availability. Therefore, we discovered a negative feedback control of the HIF-mediated response under conditions of limited iron availability. HIF2α also regulates the expression of genes involved in angiogenesis and vascularisation (i.e. VEGF, PDGF), but the effect of the IRP/IRE system on these HIF2α targets has yet to be studied. To investigate the physiological and pathophysiological role of HIF2α IRE *in vivo* and the effect of its ablation on haematopoiesis and cancer development it would be necessary to generate a knock-in mouse model, in which the IRE-IRP interaction is selectively disrupted.

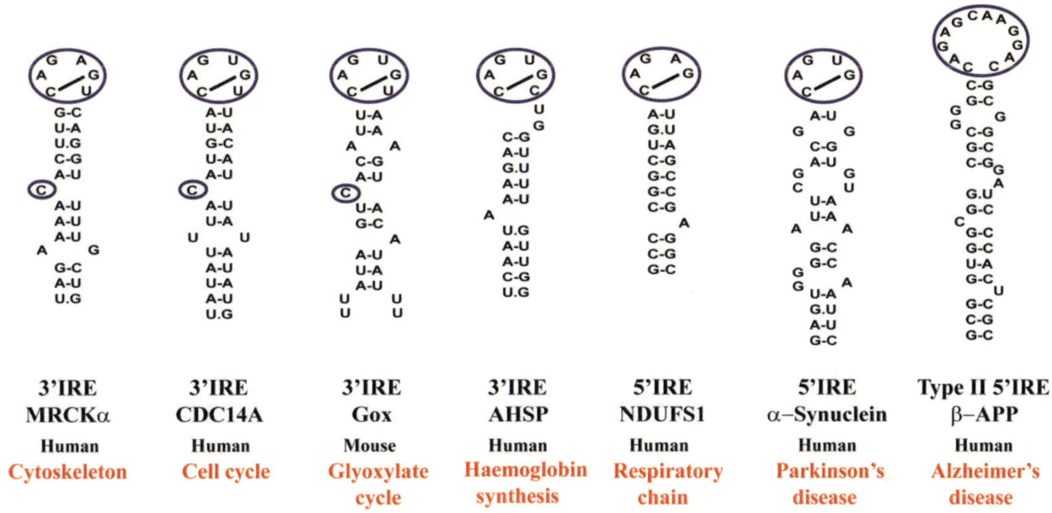

Fig. 5. Other poorly conserved IREs and the role of their encoded proteins. Apical loops and C-bulges are circled in blue. 5′ or 3′ location of the IRE and the specie where it is found are shown. The function of the encoded protein is shown in red. MRCKα: CDC42-binding protein kinase alpha, CDC14A: Cell division cycle 14A, Gox: Glycolate oxidase, AHSP: Erythroid-associated factor, NDUFS1: NADH-ubiquinone oxidoreductase Fe-S protein, β-APP: Amyloid beta A4 precursor protein.

Additional non-canonical and poorly conserved IREs have been described in different mRNAs.

An IRE-like structure is present in the 3′UTR of mouse glycolate oxidase (Gox), a liver-specific mRNA (Kohler et al., 1999) (see Figure 5). This novel IRE-containing mRNA was detected by enrichment of mRNAs using an affinity IRP1 matrix; positive mRNAs were then cloned in a cDNA library and screened by RNA-protein band shift assays. The main difference from a canonical IRE was the presence of a mismatched (A:A) nucleotide pair in the middle of the upper stem. This IRE-like sequence exhibited strong binding to IRPs at room temperature but not at 37 degrees and translational regulation in response to iron deprivation was not observed when the 3′IRE was cloned at a 5′ position of a reported construct. These observations brought the authors to claim that such an IRE is not functional in cells.

In primate sequences of the mRNA encoding for the alpha-haemoglobin-stabilizing protein (AHSP), a molecular chaperone that binds and stabilizes free alpha-globin during haemoglobin synthesis, a 3′ UTR IRE-like sequence was detected using an RNA folding program (Meehan & Connell, 2001) (see Figure 5). The main difference between this and a canonical IRE is the presence of an A8 bulge nucleotide instead of a C8 and in 2 additional unpaired nucleotides (UG) at the 3′ end of a typical CAGUGH apical loop. Although this IRE-like structure binds IRPs poorly in electrophoretic mobility shift assays, in cytoplasmic extracts the AHSP mRNA co-immunoprecipitates with IRPs via this element and this interaction is inhibited by iron. The IRP- AHSP interaction enhances AHSP mRNA stability in erythroid and heterologous cells.

The human 75-KDa subunit of mitochondrial complex I (NDUFS1) is regulated by iron at the protein but not at the mRNA level (Lin et al., 2001). In the 5′ UTR of this mRNA a motif element that resembles an IRE was identified; however this element does not contain a C8 bulged nucleotide and in it the apical loop (CAGAG) is formed by only five nucleotides instead of six (see Figure 5). Interestingly, this element is bound by a specific cytoplasmic protein, which is neither IRP1 nor IRP2 and the binding interaction can be competed with ferritin IRE and was affected by iron status. It has been suggested that NDUFS1 may be regulated by a novel IRP/IRE system.

A type II IRE motif was found in the 5′ UTR of the human mRNA encoding the Alzheimer's beta amyloid precursor protein (β-APP), which functions as a translational control element via interaction with IRP1 (Rogers et al., 2002) (see Figure 5). This IRE is structurally different from the one presented earlier. Also, a very atypical IRE motif was predicted in the 5′UTR of the human α-synuclein mRNA involved in Parkinson's disease (see Figure 5); however, no functional characterization was reported (Friedlich et al., 2007). As brain iron homeostasis is disrupted in a number of neurodegenerative disorders, a deeper understanding of the functional IRP regulation of mRNAs involved in these diseases is of great interest.

IRE-like structures were reported in the *Bacillus subtilis* genome and the aconitase of this gram-positive bacterium was described as an RNA-binding protein (Alen & Sonenshein, 1999). *B. subtilis* aconitase mutants demonstrate that its non-enzymatic activity is important for sporulation, an iron-dependent process. The authors suggest that bacterial aconitases, like their eukaryotic homologues, are bi-functional proteins, showing aconitase activity in the presence of iron and RNA binding activity in iron-deprived conditions.

A recent genome-wide study was carried out by our group to identify the whole repertoire of mRNAs that can interact with the IRPs (Sanchez et al., 2011). IRP1/IRE and IRP2/IRE mRNP complexes were immunoselected and the mRNA composition of the IRP-binding transcripts was determined using whole-genome microarrays. In this strategy we used total mRNA from five different mouse tissues relevant for iron metabolism (liver, duodenum, spleen, bone marrow and brain). Using this approach novel mRNAs that can bind to both IRPs (n=35), as well as specific-IRP1 mRNAs (n=101) and specific-IRP2 mRNAs (n=113) were detected for the first time. Bioinformatic analysis to predict IRE motifs in the novel IRP target mRNAs was carried out using the newly developed software called SIREs (Searching for IREs, (Campillos et al., 2010), see section 2.1.1.1) also designed by our group. Some of the novel IRP target mRNAs were tested *in vitro* in IRP1 competitive binding assays. We also undertook a proteomic approach to identify iron and/or IRP-modulated proteins in an iron-regulated mouse hepatic cell line and in bone marrow derived macrophages from IRP1- and IRP2-deficient mice. We are currently proceeding with the functional characterization (iron and IRP regulation) of these novel mRNAs to discover and connect known and new cellular functions that need to respond to changes in iron metabolism.

3. Diseases affecting the IRP/IRE regulatory network

In humans, several diseases are caused by the disturbance of systemic or cellular iron homeostasis. In particular for cellular iron misregulation involving the IRP/IRE regulatory system several diseases have been reported and are described in the sections below.

3.1 Hyperferritinemia-cataract syndrome (OMIM #600886)

"Hereditary Hyperferritinemia-Cataract Syndrome" (HHCS) was first described in 1995 (Bonneau et al., 1995; Girelli et al., 1995) as an autosomal dominant inherited disorder characterised by markedly elevated serum ferritin levels (≥1000 ng/ml) without iron overload and congenital early onset bilateral cataract.

The absence of iron overload in HHCS patients suggested that the elevated serum ferritin resulted from misregulation of L-ferritin expression. Analysis of the L-ferritin genetic locus in HHCS patients led to the identification of heterozygous mutations occurring within the IRE of the L-ferritin gene. An inability to block ferritin translation in this disorder has been demonstrated by experiments using cultured lymphoblastoid cells from affected patients: the mutation abolishes the binding of IRPs and leads to constitutively high levels of L-ferritin synthesis (Cazzola et al., 1997). The clinical phenotype of these mutations is only the presence of bilateral congenital cataracts. Although the mechanism of cataract formation is not clear, the deposit of excess L-ferritin in the lens seems to be responsible. A comprehensive study of cataract features in several families affected by HHCS has been performed by Craig and colleagues (Craig et al., 2003).

Since 1995, numerous mutations affecting the 5′ IRE of L-ferritin have been described, including deletions and point mutations (Millonig et al., 2010). A comprehensive revision of the described mutations in HHCS is shown in Figure 6. Most of the mutations discovered so far are located in the upper stem and the conserved hexa-nucleotide apical loop of the IRE. Historically, the L-ferritin IRE mutations have been described with the name of the city in which mutations were identified followed by the nucleotide position and change (i.e. Verona 1 (+41) C). Up to now, less than 90 families have been diagnosed with the disease around the world, so it appears to be uniformly widespread. Prevalence of this disease still needs to be precisely determined but it is estimated to be at least 1 in 200,000 according to the Orphanet database.

Our group have recently diagnosed four Spanish families (ten individuals) affected by HHCS that present four previously described single point mutations in the IRE of the L-ferritin (unpublished data, Figure 7). All our cases present high levels of serum ferritin and cataracts that were detected at a young age.

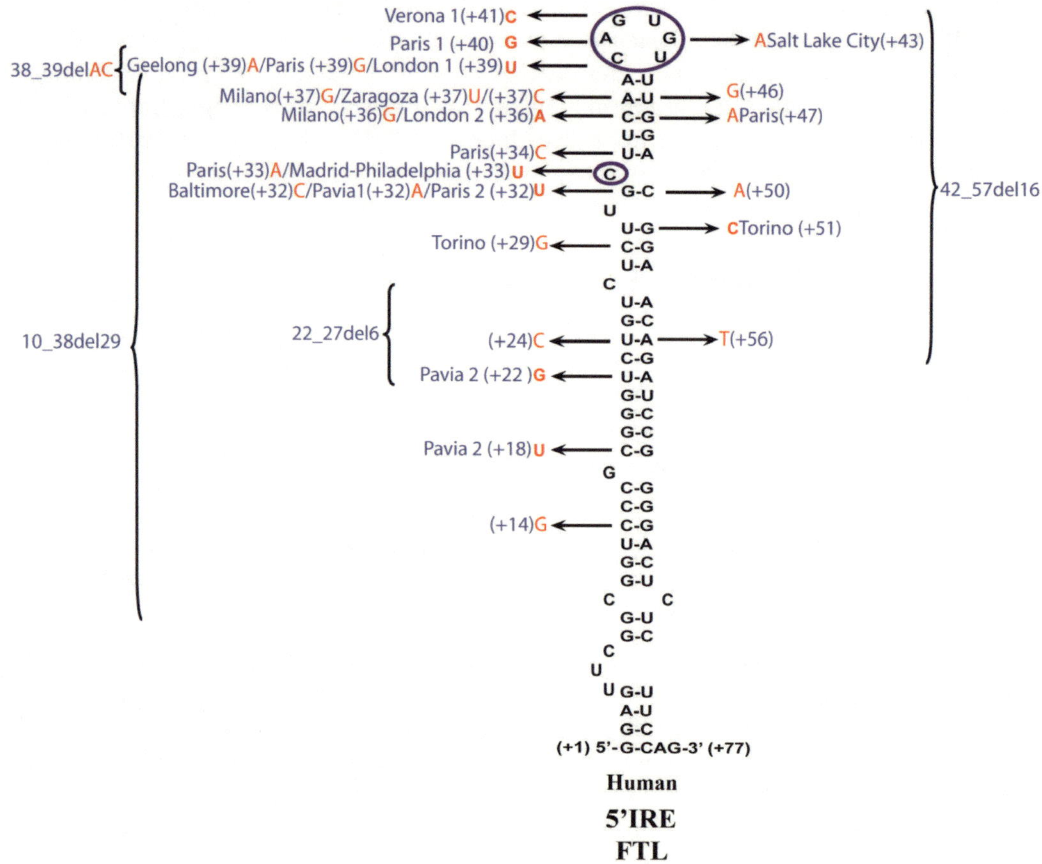

Fig. 6. Predicted secondary structure of the IRE motif in the 5′ UTR of the L-ferritin mRNA and reported mutations causing HHCS (name and position in blue and nucleotide change in red). The apical loop and the C8-bulge are circled in blue. The transcriptional start site is shown as (+1), and the first 77 nucleotides are shown in an extended stem-loop structure. Single nucleotide changes are depicted by arrows and nucleotide deletions are represented by brackets.

In HHCS patients there is a marked phenotypic variability with regard to ocular involvement, serum ferritin levels and age of cataract onset, even between subjects sharing the same mutation in the same family. This suggests that other environmental factors could be involved in the development of clinical symptoms in each person (Girelli et al., 2001). Although HHCS is an autosomal dominant disorder, a patient without family history has recently been reported (Cao et al., 2010).

Because of the high levels of serum ferritin, some HHCS patients have been misdiagnosed with the iron-overload genetic disease Hereditary Hemochromatosis. These HHCS patients have been studied by liver biopsy and have developed iron-deficiency anemia after repeated venesections. A correct genetic diagnosis in HHCS patients is very important, as it will prevent unnecessary clinical tests and the implementation of inadequate treatments. For this reason, it is important to increase awareness of this rare pathology among pediatricians, ophthalmologists, gastroenterologists, haematologists and general practitioners. Patients diagnosed with HHCS should be counselled regarding the relative harmlessness of this genetic disease, with early cataract surgery as the only clinical consequence.

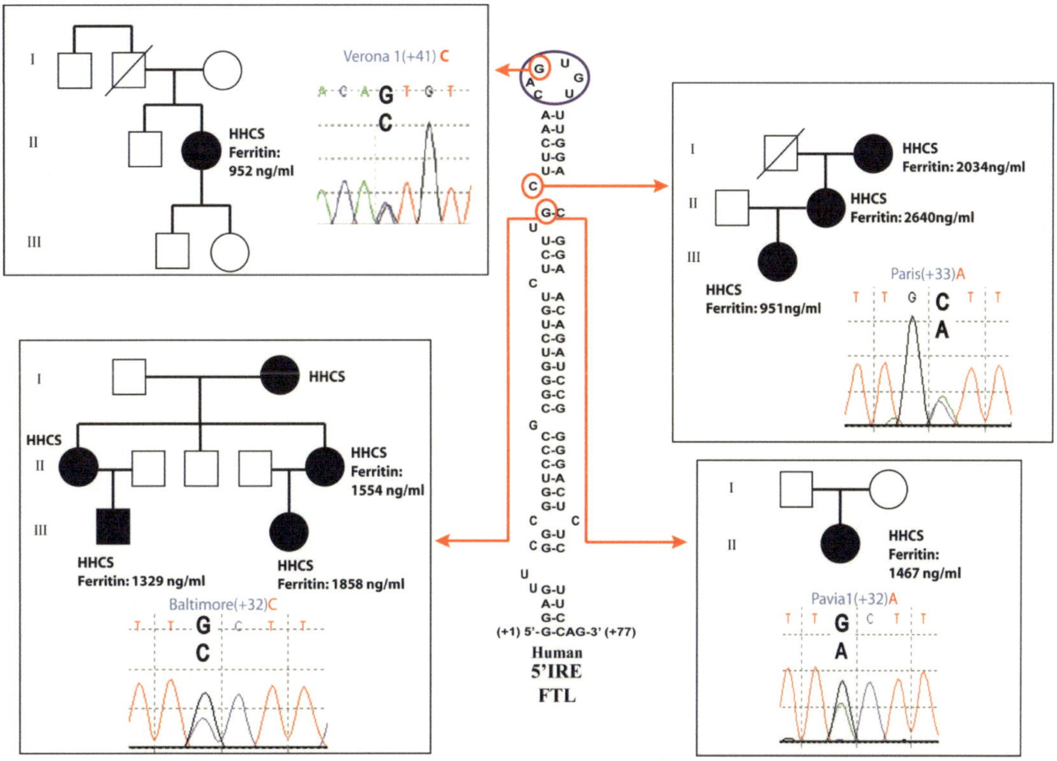

Fig. 7. Four Spanish families affected by hyperferritinemia-cataract syndrome reported in our laboratory. Family pedigrees are shown together with histograms reporting the nucleotide change and the mutation name and position. In the pedigrees, squares and circles symbolize males and females, respectively, and black symbols denote affected patients with hyperferritinemia and cataracts. Serum ferritin (ng/ml) values are indicated in affected individuals. Dashed symbols represent deceased individuals. Roman numerals indicate generations. Point mutations are located in the IRE structure of L-ferritin.

3.2 Autosomal dominant Iron overload syndrome (OMIM +134770)

An autosomal dominant iron overload syndrome has been described in a unique Japanese family by Kato and colleagues (Kato et al., 2001). In this family a point mutation (A49U) in the IRE of the H-ferritin gene was found. However, no other mutations in the IRE of the H-Ferritin that affects the IRP/IRE binding have been reported by any other researchers, including a large study with subjects presenting abnormal serum ferritin values and abnormal iron status (Cremonesi et al., 2003).

The proband described by Kato and collaborators was a woman showing high serum ferritin levels, iron overload and increased transferrin saturation. Authors also studied seven family members and found that three of them showed an iron overload phenotype defined by elevated serum iron values and excessive iron deposition in liver and bone marrow evidenced by magnetic resonance imaging. Two of these three relatives also had elevated serum ferritin levels, but the proband's daughter did not (Figure 8A).

After excluding other causes of iron overload, they sequenced H- and L-ferritin cDNAs in the proband. A heterozygous single A-to-U conversion at position 49 inside the IRE was found in the sequence of the H-ferritin gene (see Figure 8B and 8C).

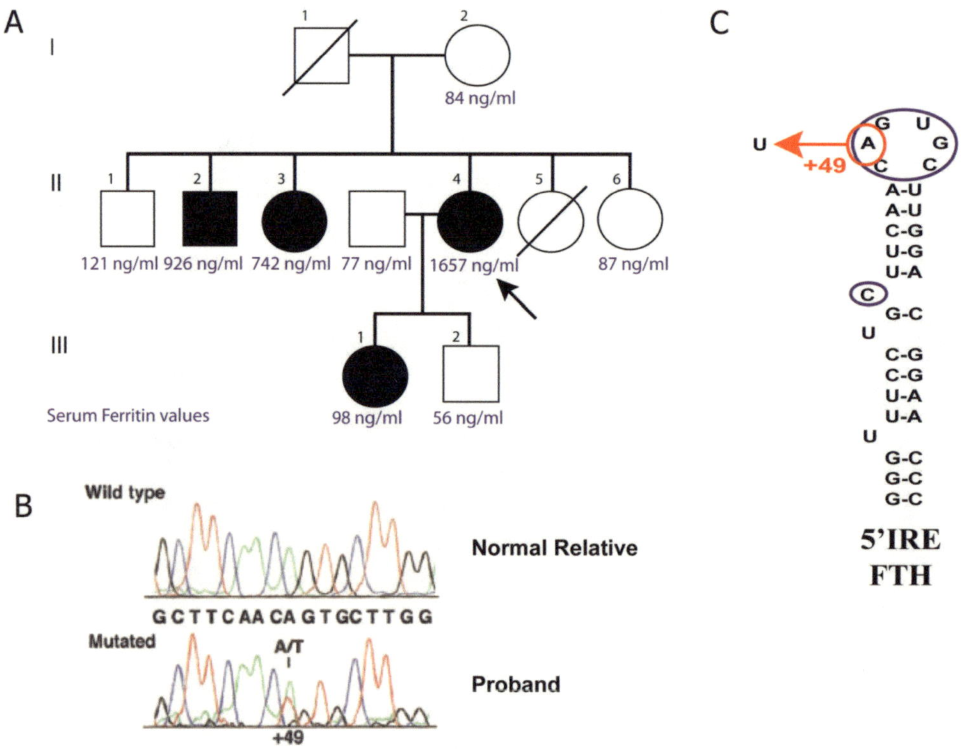

Fig. 8. A mutation in the IRE of H-ferritin mRNA causes autosomal dominant iron overload. A. Pedigree of a family with dominant primary iron overload. Black symbols denote individuals showing the A49T genotype. Serum ferritin (ng/ml) values are indicated. The arrow indicates the proband (II-4). B. Histograms for a normal relative and the proband showing the sequence of H-ferritin where the mutation (+49A>T) was found in heterozygous state. C. Predicted secondary structure of the 5' IRE in H-ferritin subunit mRNA. The mutation position (+49) is based on the human H-ferritin chain mRNA sequence L20941. The A49U mutation affects the second nucleotide of the IRE loop. Adapted from Kato et. al. 2001.

The A49U mutation affects the second base of the IRE apical loop (CAGUG), a nucleotide that was reported to have direct protein contact with IRP1 in the IRP1/IRE crystallography structure (Walden et al., 2006). This mutation was also detected in the genomic DNA of the four relatives who had iron overload, but not in the genomic DNA of 42 unrelated control subjects. The segregation of the mutation and iron overload in the family members was consistent with an autosomal dominant pattern of inheritance. The +49A>T mutation was considered a novel cause of hereditary iron overload, most likely related to an impairment of the ferroxidase activity generated by H subunit (Kato et al., 2001).

3.3 Mutations in the ferroportin 5' IRE

A radiation-induced mouse model with a 58 bp deletion in the 5' UTR of ferroportin gene, including the IRE motif, has been described (Mok et al., 2004). These mice present erythropoietin-dependent polycythaemia when the mutation is in the heterozygous state and microcytic hypochromic anaemia in homozygosity. Both defects in erythropoiesis were transient and corrected in early adulthood by the action of hepcidin.

A 5' UTR mutation has been detected in a patient with iron overload due to Hereditary Hemochromatosis type 4, also known as ferroportin disease (Liu et al., 2005). The mutation is located seven nucleotides downstream of the ferroportin IRE and may alter the IRE-IRP recognition, although this has not been proven.

3.4 IRPs in iron-sulphur cluster deficiency anaemias

As mentioned in section 2.1.2.1, IRP1 has a dual function; firstly as a cytosolic aconitase when it incorporates an iron-sulphur cluster, and secondly as an RNA-binding protein when this cluster is removed in iron-deprived conditions. The formation and assembly of iron-sulphur clusters in the cell is therefore very important for the regulation of IRP1 activity.

A novel disorder affecting the iron/sulphur cluster biogenesis has been described in a patient with a recessive form of inherited sideroblastic anaemias and a zebrafish model with severe hypochromic anaemia, the *shiraz* mutant (Camaschella et al., 2007; Wingert et al., 2005). Both phenotypes are due to a mutation in the GLRX5 gene, which encodes for a mitochondrial protein important for iron/sulphur cluster biogenesis. The observed anaemia is the result of GLRX5 deficiency that increases IRP1 activity in the absence of iron/sulfur clusters which hampers its conversion to an aconitase. Increased IRP1 IRE binding activity leads to Alas2 translational repression and cytosolic iron depletion that also activates IRP2, which further contributes to Alas2 blocking. The described patient bears a homozygous mutation that interferes with intron 1 splicing and drastically reduces GLRX5 mRNA levels. Clinically this patient presents with iron overload and mild sideroblastic anaemia (Camaschella et al., 2007). Surprisingly, the anaemia in the patient was worsened by blood transfusions but partially reversed by iron chelation, presumably because iron chelation will redistribute iron to the cytosol, which might decrease IRP2 excess, improving haem synthesis and anaemia. The discovery of this disease establishes a link between two pathways of mitochondria iron utilization: haem biosynthesis and iron/sulphur cluster biogenesis.

X-linked sideroblastic anaemia with ataxia (XLSA/A) is another disease affecting the iron/sulphur cluster (ISC) pathway. XLSA/A is a rare inherited disorder characterized by mild anaemia and ataxia and is caused by mutations in the ABCB7 gene, which encodes a member of the ATP-binding cassette transporter family involved in the transport of ISC from the mitochondria to the cytoplasm. The liver-specific conditional knockout of Abcb7 results in strong decrease of cytosolic aconitase activity and a 6-fold reciprocal increase in

IRP1 RNA binding activity, with concomitant increase in TFR1 expression and hepatic iron overload (Pondarre et al., 2006). However, increased levels of TFR1 proteins were attributed to IRP2 stabilizing effects rather than IRP1, as surprisingly it was found that IRP1 protein levels were reduced in these mice due to an iron-dependent IRP1 protein degradation. RNA binding activity and protein levels of IRP2 were found to increase, despite the apparent cellular iron overload that does not seem to be appropriately sensed by IRP2.

In conclusion, ISC deficiency leads to dysregulated activation of IRP1 and IRP2 and it seems that IRP RNA binding activity may respond more to the flux of iron through a specific metabolic pathway, such as the ISC assembly, than to the absolute levels of cellular iron. Therefore, major problems associated with these disorders seem to be a consequence of inappropriate regulation of downstream targets of cytosolic IRPs, rather than ISC deficiency *per se*.

3.5 Other pathophysiological roles for IRPs

Brain homeostasis of trace metals such as copper and iron is dysregulated in neurological disorders such as Alzheimer's disease, where increased iron and decreased copper levels are observed. Young mice with targeted deletion of IRP2 have significantly less brain copper and the expression of β-APP is significantly up-regulated in the hippocampus (Mueller et al., 2009). In humans, polymorphisms in the promoter region of IRP2 gene are statistically associated with Alzheimer's disease (Coon et al., 2006). This finding awaits further confirmation in independent and larger studies, and also the functional significance of these polymorphisms needs to be clarified. Mouse work on the role of IRP2 in neuropathology is somewhat controversial. One group have reported that aging IRP2 KO mice develop a progressive neurodegenerative disorder (LaVaute et al., 2001), while the IRP2 KO mice generated by an independent group using a different targeting strategy do not manifest severe neurodegeneration, despite performing poorly in neurobehavioural tests (Galy et al., 2006). In spite of the observed iron accumulation in the neurons of the substantia nigra of Parkinson's patients, ferritin levels are not up-regulated. This effect was attributed to high levels of IRP1-IRE binding activity, which is insensitive to iron concentration, probably because of a different compartmentalization of the iron (Faucheux et al., 2002). IRP-1 and -2 activities were found to be increased in brain cells in a Transmissible Spongiform Encephalopathy mouse model (Kim et al., 2007).

Genome-wide association studies in combination with expression profiling implicate IRP2 as a susceptibility gene in chronic obstructive pulmonary disease (COPD) (DeMeo et al., 2009). This study also found that IRP2 protein and mRNA were increased in lung-tissue samples from COPD subjects in comparison with controls. The association of IRP2 SNPs with COPD has been recently replicated by a second group (Chappell et al., 2011).

IRPs have been involved in cancer biology. The over-expression of IRP1 suppresses growth of tumour xenografts in nude mice (Chen et al., 2007). In these experiments, stable transfected and tetracycline inducible (tet-off system) H1299 lung cancer cells with IRP1 wild-type or a mutated IRP1 version that constitutively binds IRE were used; these cells and control cells were then transplanted into nude mice to study their tumourogenic effects. Interestingly, similar experiments with IRP2 showed the opposite behaviour, a pro-oncogenic activity of the over-expression of IRP2 that was attributed to an IRP2-specific domain of 73 amino acids (Maffettone et al., 2010). In both systems the expression of ferritin and TFR1 was similar; however, tumours over-expressing IRP1 and IRP2 exhibited distinct gene-expression profiles, suggesting that IRPs may differentially modulate cancer growth by regulating a different subset of genes, which could be related or not to iron homeostasis. Indeed, the IRP2 pro-oncogenic activity was associated with an increase in the phosphorylation of ERK ½, an extracellular signal-regulated kinase, and with high levels of the proto-oncogene c-myc that was previously implicated in the transcriptional activation of IRP2 (Wu et al., 1999). The understanding of the molecular pathways that involves IRPs in cancer biology is very incipient and further work is required.

4. Small molecules and drugs affecting the IRP/IRE regulatory network

Small-molecules that selectively bind to and modulate the IRP-IRE interaction, by inhibiting or enhancing it, have been described in two studies.

By chemical footprinting assay the natural product yohimbine was found to selectively interfere with the ferritin IRE and inhibit IRP-ferritin IRE binding, increasing the rate of ferritin biosynthesis in cell-free extracts (Tibodeau et al., 2006). The selective effect of this compound proved that small-molecules can distinguish between different members of the IRE family. Further development of therapeutic approaches, with this or similar compounds, could be used to increase iron-storage capacity in pathological conditions that require it, such as iron-overload diseases.

Using a cell-based screen method several small molecules that decrease HIF2α translation by enhancing the binding of preferentially IRP1 to the 5′ IRE present in HIF2α were described by Zimmer and collaborators (Zimmer et al., 2008). An enhancer effect of these compounds on the IRP-IRE binding was also observed for transferrin receptor 1 (TFR1), increasing its mRNA stability. As hypoxia inducible factors (HIFs) are linked to cancer progression, angiogenesis and inflammation, HIF inhibitors (like these compounds) could be used in antineoplastic and anti-inflammatory therapies.

Other small molecules and drugs that interfere with iron uptake via DMT1 or transferrin receptor 1 have been reported but their mechanism of action does not seem to be related with the modulation of the IRP-IRE regulatory system (Brown et al., 2004; Horonchik & Wessling-Resnick, 2008; Wetli et al., 2006).

5. Conclusions and future perspectives

In recent years, impressive progress has been made in unraveling the control of iron homeostasis by the IRP/IRE regulatory system. However, many details remain unanswered and require further investigation. For instance, a recent high-throughput screening study has considerably enlarged the number of known IRP-binding mRNAs, extending the IRP functions to multiple pathways, including cancer biology (Sanchez et al., 2011). Now the challenge is to uncover the role and mechanisms of action of these new mRNAs regulated by IRPs with studies ranging from basic research to medical and applied physiology.

Additional IRP mouse models with cell-specific ablation or over-expression in an inducible or non-inducible system will provide valuable information concerning the pathophysiological role of IRPs. To elucidate the specific role of mRNA isoforms containing an IRE and the physiological role that IRPs exert on them *in vivo*, the generation of animal models with a particular disrupted IRE would be of great interest. A deeper study into several research fields affecting iron and IRP misregulation (such as iron brain homeostasis, iron in cancer biology and iron implication in immunity and infection) will have implications for the development of therapies for common and rare disorders related to the IRP/IRE regulatory system.

6. Acknowledgements

Dr. Mayka Sanchez's group is supported by by 'Instituto de Salud Carlos III', Spanish Health Program (Ministry of Science and Innovation; PS09/00341); Spanish Ministry of Science and Innovation (RYC−2008−02352 research contract under the Ramon y Cajal program). Dr. Mayka Sanchez's group was also awarded with a European Union programme for research in rare diseases (ERA-Net on rare diseases) project, ERARE-115, HMA-IRON, co-ordinated by Dr. Carole Beaumont.

7. References

Alen, C., & Sonenshein, A. L. (1999). Bacillus subtilis aconitase is an RNA-binding protein. *Proc Natl Acad Sci U S A,* 96(18), 10412-10417.

Andrews, N. C. (2010). Ferrit(in)ing out new mechanisms in iron homeostasis. *Cell Metab,* 12(3), 203-204.

Arosio, P., Ingrassia, R., & Cavadini, P. (2009). Ferritins: a family of molecules for iron storage, antioxidation and more. *Biochim Biophys Acta,* 1790(7), 589-599.

Bengert, P., & Dandekar, T. (2003). A software tool-box for analysis of regulatory RNA elements. *Nucleic Acids Res,* 31(13), 3441-3445.

Bianchi, L., Tacchini, L., & Cairo, G. (1999). HIF-1-mediated activation of transferrin receptor gene transcription by iron chelation. *Nucleic Acids Res,* 27(21), 4223-4227.

Binder, R., Horowitz, J. A., Basilion, J. P., et al. (1994). Evidence that the pathway of transferrin receptor mRNA degradation involves an endonucleolytic cleavage within the 3' UTR and does not involve poly(A) tail shortening. *EMBO J,* 13(8), 1969-1980.

Bonneau, D., Winter-Fuseau, I., Loiseau, M. N., et al. (1995). Bilateral cataract and high serum ferritin: a new dominant genetic disorder? *J Med Genet,* 32(10), 778-779.

Brazzolotto, X., Andriollo, M., Guiraud, P., et al. (2003). Interactions between doxorubicin and the human iron regulatory system. *Biochim Biophys Acta,* 1593(2-3), 209-218.

Brown, J. X., Buckett, P. D., & Wessling-Resnick, M. (2004). Identification of small molecule inhibitors that distinguish between non-transferrin bound iron uptake and transferrin-mediated iron transport. *Chem Biol,* 11(3), 407-416.

Butt, J., Kim, H. Y., Basilion, J. P., et al. (1996). Differences in the RNA binding sites of iron regulatory proteins and potential target diversity. *Proc Natl Acad Sci U S A,* 93(9), 4345-4349.

Cairo, G., & Pietrangelo, A. (1994). Transferrin receptor gene expression during rat liver regeneration. Evidence for post-transcriptional regulation by iron regulatory factorB, a second iron-responsive element-binding protein. *J Biol Chem,* 269(9), 6405-6409.

Cairo, G., & Pietrangelo, A. (2000). Iron regulatory proteins in pathobiology. *Biochem J,* 352 Pt 2, 241-250.

Caltagirone, A., Weiss, G., & Pantopoulos, K. (2001). Modulation of cellular iron metabolism by hydrogen peroxide. Effects of H2O2 on the expression and function of iron-responsive element-containing mRNAs in B6 fibroblasts. *J Biol Chem, 276*(23), 19738-19745.

Camaschella, C., Campanella, A., De Falco, L., et al. (2007). The human counterpart of zebrafish shiraz shows sideroblastic-like microcytic anemia and iron overload. *Blood, 110*(4), 1353-1358.

Campillos, M., Cases, I., Hentze, M. W., et al. (2010). SIREs: searching for iron-responsive elements. *Nucleic Acids Res, 38* Suppl, W360-367.

Cao, W., McMahon, M., Wang, B., et al. (2010). A case report of spontaneous mutation (C33>U) in the iron-responsive element of L-ferritin causing hyperferritinemia-cataract syndrome. *Blood Cells Mol Dis, 44*(1), 22-27.

Cazzola, M., Bergamaschi, G., Tonon, L., et al. (1997). Hereditary hyperferritinemia-cataract syndrome: relationship between phenotypes and specific mutations in the iron-responsive element of ferritin light-chain mRNA. *Blood, 90*(2), 814-821.

Cmejla, R., Petrak, J., & Cmejlova, J. (2006). A novel iron responsive element in the 3'UTR of human MRCKalpha. *Biochem Biophys Res Commun, 341*(1), 158-166.

Coon, K. D., Siegel, A. M., Yee, S. J., et al. (2006). Preliminary demonstration of an allelic association of the IREB2 gene with Alzheimer's disease. *J Alzheimers Dis, 9*(3), 225-233.

Craig, J. E., Clark, J. B., McLeod, J. L., et al. (2003). Hereditary hyperferritinemia-cataract syndrome: prevalence, lens morphology, spectrum of mutations, and clinical presentations. *Arch Ophthalmol, 121*(12), 1753-1761.

Cremonesi, L., Foglieni, B., Fermo, I., et al. (2003). Identification of two novel mutations in the 5'-untranslated region of H-ferritin using denaturing high performance liquid chromatography scanning. *Haematologica, 88*(10), 1110-1116.

Crichton, R. R. (2009). *Iron metabolism : from molecular mechanisms to clinical consequences* (3rd ed.). Chichester, UK: John Wiley & Sons.

Chappell, S. L., Daly, L., Lotya, J., et al. (2011). The role of IREB2 and transforming growth factor beta-1 genetic variants in COPD: a replication case-control study. *BMC Med Genet, 12*, 24.

Chen, G., Fillebeen, C., Wang, J., et al. (2007). Overexpression of iron regulatory protein 1 suppresses growth of tumor xenografts. *Carcinogenesis, 28*(4), 785-791.

Dandekar, T., Stripecke, R., Gray, N. K., et al. (1991). Identification of a novel iron-responsive element in murine and human erythroid delta-aminolevulinic acid synthase mRNA. *EMBO J, 10*(7), 1903-1909.

De Domenico, I., Ward, D. M., & Kaplan, J. (2007). Hepcidin regulation: ironing out the details. *J Clin Invest, 117*(7), 1755-1758.

Delaby, C., Pilard, N., Puy, H., et al. (2008). Sequential regulation of ferroportin expression after erythrophagocytosis in murine macrophages: early mRNA induction by haem, followed by iron-dependent protein expression. *Biochem J, 411*(1), 123-131.

DeMeo, D. L., Mariani, T., Bhattacharya, S., et al. (2009). Integration of genomic and genetic approaches implicates IREB2 as a COPD susceptibility gene. *Am J Hum Genet, 85*(4), 493-502.

Donovan, A., Brownlie, A., Dorschner, M. O., et al. (2002). The zebrafish mutant gene chardonnay (cdy) encodes divalent metal transporter 1 (DMT1). *Blood, 100*(13), 4655-4659.

Donovan, A., Lima, C. A., Pinkus, J. L., et al. (2005). The iron exporter ferroportin/Slc40a1 is essential for iron homeostasis. *Cell Metab,* 1(3), 191-200.
Drakesmith, H., & Prentice, A. (2008). Viral infection and iron metabolism. *Nat Rev Microbiol,* 6(7), 541-552.
Drapier, J. C. (1997). Interplay between NO and [Fe-S] clusters: relevance to biological systems. *Methods,* 11(3), 319-329.
Eisenstein, R. S. (2000). Iron regulatory proteins and the molecular control of mammalian iron metabolism. *Annu Rev Nutr,* 20, 627-662.
Faucheux, B. A., Martin, M. E., Beaumont, C., et al. (2002). Lack of up-regulation of ferritin is associated with sustained iron regulatory protein-1 binding activity in the substantia nigra of patients with Parkinson's disease. *J Neurochem,* 83(2), 320-330.
Ferreira, C., Bucchini, D., Martin, M. E., et al. (2000). Early embryonic lethality of H ferritin gene deletion in mice. *J Biol Chem,* 275(5), 3021-3024.
Fillebeen, C., Muckenthaler, M., Andriopoulos, B., et al. (2007). Expression of the subgenomic hepatitis C virus replicon alters iron homeostasis in Huh7 cells. *J Hepatol,* 47(1), 12-22.
Fleming, M. D., Romano, M. A., Su, M. A., et al. (1998). Nramp2 is mutated in the anemic Belgrade (b) rat: evidence of a role for Nramp2 in endosomal iron transport. *Proc Natl Acad Sci U S A,* 95(3), 1148-1153.
Fleming, M. D., Trenor, C. C., 3rd, Su, M. A., et al. (1997). Microcytic anaemia mice have a mutation in Nramp2, a candidate iron transporter gene. *Nat Genet,* 16(4), 383-386.
Friedlich, A. L., Tanzi, R. E., & Rogers, J. T. (2007). The 5'-untranslated region of Parkinson's disease alpha-synuclein messengerRNA contains a predicted iron responsive element. *Mol Psychiatry,* 12(3), 222-223.
Galy, B., Ferring-Appel, D., Kaden, S., et al. (2008). Iron regulatory proteins are essential for intestinal function and control key iron absorption molecules in the duodenum. *Cell Metab,* 7(1), 79-85.
Galy, B., Ferring-Appel, D., Sauer, S. W., et al. (2010). Iron regulatory proteins secure mitochondrial iron sufficiency and function. *Cell Metab,* 12(2), 194-201.
Galy, B., Holter, S. M., Klopstock, T., et al. (2006). Iron homeostasis in the brain: complete iron regulatory protein 2 deficiency without symptomatic neurodegeneration in the mouse. *Nat Genet,* 38(9), 967-969; discussion 969-970.
Ganz, T., & Nemeth, E. (2011). Hepcidin and disorders of iron metabolism. *Annu Rev Med,* 62, 347-360.
Gao, J., Lovejoy, D., & Richardson, D. R. (1999). Effect of iron chelators with potent anti-proliferative activity on the expression of molecules involved in cell cycle progression and growth. *Redox Rep,* 4(6), 311-312.
Girelli, D., Bozzini, C., Zecchina, G., et al. (2001). Clinical, biochemical and molecular findings in a series of families with hereditary hyperferritinaemia-cataract syndrome. *Br J Haematol,* 115(2), 334-340.
Girelli, D., Olivieri, O., De Franceschi, L., et al. (1995). A linkage between hereditary hyperferritinaemia not related to iron overload and autosomal dominant congenital cataract. *Br J Haematol,* 90(4), 931-934.
Goforth, J. B., Anderson, S. A., Nizzi, C. P., et al. (2010). Multiple determinants within iron-responsive elements dictate iron regulatory protein binding and regulatory hierarchy. *RNA,* 16(1), 154-169.

Gray, N. K., Pantopoulos, K., Dandekar, T., et al. (1996). Translational regulation of mammalian and Drosophila citric acid cycle enzymes via iron-responsive elements. *Proc Natl Acad Sci U S A*, 93(10), 4925-4930.

Gu, J. M., Lim, S. O., Oh, S. J., et al. (2008). HBx modulates iron regulatory protein 1-mediated iron metabolism via reactive oxygen species. *Virus Res*, 133(2), 167-177.

Hausmann, A., Lee, J., & Pantopoulos, K. (2011). Redox control of iron regulatory protein 2 stability. *FEBS Lett*, 585(4), 687-692.

Henderson, B. R., Menotti, E., & Kuhn, L. C. (1996). Iron regulatory proteins 1 and 2 bind distinct sets of RNA target sequences. *J Biol Chem*, 271(9), 4900-4908.

Henderson, B. R., Seiser, C., & Kuhn, L. C. (1993). Characterization of a second RNA-binding protein in rodents with specificity for iron-responsive elements. *J Biol Chem*, 268(36), 27327-27334.

Hentze, M. W., Muckenthaler, M. U., Galy, B., et al. (2010). Two to tango: regulation of Mammalian iron metabolism. *Cell*, 142(1), 24-38.

Horonchik, L., & Wessling-Resnick, M. (2008). The small-molecule iron transport inhibitor ferristatin/NSC306711 promotes degradation of the transferrin receptor. *Chem Biol*, 15(7), 647-653.

Hubert, N., & Hentze, M. W. (2002). Previously uncharacterized isoforms of divalent metal transporter (DMT)-1: implications for regulation and cellular function. *Proc Natl Acad Sci U S A*, 99(19), 12345-12350.

Iwai, K., Drake, S. K., Wehr, N. B., et al. (1998). Iron-dependent oxidation, ubiquitination, and degradation of iron regulatory protein 2: implications for degradation of oxidized proteins. *Proc Natl Acad Sci U S A*, 95(9), 4924-4928.

Kannengiesser, C., Jouanolle, A. M., Hetet, G., et al. (2009). A new missense mutation in the L ferritin coding sequence associated with elevated levels of glycosylated ferritin in serum and absence of iron overload. *Haematologica*, 94(3), 335-339.

Kato, J., Fujikawa, K., Kanda, M., et al. (2001). A mutation, in the iron-responsive element of H ferritin mRNA, causing autosomal dominant iron overload. *Am J Hum Genet*, 69(1), 191-197.

Kim, B. H., Jun, Y. C., Jin, J. K., et al. (2007). Alteration of iron regulatory proteins (IRP1 and IRP2) and ferritin in the brains of scrapie-infected mice. *Neurosci Lett*, 422(3), 158-163.

Kim, S., & Ponka, P. (2002). Nitric oxide-mediated modulation of iron regulatory proteins: implication for cellular iron homeostasis. *Blood Cells Mol Dis*, 29(3), 400-410.

Kim, S., Wing, S. S., & Ponka, P. (2004). S-nitrosylation of IRP2 regulates its stability via the ubiquitin-proteasome pathway. *Mol Cell Biol*, 24(1), 330-337.

Kohler, S. A., Menotti, E., & Kuhn, L. C. (1999). Molecular cloning of mouse glycolate oxidase. High evolutionary conservation and presence of an iron-responsive element-like sequence in the mRNA. *J Biol Chem*, 274(4), 2401-2407.

Kwok, J. C., & Richardson, D. R. (2002). Unexpected anthracycline-mediated alterations in iron-regulatory protein-RNA-binding activity: the iron and copper complexes of anthracyclines decrease RNA-binding activity. *Mol Pharmacol*, 62(4), 888-900.

LaVaute, T., Smith, S., Cooperman, S., et al. (2001). Targeted deletion of the gene encoding iron regulatory protein-2 causes misregulation of iron metabolism and neurodegenerative disease in mice. *Nat Genet*, 27(2), 209-214.

Leedman, P. J., Stein, A. R., Chin, W. W., et al. (1996). Thyroid hormone modulates the interaction between iron regulatory proteins and the ferritin mRNA iron-responsive element. *J Biol Chem*, 271(20), 12017-12023.

Levy, J. E., Jin, O., Fujiwara, Y., et al. (1999). Transferrin receptor is necessary for development of erythrocytes and the nervous system. *Nat Genet,* 21(4), 396-399.

Lin, E., Graziano, J. H., & Freyer, G. A. (2001). Regulation of the 75-kDa subunit of mitochondrial complex I by iron. *J Biol Chem,* 276(29), 27685-27692.

Liu, W., Shimomura, S., Imanishi, H., et al. (2005). Hemochromatosis with mutation of the ferroportin 1 (IREG1) gene. *Intern Med,* 44(4), 285-289.

Liu, X. B., Hill, P., & Haile, D. J. (2002). Role of the ferroportin iron-responsive element in iron and nitric oxide dependent gene regulation. *Blood Cells Mol Dis,* 29(3), 315-326.

Lok, C. N., & Ponka, P. (2000). Identification of an erythroid active element in the transferrin receptor gene. *J Biol Chem,* 275(31), 24185-24190.

Lymboussaki, A., Pignatti, E., Montosi, G., et al. (2003). The role of the iron responsive element in the control of ferroportin1/IREG1/MTP1 gene expression. *J Hepatol,* 39(5), 710-715.

Macke, T. J., Ecker, D. J., Gutell, R. R., et al. (2001). RNAMotif, an RNA secondary structure definition and search algorithm. *Nucleic Acids Res,* 29(22), 4724-4735.

Mackenzie, B., & Garrick, M. D. (2005). Iron Imports. II. Iron uptake at the apical membrane in the intestine. *Am J Physiol Gastrointest Liver Physiol,* 289(6), G981-986.

Maffettone, C., Chen, G., Drozdov, I., et al. (2010). Tumorigenic properties of iron regulatory protein 2 (IRP2) mediated by its specific 73-amino acids insert. *PLoS One,* 5(4), e10163.

Maffettone, C., De Martino, L., Irace, C., et al. (2008). Expression of iron-related proteins during infection by bovine herpes virus type-1. *J Cell Biochem,* 104(1), 213-223.

Mastrogiannaki, M., Matak, P., Keith, B., et al. (2009). HIF-2alpha, but not HIF-1alpha, promotes iron absorption in mice. *J Clin Invest,* 119(5), 1159-1166.

Mattace Raso, G., Irace, C., Esposito, E., et al. (2009). Ovariectomy and estrogen treatment modulate iron metabolism in rat adipose tissue. *Biochem Pharmacol,* 78(8), 1001-1007.

Meehan, H. A., & Connell, G. J. (2001). The hairpin loop but not the bulged C of the iron responsive element is essential for high affinity binding to iron regulatory protein-1. *J Biol Chem,* 276(18), 14791-14796.

Meyron-Holtz, E. G., Ghosh, M. C., & Rouault, T. A. (2004). Mammalian tissue oxygen levels modulate iron-regulatory protein activities in vivo. *Science,* 306(5704), 2087-2090.

Mignone, F., Grillo, G., Licciulli, F., et al. (2005). UTRdb and UTRsite: a collection of sequences and regulatory motifs of the untranslated regions of eukaryotic mRNAs. *Nucleic Acids Res,* 33(Database issue), D141-146.

Millonig, G., Muckenthaler, M. U., & Mueller, S. (2010). Hyperferritinaemia-cataract syndrome: worldwide mutations and phenotype of an increasingly diagnosed genetic disorder. *Hum Genomics,* 4(4), 250-262.

Minotti, G., Ronchi, R., Salvatorelli, E., et al. (2001). Doxorubicin irreversibly inactivates iron regulatory proteins 1 and 2 in cardiomyocytes: evidence for distinct metabolic pathways and implications for iron-mediated cardiotoxicity of antitumor therapy. *Cancer Res,* 61(23), 8422-8428.

Mok, H., Jelinek, J., Pai, S., et al. (2004). Disruption of ferroportin 1 regulation causes dynamic alterations in iron homeostasis and erythropoiesis in polycythaemia mice. *Development,* 131(8), 1859-1868.

Muckenthaler, M., Gray, N. K., & Hentze, M. W. (1998). IRP-1 binding to ferritin mRNA prevents the recruitment of the small ribosomal subunit by the cap-binding complex eIF4F. *Mol Cell,* 2(3), 383-388.

Muckenthaler, M. U., Galy, B., & Hentze, M. W. (2008). Systemic iron homeostasis and the iron-responsive element/iron-regulatory protein (IRE/IRP) regulatory network. *Annu Rev Nutr,* 28, 197-213.

Mueller, C., Magaki, S., Schrag, M., et al. (2009). Iron regulatory protein 2 is involved in brain copper homeostasis. *J Alzheimers Dis,* 18(1), 201-210.

Mulero, V., & Brock, J. H. (1999). Regulation of iron metabolism in murine J774 macrophages: role of nitric oxide-dependent and -independent pathways following activation with gamma interferon and lipopolysaccharide. *Blood,* 94(7), 2383-2389.

Mutze, S., Hebling, U., Stremmel, W., et al. (2003). Myeloperoxidase-derived hypochlorous acid antagonizes the oxidative stress-mediated activation of iron regulatory protein 1. *J Biol Chem,* 278(42), 40542-40549.

Nemeth, E., Tuttle, M. S., Powelson, J., et al. (2004). Hepcidin regulates cellular iron efflux by binding to ferroportin and inducing its internalization. *Science,* 306(5704), 2090-2093.

Nurtjahja-Tjendraputra, E., Fu, D., Phang, J. M., et al. (2007). Iron chelation regulates cyclin D1 expression via the proteasome: a link to iron deficiency-mediated growth suppression. *Blood,* 109(9), 4045-4054.

O'Donnell, K. A., Yu, D., Zeller, K. I., et al. (2006). Activation of transferrin receptor 1 by c-Myc enhances cellular proliferation and tumorigenesis. *Mol Cell Biol,* 26(6), 2373-2386.

Pantopoulos, K., & Hentze, M. W. (1995). Nitric oxide signaling to iron-regulatory protein: direct control of ferritin mRNA translation and transferrin receptor mRNA stability in transfected fibroblasts. *Proc Natl Acad Sci U S A,* 92(5), 1267-1271.

Pondarre, C., Antiochos, B. B., Campagna, D. R., et al. (2006). The mitochondrial ATP-binding cassette transporter Abcb7 is essential in mice and participates in cytosolic iron-sulfur cluster biogenesis. *Hum Mol Genet,* 15(6), 953-964.

Ponka, P., Beaumont, C., & Richardson, D. R. (1998). Function and regulation of transferrin and ferritin. *Semin Hematol,* 35(1), 35-54.

Recalcati, S., Conte, D., & Cairo, G. (1999). Preferential activation of iron regulatory protein-2 in cell lines as a result of higher sensitivity to iron. *Eur J Biochem,* 259(1-2), 304-309.

Recalcati, S., Minotti, G., & Cairo, G. (2010). Iron regulatory proteins: from molecular mechanisms to drug development. *Antioxid Redox Signal,* 13(10), 1593-1616.

Rogers, J. T., Randall, J. D., Cahill, C. M., et al. (2002). An iron-responsive element type II in the 5'-untranslated region of the Alzheimer's amyloid precursor protein transcript. *J Biol Chem,* 277(47), 45518-45528.

Rouault, T. A. (2006). The role of iron regulatory proteins in mammalian iron homeostasis and disease. *Nat Chem Biol,* 2(8), 406-414.

Salahudeen, A. A., Thompson, J. W., Ruiz, J. C., et al. (2009). An E3 Ligase Possessing an Iron Responsive Hemerythrin Domain Is a Regulator of Iron Homeostasis. *Science.*

Sanchez, M., Galy, B., Dandekar, T., et al. (2006). Iron regulation and the cell cycle: identification of an iron-responsive element in the 3'-untranslated region of human cell division cycle 14A mRNA by a refined microarray-based screening strategy. *J Biol Chem,* 281(32), 22865-22874.

Sanchez, M., Galy, B., Muckenthaler, M. U., et al. (2007). Iron-regulatory proteins limit hypoxia-inducible factor-2alpha expression in iron deficiency. *Nat Struct Mol Biol,* 14(5), 420-426.

Sanchez, M., Galy, B., Schwanhaeusser, B., et al. (2011). Iron regulatory protein-1 and -2: transcriptome-wide definition of binding mRNAs and shaping of the cellular proteome by IRPs. *Blood, In press.*

Schalinske, K. L., Chen, O. S., & Eisenstein, R. S. (1998). Iron differentially stimulates translation of mitochondrial aconitase and ferritin mRNAs in mammalian cells. Implications for iron regulatory proteins as regulators of mitochondrial citrate utilization. *J Biol Chem,* 273(6), 3740-3746.

Smith, S. R., Ghosh, M. C., Ollivierre-Wilson, H., et al. (2006). Complete loss of iron regulatory proteins 1 and 2 prevents viability of murine zygotes beyond the blastocyst stage of embryonic development. *Blood Cells Mol Dis,* 36(2), 283-287.

Tibodeau, J. D., Fox, P. M., Ropp, P. A., et al. (2006). The up-regulation of ferritin expression using a small-molecule ligand to the native mRNA. *Proc Natl Acad Sci U S A,* 103(2), 253-257.

Vanoaica, L., Darshan, D., Richman, L., et al. (2010). Intestinal ferritin H is required for an accurate control of iron absorption. *Cell Metab,* 12(3), 273-282.

Vashisht, A. A., Zumbrennen, K. B., Huang, X., et al. (2009). Control of Iron Homeostasis by an Iron-Regulated Ubiquitin Ligase. *Science.*

Walden, W. E., Selezneva, A. I., Dupuy, J., et al. (2006). Structure of dual function iron regulatory protein 1 complexed with ferritin IRE-RNA. *Science,* 314(5807), 1903-1908.

Wallander, M. L., Leibold, E. A., & Eisenstein, R. S. (2006). Molecular control of vertebrate iron homeostasis by iron regulatory proteins. *Biochim Biophys Acta,* 1763(7), 668-689.

Wallander, M. L., Zumbrennen, K. B., Rodansky, E. S., et al. (2008). Iron-independent phosphorylation of iron regulatory protein 2 regulates ferritin during the cell cycle. *J Biol Chem,* 283(35), 23589-23598.

Wang, J., Chen, G., Muckenthaler, M., et al. (2004). Iron-mediated degradation of IRP2, an unexpected pathway involving a 2-oxoglutarate-dependent oxygenase activity. *Mol Cell Biol,* 24(3), 954-965.

Wang, J., Chen, G., & Pantopoulos, K. (2005). Nitric oxide inhibits the degradation of IRP2. *Mol Cell Biol,* 25(4), 1347-1353.

Wang, J., & Pantopoulos, K. (2011). Regulation of cellular iron metabolism. *Biochem J,* 434(3), 365-381.

Wetli, H. A., Buckett, P. D., & Wessling-Resnick, M. (2006). Small-molecule screening identifies the selanazal drug ebselen as a potent inhibitor of DMT1-mediated iron uptake. *Chem Biol,* 13(9), 965-972.

Wingert, R. A., Galloway, J. L., Barut, B., et al. (2005). Deficiency of glutaredoxin 5 reveals Fe-S clusters are required for vertebrate haem synthesis. *Nature,* 436(7053), 1035-1039.

Wu, K. J., Polack, A., & Dalla-Favera, R. (1999). Coordinated regulation of iron-controlling genes, H-ferritin and IRP2, by c-MYC. *Science,* 283(5402), 676-679.

Zhang, D. L., Hughes, R. M., Ollivierre-Wilson, H., et al. (2009). A ferroportin transcript that lacks an iron-responsive element enables duodenal and erythroid precursor cells to evade translational repression. *Cell Metab,* 9(5), 461-473.

Zimmer, M., Ebert, B. L., Neil, C., et al. (2008). Small-molecule inhibitors of HIF-2a translation link its 5'UTR iron-responsive element to oxygen sensing. *Mol Cell,* 32(6), 838-848.

Section 3

Functional Role of Iron

3

Relationship Between Iron and Erythropoiesis

Nadia Maria Sposi
Department of Hematology, Oncology and Molecular Medicine,
Istituto Superiore di Sanità, Rome,
Italy

1. Introduction

In recent years there has been important advancement in our knowledge of iron metabolism regulation that also has implications for understanding the physiopathology of some human disorders like beta-thalassemia and other iron overload diseases. In fact, progressive iron overload is the most salient and ultimately fatal complication of beta-thalassemia. Iron deposition occurs in visceral organs (mainly in the heart, liver and endocrine glands), causing tissue damage and ultimately organ dysfunction and failure. Both transfusional iron overload and excess gastrointestinal absorption are contributory. Paradoxically, excess gastrointestinal iron absorption persists despite massive increases in total body iron load. However, little is known about the relationship among ineffective erythropoiesis, the role of iron-regulatory genes, and tissue iron distribution in beta-thalassemia. The focus of this chapter is an update about iron homeostasis and erythroid differentiation with a particular attention to the molecular mechanisms of iron homeostasis deregulation in thalassemia and to the GDF15-BMP-Hepcidin-Ferroportin regulatory pathway in order to understand the contribution to iron overload. The chapter describes evidences for these relationships and discusses how recent discoveries on iron metabolism and erythropoiesis could lead to new therapeutic strategies and better clinical care of these diseases, thereby yielding a much better quality of life for the patients.

2. Overall view on erythroid cells differentiation and importance of iron homeostasis

Iron homeostasis depends on a coordinated regulation of molecules involved in the import of this element and those exporting it out of the cells. In some cell types, such as erythroid cells, iron import mechanisms are highly expressed, thus allowing massive iron uptake (Pietrangelo, 2002; Testa et al.,1995). Excessive iron, however, may be toxic for these cells, particularly in view of its capacity to generate superoxide radicals and H_2O_2, which may freely diffuse into the nucleus resulting in cell damage (Karthikeyan, 2002) and it seemed therefore of interest to investigate whether erythroid cells possess specific mechanisms for iron export. Within the hematopoietic differentiation, the maintenance of iron homeostasis is essential for erythroid cells and macrophages. Erythroid cells need to incorporate very high amounts of iron to support the continued synthesis of heme and hemoglobin, while the macrophage cells play a key role in iron storage and recycling (Ponka, 1997; Testa et al.,1993; Testa, 2002). Human erythropoiesis is a dynamic complex multistep process that involves differentiation of pluripotent hematopoietic stem cells (HSCs) and early multipotent progenitors (MPP) to generate committed erythroid precursors, the erythroblasts, which then give birth to mature erythrocytes, i.e. the red blood cells (RBCs) (Orkin & Zon, 2008; Palis, 2008; Tsiftsoglou et al., 2009; Weissman, 2000). Briefly, the early erythroid progenitors (BFU-E, burst-forming units-erythroid) differentiate into late colony-forming units erythroid (CFU-E) and proerythroblasts followed by a progressive wave of erythroblast maturation in polychromatic and orthochromatic erythroblasts coupled with a gradual increase of erythroid-specific markers (Fig.1). As the hematopoietic process progresses from the early stages into erythroid cell maturation, cells gradually lose their potential for cell proliferation and become mature enucleated cells(Fig.1). Mature erythrocytes are biconcave disks without mithocondria and other organelles but full of hemoglobin able to bind and deliver O_2 (Ingley et al., 2004; Koury et al., 2002; Stamatoyannopoulos, 2005; Tsiftsoglou et al., 2009). The hematopoietic differentiation is a highly complex system in which, from a pool of totipotent stem cells, originate all the cells of peripheral blood (Golde, 1991; Metcalf, 1989; Orkin, 1996; Smith, 2003). The blood has a very important role in the functions of the organism from the earliest moments of its development, so that during embryonic life the various stages of the hematopoietic process alternate at different sites according to the different stages of development (Emerson et al., 1989). The embryonic→fetal hematopoiesis is characterized by three fundamental periods of activity progressively involving the yolk sac, liver and bone marrow. The first period, during which hematopoiesis is localized at the yolk sac, begins between the 14th and 19th days of embryonic life and continues until the completion of 3rd month (Emerson et al., 1989). Starting from the third month, the second phase of hematopoiesis takes place in the liver where it reaches its maximum during the 3rd-4th month and remains active until a few weeks before birth, when the definitive hematopoiesis (third phase) is concentrated only in the bone marrow and it will continue throughout adult life (Emerson et al., 1989). In this system of hematopoietic differentiation four compartments may be identified: stem cells and the progenitors (cellular compartments), precursors and mature elements of circulating blood (maturation compartments). Hematopoietic stem cells are characterized by the ability to self-renew (i.e. to generate other totipotent stem cells) and differentiate into hematopoietic progenitor cells. Stem cells also show the important property to remain for long time in a state of quiescence during adult life (Domen,1999;Metcalf,1989; Orkin, 1996; Smith, 2003). Primitive progenitors are able to generate blast colonies (CFU-B), the progenitors of high proliferative potential (HPP-CFC, colony-forming cells that power high-proliferative), and finally the multipotent progenitors that are still capable of generating mixed colonies, belonging to the different types of hematopoietic differentiation: erythroid, granulocyte, monocyte, and megakaryocytic (the CFU-GEMM) (Orkin, 1996; Ogawa, 1993; Grover, 1994). Mature progenitors are committed to the differentiation towards a singular hematopoietic lineage and are functionally defined as early burst forming units (BFUs) or more differentiated colony forming units (CFUs): erythroid progenitors are BFU-E and CFU-E; granulocytic-macrophagic progenitors are CFU-GM, CFU-G and CFU-M; finally megakaryocitc progenitors are BFU-Mk and CFU-Mk (Grover, 1994; Ogawa, 1993; Orkin, 1996; Smith, 2003). The survival, proliferation and differentiation of hematopoietic stem and progenitor cells are regulated by a complex network of hematopoietic growth factors collectively known as colony stimulating factors (CSFs), interleukins (ILs) or hemopoietins that are released from accessory cells such as fibroblasts, macrophages, lymphocytes and endothelial cells. Depending on their mechanism of action during hematopoietic differentiation, these factors can be classified into three categories: the first category includes growth factors that exert their action at the earliest stages of hematopoiesis, e.g. the c-kit receptor ligand (KL) or stem cell factor (SCF) (Bernstein,1991), FLT-3 ligand (FL) (Gabbianelli, 1995;Lyman,1994;), the basic fibroblast growth factor (bFGF) (Berardi, 1995; Gabbianelli, 1990) and interleukin-6 (IL-6) [Leary, 1988]; in the second category are growth factors acting as multilineage, whose prototypes are the IL-3 and GM-CSF that are able to stimulate primitive progenitors to proliferate and differentiate into all hematopoietic lineage (Metcalf, 1993); and finally in the third category are included the growth factors acting as unilineage, i.e. those that stimulate the differentiation and proliferation of a single lineage and include erythropoietin (EPO) [Fried, 1995; Krantz, 1991], the granulocytic growth factor (G-CSF) [Demetri & Griffin, 1991], monocytic growth factor (M-CSF) [Sherr, 1990] and thrombopoietin (TPO) [Kaushanky et al., 1994]. These unilineage factors act on progenitors already moving towards hematopoietic lineage and promote the production of mature cells in the circulating blood, i.e. erythrocytes, neutrophils, eosinophils, monocytes/macrophages and megakaryocytes. During the hematopoietic differentiation, the maintenance of iron homeostasis is essential for erythrocytes and macrophages. Erythroid cells need to incorporate very high amounts of iron to support the continued synthesis of heme and hemoglobin, while the macrophage cells play a key role in the storage and recycling of iron (Testa et al., 1993; Testa, 2002; Tsiftsoglou,2009). During the differentiation of erythroid progenitors towards mature red cells the following morphologically recognizable stages can be distinguished: 1) the earlier stage of proerythroblast, that presents a nucleus relatively large in respect to the cytoplasm, and one or two nucleoli; 2) the more advanced basophilic erythroblast, characterized by a reduced cellular diameter, a nuclear volume reduced more rapidly than the cytoplasm, and a cytoplasm uniformly basophilic; 3) the polychromatophilic erythroblast, that shows the initial condensation of the nucleus, nucleoli no longer visible and the cytoplasm with acidophilic areas; 4) the orthochromatic erythroblast, with a nucleus:cytoplasm ratio of approximately 1:4, nucleus darker and subject to pyknotic degeneration, and cytoplasm slightly pink as a consequence of the progressive increase in hemoglobin concentration; 5) and finally the reticulocyte that has lost its nucleus and, through the complete degradation of ribosomes and mitochondria, proceeds to the transformation in mature erythrocyte (Grover, 1994; Loken et al., 1987; Okumura et al., 1992; Orkin, 1996) (Fig.1). In adult mammalian bone marrow erythroblasts are always associated to the erythroblastic islets, that represent the drive amplification stage anatomy of erythropoiesis and consists of 1 or 2 histiocytic crown cells surrounded by erythroblasts at all stages of maturation. The histiocytes have thin cytoplasmic extensions that insert between erythroblasts suggesting that factors of nutrition can be provided by the histiocytic cell, centrally located, to the peripheral maturing erythroblasts (Grover, 1994; Orkin, 1996). The circulating red cell mass is maintained constant by a homeostatic mechanism regulating erythropoiesis, based on an erythropoietic stimulus which ensures that, under physiological conditions, the production of red blood cells equals their destruction. Moreover, in response to hypoxia, hemorrhage or hemolysis, this stimulus causes increase in the production of red blood cells (Ponka, 1997). The most important factor involved in the control of erythropoiesis is erythropoietin, but other substances, particularly hormones, contribute to the regulation of this process [Fried, 1995; Ponka, 1997]. Transferrin comes out from the bone marrow sinusoids using ample fenestrature exits, and binds to surface receptors carried by erythroblasts. The iron transferred from transferrin and transported to the mitochondria is reduced from $Fe3+$ to $Fe2+$ and then inserted into protoporphyrin IX by tetrapyrroles heme synthetase (Heme synthetase HS) for the synthesis of heme (Ponka, 1997; Testa et al., 1993; Testa, 2002). The reticuloendothelial system is a functional unit that includes cells having heterogeneous histologically different identities and a widespread distribution throughout the body, which share the common property of phagocytic activity, e.g. endothelial cells of blood capillaries of liver, spleen, bone marrow and lymph nodes, tissue and circulating macrophages (Andrews, 2000; Ponka, 1997). Reticuloendothelial system is the most important source of iron that enters the blood compartment. The flow of iron from reticuloendothelial plasma is unidirectional, as the reticuloendothelial cells are not able to pick up the metal from transferrin, but receive only hemoglobin or ferritin iron (Ponka, 1997; Andrews, 2000).Senescent erythrocytes at the end of their life (approximately 120 days) are phagocytized by endothelial cells and represent the largest source of iron entering the reticuloendothelial system. About 85% of the iron that enters the reticuloendothelial cells is promptly transferred to plasma transferrin and the remaining 15% is stored as intracellular ferritin, and transferred to plasma much more slowly [(Andrews, 2000; Grover, 1994; Ponka, 1997).

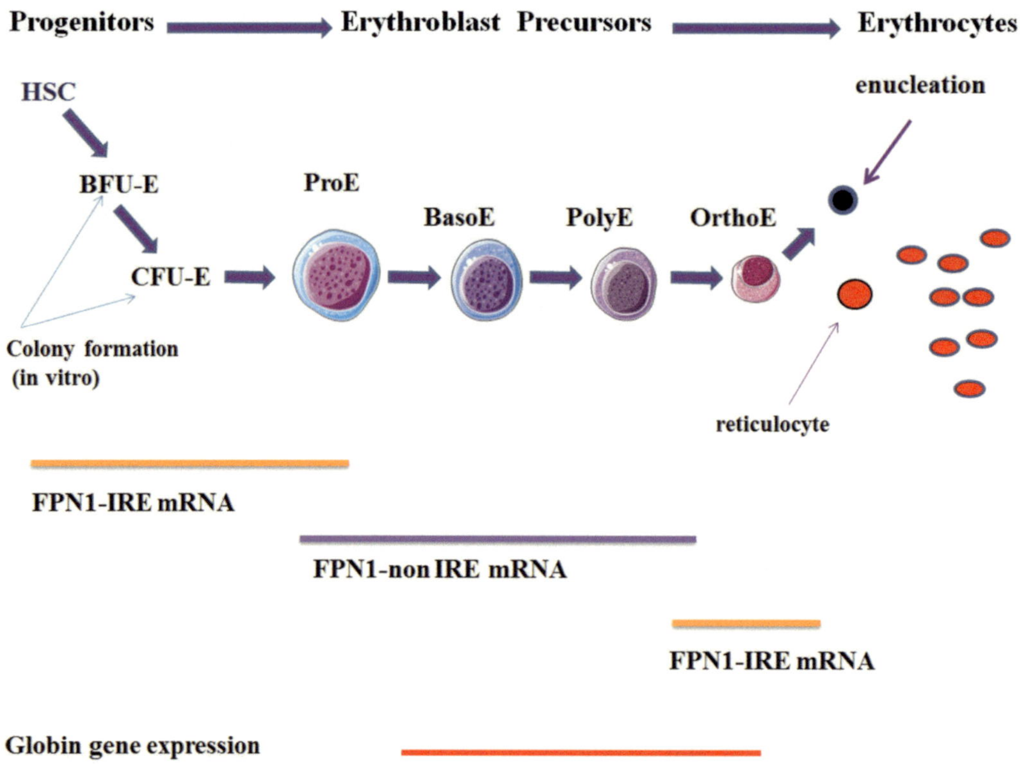

Fig. 1. **Pathway of the erythropoiesis from progenitors to mature cells.** Different stages are indicated: hematopoietic stem cell (HSC), burst-forming unit erythroid (BFU-E), colony-forming unit erythroid (CFU-E), proerythroblast (ProE), basophylic (BasoE), polychromatic (PolyE) and orthochromatic erythroblast (OrthoE). Coloured bars indicate timing of FPN1 alternative transcript expression (bottom) and hemoglobin synthesis referred to stages of erythropoiesis (bottom).

3. Iron acquisition by erythroid cells

Most of the iron in the plasma is bound to transferrin, an 80-kDa glycoprotein with homologous N-terminal and C-terminal iron-binding domains that is synthesized in the liver(De Domenico et al., 2008). Plasma transferrin has two important roles in iron physiology: first, the high iron-binding affinity of transferrin and the presence of a high concentration of apotransferrin (the iron-free form of transferrin) ensure that when iron enters plasma it is chelated , so limiting the ability of iron to generate toxic radicals; second, transferrin also directs iron towards cells that express transferrin receptors(De Domenico et al., 2008). Erythroid precursors require efficient iron uptake from Tf so that hemoglobin can be produced. TfR1 mediates erythroid iron acquisition, and its expression paralleles the maturation of erythroid progenitors (Hentze et al.,2004). The number of TfRs on erythroid cell, markedly higher than on other cell types (Sposi et al., 2000) is directly related to hemoglobin (Hb) production (Horton, 1983; Iacopetta et al., 1982; Nunez et al., 1977). In normal erythropoiesis, the hyperexpression of TfR1, starting from early erythroid HPC differentiation, is Epo-dependent and mediated via transcriptional and post-transcriptional mechanisms (Sposi et al., 2000). Both the number of TfRs present on the membrane and cellular ferritin concentration are regulated by intracellular iron level. Coordinate regulation of TfRs and ferritin is one of the most extensively studied mechanisms of post-transcriptional control of gene expression. In response to iron deprivation, the cytoplasmic stability of *TfR* mRNA is increased and ferritin mRNA translation inhibited (Klausner et al., 1993). As a consequence, enhanced iron uptake and diminished iron storage compensate for the lack of iron. The feedback regulation can be considered as a protective mechanism that prevents nutritional starvation and permits the biosynthesis of essential iron or heme-containing proteins. Under conditions of high iron supply, when cells need to store excess iron in order to prevent adverse effects of iron overload, the regulatory balance is inversed: *TfR* mRNA decays more rapidly and ferritin translation is no longer inhibited(Klausner et al., 1993). After binding to its receptor, the complex of Fe(III)-transferrin-TfR1 is rapidly internalized by receptor-mediated endocytosis through clathrin-coated pits (De Domenico et al., 2008 ; Ponka et al,1998). Acidification of the endosome produces a conformational change in both transferrin-Fe(III) and TfR1 with the consequent release of iron (Bali et al., 1991; De Domenico et al., 2008; Sipe & Murphy, 1991). The endosomal Fe(III) is converted into Fe(II) by a STEAP3, an erythroid-specific reductase (Ohgami et al., 2005). DMT1/Nramp2, a protons and Fe(II) co-transporter present in the endosomal membrane, transports iron into the cytosol (De Domenico et al., 2008; Gunshin et al., 2001). DMT1/Nramp2 is a member of the natural resistance-associate-macrophage protein (Nramp) family (Cellier et al., 1995). Several isoforms of the DMT1/Nramp2 mRNA are known, resulting from alternative splicing and/or the use of two alternative upstream promoter regions (Hubert & Hentze, 2002; Millot et al., 2009; Tabuchi et al., 2002). The isoform I is localized mainly at the apical site of the enterocytes and other epithelial cells whereas isoform II is found on the endosomal membrane of peripheral tissues and erythroid cells (Canonne-Hergaux et al., 2001; Millot et al., 2009). At acidic pH, apotransferrin remains bound to TfR1 and the complex is recycled to the cell surface (De Domenico et al., 2008). At the more neutral pH of plasma, apotransferrin dissociates from TfR1 and is free to bind iron and initiate further rounds of receptor-mediated endocytosis (De Domenico et al., 2008).

4. Iron utilization by erythroid cells

Erythroblasts also handle large amounts of iron. In these cells, most of the iron leaving the endosome is then transported to the mitochondria for heme synthesis and iron-sulfur cluster assembly (Napier et al., 2005). Potentially, iron may be directly transported from endosome into mitochondria by a "kiss-and-run mechanism" through a direct contact between both organelles, effectively bypassing the cytosol (Sheftel et al., 2007).Mitoferrin (Mfrn1, SLC25a37), a protein belonging to the family of mitochondrial solute carrier proteins expressed in the inner mitochondrial membrane, is thought to be implicated in shuttling iron across mitochondrial membrane (Millot et al., 2009; Shaw et al., 2006). The zebra fish mutant *frascati* with a mutated Mfrn1 gene shows profound hypochromic anaemia due to defective iron uptake by mitochondria (Shaw et al., 2006). Mfrn1 has a paralogue in mammals, Mrfn2 that is ubiquitously expressed. Silencing of both Mrfn1 and Mrfn2 induces reduction in heme synthesis by 90% (Paradkar et al., 2009). Most of heme in the body is synthesized in erythroid cells, as a precursor to hemoglobin formation, although heme is also the prosthetic group of various types of proteins, such as cytosolic or mitochondrial cytochromes, catalase, peroxidase and NO synthase (Millot et al., 2009). The erythroid-specific first enzyme of protoporphyrin IX synthesis, 5-aminolaevulinate synthase (ALAS), is encoded by two different genes: ALAS1 which is ubiquitously expressed and ALAS2, which is expressed only in erythroid cells (Furuyama et al., 2007). Regulation mechanisms differ widely between the two isoforms, i.e ALAS1 expression is negatively regulated by heme, whereas ALAS2 expression is only dependent on iron (Furuyama et al., 2007). Ferrochelatase, the last enzyme of the pathway, synthesizes heme from Fe(II) and protoporphyrin IX (PIX). Heme is then transported out of the mitochondria to be associated to globin chains and apocytochromes (Furuyama et al., 2007). Three molecules have been identified as possible mitochondrial heme exporters or transporters: the breast cancer resistance protein (ABCG2) (Jonker et al., 2002), the ABC-mitochondrial erythroid (ABC-me) transporter (Shirihai et al., 2000) and the feline leukemic virus subgroup C receptor (FLVCR)(Quigley et al., 2004). Heme export from mitochondria is thought to be mediated by ATP-Binding Cassette (ABC) transporters, i.e. ABCG2 and ABC-me (Shirihai et al., 2000), although the exact nature of the transporter has not been elucidated. FLVCR could be required for differentiation of erythroid precursors into colony forming units, potentially protecting cells against heme toxicity by exporting excess heme that can otherwise result in oxidative stress (Dunn et al., 2008; Quigley et al., 2004). However, the heme transporters responsible for heme release remain unclear. Another important function of iron in the mitochondria is to ensure the [Fe-S] cluster synthesis. It has been proposed that frataxin acts as a metabolic switch between [Fe-S] cluster and heme synthesis (Becker et al., 2002; Dunn et al., 2006). Frataxin expression is much decreased in the disease Friedreich's ataxia, in which iron loading occurs in the mitochondria (Dunn et al., 2006; Puccio et al., 2001). The molecular form of this excess iron remains unknown, but it could be unbound iron or iron stored in mitochondrial ferritin or other proteins (Dunn et al., 2006). Ferritin mitochondrial (FtMt) mRNA does not contain IRE, contrary to the H and L ferritin mRNAs, and therefore the FtMt synthesis is not regulated by the IRE/IRP system (Drysdale et al., 2002; Levi et al., 2001). The role of this FtMt is not fully elucidated but is thought to be a protective molecule against iron-mediated oxidative damage rather than an iron-storage molecule (Millot at al.,

2009). Although erythroid cells consume large amounts of iron, they have to maintain safety mechanisms to avoid iron and/or heme excess. It can be stored in ferritin or exported by ferroportin. Additionally, erythroblasts also have the capacity to export excess heme by FLVCR (Keel et al., 2008).

5. Iron- and haem-dependent regulation in erythroid cells

Iron metabolism and cellular heme represent two of the most key regulators of erythropoiesis (Andrews, 2008; Nemeth et al., 2008; Tsiftsoglou et al., 2009). The principal source of iron for erythrocyte precursors is plasma iron-transferrin (Fe-Tf), whereas heme derives from plasma as well as "de novo" biosynthesis inside the mitochondria as protoporphyrin IX first and then as iron-protoporphyrin IX (heme) after incorporation of iron with ferrochelatase (Tsiftsoglou et al., 2009). Trafficking and storage of iron in the mitochondria is tightly regulated as excess free iron promotes the generation of harmful reactive oxygen species whereas an inadequate supply of iron prevents haemoglobin synthesis leading to microcytic hypochromic anaemia (Martin et al., 2006; Millot et al., 2009). Cellular iron homeostasis is coordinately regulated posttranscriptionally by IRE/IRP system during erythroid differentiation. The analysis of IRP expression in hemopoietic cells provided some potentially interesting findings. It is well established that two different IRPs, IRP-1 and IRP-2, exist in mammalian cells (Henderson et al., 1993; Sposi et al., 2000). Both these proteins interact with the IRE sequence, six nucleotide loops, present in the certain mRNA 5' or 3' untranslated regions. The binding of IRP to ferritin mRNA results in translational block, while the binding to TfR mRNA results in mRNA stabilization (Sposi et al., 2000; Thomson et al., 1999). In spite of these similarities, however, IRP-1 and IRP-2 exhibit some important differences. In fact IRP-1 is related to mitochondrial aconitase, an enzyme of the Krebs cycle. Under high iron conditions IRP-1 dissociates from the IRE and is converted to a cytoplasmic aconitase through insertion of a [4Fe-4S] cluster (Haile et al., 1992). IRP-2 shares 60% amino-acid homology with IRP-1, but differs having a 73-amino-acid insertion in its N-terminal region, which confers a sensitivity to degradation via the ubiquitin–proteasome pathway in iron loading conditions (Guo et al., 1995; Henderson et al., 1993). IRP-2 is unable to assemble a [4Fe-4S] cluster and thus lacks aconitase activity. IRP-1 and IRP-2 are differentially expressed in hemopoietic cells and their expression is modulated during differentiation/proliferation of these cells. Thus, during differentiation of Hemopoietic Progenitor Cells (HPCs) from progenitor cells to mature cells it was observed that, during the initial stages of hemopoietic cell differentiation both IRP-1 and IRP-2 mRNAs are induced in all hemopoietic lineages; however, at later stages of differentiation, IRP-2 is expressed in all hemopoietic lineages at different stages of differentiation/maturation, IRP-1 is selectively expressed only in erythroid cells, while its expression is lost in all the other hemopoietic lineages (Sposi et al., 2000). It is not clear whether both IRP1 and IRP2 contribute to stabilization of TfR1 mRNA but several lines of evidence suggest that IRP2 is the main iron-sensor in erythroid cells: i.e., heme deficiency stabilizes IRP2 whereas accumulation of free heme induces its ubiquitination and degradation by the proteasome (Ishikawa et al., 2005; Millot et al., 2009); IRP2 knock-out mice develop microcytic hypochromic anaemia with reduced TfR1 expression in bone marrow cells (Cooperman et al. 2005; Galy et al., 2005; Millot et al., 2009); primary erythroblasts deficient in Stat5 showed a reduction in IRP2 expression, with a concomitant reduction in TfR1 mRNA and increasing of IRP1 (Kerenyi et al., 2008). The observation that in differentiating erythroblasts, TfR1 mRNA stability and IRP mRNA-binding affinity are no longer modulated by iron supply, has recently challenged the implication of the IRE/IRP system in iron homeostasis regulation in erythroid cells (Schranzhofer et al., 2006). This would be in agreement with the so called "kiss-and-run" hypothesis (Ponka et al., 1997; Richardson et al., 1996). It suggests that during terminal erythropoiesis endosomes come into close vicinity/physical contact with mitochondria to directly shuttle iron into this organelle for heme synthesis without modulating the mRNA-binding activity of the IRPs (Ponka et al., 2002; Zhang et al., 2005). This dual mechanism contributes to maintaining the high flux of incoming iron available for heme synthesis rather than being sequestered into ferritin (Millot et al., 2009). The level of cellular heme is very critical in the regulation of erythropoiesis. Heme biosynthesis is increased dramatically during Epo-moderated erythropoiesis to meet extra demand for red blood cell production under hypoxic conditions or stress erythropoiesis (Tsiftsoglou et al., 2009). Heme is needed for the production of large number of hemoproteins involved in cell respiration, O_2 tension sensing and metabolism (Tsiftsoglou et al., 2009). Heme is also needed to regulate the transcription of globin and nonglobin genes, because it has been found to regulate the action of transcription factors at nuclear level (Tsiftsoglou et al., 2009). Heme itself functions as a transcriptional regulator. It can induce heme oxygenase 1, HO-1, a molecule which reciprocally induces heme degradation (Huihui and Ginzburg, 2010). Heme strongly stimulates HO-1 expression by inhibiting the transcriptional repressor Bach 1. Binding of a heterodimer of the small maf transcription factor and Bach 1 to the multiple MARE (maf recognition element) sites in HO-1 enhancer represses HO-1 gene expression (Millot et al., 2009). It has been shown that HO-1 mRNA decreases following erythroid differentiation of Friend erythroleukemia cells, while mRNAs coding for the enzymes of the heme biosynthetic pathway increase (Millot et al., 2009; Fujita and Sassa, 1989). Heme non participating in hemoglobin synthesis results in a downregulation of IRP2 which reduces TfR1 expression on the cell surface and thus the amount of iron entering cells so preventing excess heme from accumulating in erythroid precursors (Huihui and Ginzburg, 2010; Ishikawa et al., 2005). In order to prevent excess globin synthesis, heme deficiency represses globin synthesis by activating a stress protein kinase named heme regulated inhibitor (HRI) which phosphorylates eIF2α (McEwen et al., 2005; Millot et al., 2009). Finally heme export has also recently been demonstrated in erythroid precursors. It has been shown that the feline leukemia virus, subgroup C, receptor (FLVCR) could function as a heme exporter (Quigly et al., 2004; Taylor et al., 1999). FLVCR is a member of the family of MFS (major facilitator superfamily) proteins which transport small solutes across membranes by using the energy of ion-proton gradient (Millot et al., 2009; Taylor et al., 1999). The absence of FLVCR results in arrest of proerythroblast differentiation and apoptosis, likely due to heme toxicity, whereas FLCVR overexpression in mice results in a mild microcytic hypocromic anemia suggesting that it is needed to maintain heme and globin balance and avoid accumulation of free heme or excess globin in the cytoplasm (Huihui and Ginzburg, 2010; Keel et al., 2008). In conclusion during erythroid differentiation the existence of an interplay of positive and negative feedback mechanisms maintains sufficient iron supply for heme synthesis and prevents formation or accumulation of heme in excess of globin chains.

6. Iron deficiency and anemia

Under physiological conditions, there is a balance between iron absorption, iron transport and iron storage in the human body. Iron deficiency anemia may result from the interplay of three distinct risk factors: increased iron requirements, limited external supply and increased blood loss (Munoz et al., 2010). Likewise, inappropriately high levels of hepcidin expression lower plasma iron levels and cause anemia. In this context, the common acquired anemia of chronic diseases (ACD) and the genetic iron-refractory iron deficiency anemia (IRIDA) are the most interesting examples. Several physiopathological features contribute to the anemia of chronic diseases, also known as the anemia of inflammation: impaired proliferation of erythroid progenitors and blunted response to erythropoietin, reduced erythropoietin synthesis as well as reduced life span of red blood cells (Millot et al., 2009). The basis of the disorder is that inflammatory stimuli, such as those caused by bacterial infections, cause acute hypoferremia presumably in an attempt to limit the growth of bacteria by limiting iron (De Domenico et al., 2008; Schaible and Kaufmann, 2004). During inflammation IL-6 seems to be the major pro-inflammatory cytokine implicated in hepcidin activation through a Stat3 dependent signaling pathway, so allowing the identification of a link between iron homeostasis and inflammation (Millot et al., 2009; Wrighting and Andrews. 2006). Hypoferremia develops rapidly as a result of decreased macrophage iron release leading to iron-limited erythropoiesis. Increased cellular iron retention is the result of decreased levels of cell-surface ferroportin, which, in turn, results from sustained secretion of hepcidin (De Domenico et al., 2008). Low or undetectable levels of hepcidin are normally observed in patients with iron deficiency. On the contrary, patients with IRIDA show very low iron stores and microcytic anemia refractory to iron treatment in consequence of inappropriately high hepcidin levels. IRIDA is caused by mutations in TMPRSS6 (matriptase-2), a gene that encodes a protease that negatively regulates hepcidin expression (Du et al., 2008). Recently it has been observed that genetic variants in TMPRSS6, frequent in the general population, may modulate the ability to absorb iron and to synthesize hemoglobin for maturing erythroid cells (Andrews, 2009). Recent study suggest that TMPRSS6 normally acts to down-regulate hepcidin expression by cleaving membrane-bound hemojuvelin, HJV, (Silvestri et al., 2008).

7. Iron overload and hereditary hemochromatosis

Hereditary hemochromatosis is an iron overload disease characterized by excessive body iron that causes tissue damage in the liver, pancreas and heart (Pietrangelo A, 2004). Currently four types have been identified in Caucasian populations: type 1 is the common form and is an autosomal recessive disorder of low penetrance strongly associated with mutations in the HFE gene ; type 2 (juvenile hemochromatosis) is autosomal recessive, of high penetrance with causative mutations identified in the HFE2 and HAMP genes; type 3 is also autosomal recessive with mutations in the TfR2 gene; type 4, or HFE4 (OMIM 606069), or ferroportin disease, is an autosomal dominant condition with heterozygous mutations in the ferroportin 1 (FPN1) gene (Worwood, 2005). FPN1(also known as Ireg1 and MTP1), the product of the Slc40a1 gene, was independently identified by three groups, using different approaches (Abboud & Haile, 2000; Donovan et al, 2000; McKie et al., 2000) and has been reported to be expressed and to play a critical role in several different tissue involved in mammalian iron homeostasis, including duodenal enterocytes (iron uptake and export into the circulation; hepatocytes (storage); syncytiotrophoblasts (transfer to embryo) and reticuloendothelial macrophages (iron recycling from senescent red blood cells). FPN1 appears to act as an iron exporter (Donovan et al., 2000; McKie et al., 2000) and to be specifically regulated according to body iron requirements (Donovan et al., 2000; Martini et al., 2002; McKie & Barlow, 2004; Mok et al., 2004; Pietrangelo et al., 2004; Yang et al., 2002; Zoller et al., 2001) in these tissues. The FPN1 gene has been highly conserved during evolution and encodes for a protein composed of 571 aminoacids with a predict mass of 62 kDa (for review see Cianetti et al., 2010).The presence of a well-conserved IRE in the 5′-UTR of FPN1 mRNA indicated the possibility of post-transcriptional control through the IRP-IRE systems (Donovan et al., 2000; Liu et al, 2002; Lymboussaki et al., 2003; McKie & Barlow, 2004) but several recent observation have indicated a more complex regulation of FPN1 expression by iron (Cianetti et al., 2010). Hemochromatosis associated with mutations in FPN1 can result in two different types of iron loading: one type is phenotypically indistinguishable from classical HFE hemochromatosis (or hemochromatosis type 1) (Spelling), in that the patients have both an elevated transferrin saturation and serum ferritin, while the other type termed "ferroportin disease" is associated with microcytic anemia, a raised serum ferritin and iron deposition in macrophages rather than hepatocytes (Pietrangelo, 2004). FPN1 mutations have two effects, either causing misfolding of the protein and failure to reach the cell surface ("loss of function")(Schimanski, 2005), or the mutant protein is expressed at the cell surface but is not inhibited by hepcidin ("loss of regulation")(Drakesmith, 2005). Briefly it was shown that A77D, V162del, and G490D mutations, that are associated with typical pattern of disease in vivo, cause a loss of iron export function in vitro, but do not physically or functionally impede wild-type FPN1 (Drakesmith, 2005; Schimanski, 2005). These mutations may, therefore, lead to disease by haploinsufficieny. By contrast the Y64N, N144D, Q248H and C326Y mutations, which can be associated with greater transferrin saturation and more prominent iron deposition in liver parenchyma in vivo, retained iron export function in vitro (Drakesmith, 2005; Schimanski, 2005). Because the peptide hormone hepcidin inhibits ferroportin as part of a homeostatic negative feedback loop, it was postulated that this group of mutations may resist inhibition to hepcidin resulting in a permanently "turned on" iron exporter (Drakesmith, 2005; Schimanski, 2005). All these results with A77D, V162del and G490D mutations of FPN1 are consistent with the scheme proposed by Montosi et al (Montosi et al., 2001)) to explain the macrophage iron loading observed in patients with these mutations (Schimanski et al., 2005): lower serum iron resulting from iron sequestration in macrophages reduces availability to the bone marrow for erythropoiesis thus leading to anemia that was effectively observed in some patients with mild anemia in the early stages of disease and that respond poorly to phlebotomy (Pietrangelo,2004; Schimanski et al, 2005). So iron overload may be a consequence of the erythron signalling to the gut enterocyte to increase iron uptake from the diet to compensate for the anemia. According to recent progress in this field it is likely that the erythron signalling is directly working through hepcidin-ferroportin interaction. By contrast the Y64N, N144D, Q248H and C326Y mutations, which can be associated with greater transferrin saturation and more prominent iron deposition in liver parenchyma in vivo, retain iron export function in vitro (Schimanski et al., 2005; Drakesmith et al., 2005). It was postulated that this group of mutations may resist inhibition by hepcidin, so interfering with its homeostatic negative feedback loop and resulting in a permanently "turned on" iron exporter (Schimanski et al., 2005; Drakesmith et al., 2005).

8. Ineffective erythropoiesis and thalassemia

In recent years there has been important advancement in our understanding of iron metabolism, mainly as a result of the discovery of hepcidin , a key regulator of whole-body iron homeostasis (for an exhaustive review see Ganz& Nemeth, 2006; Piperno et al, 2009; Lee & Beutler, 2009). Increasing experimental evidence suggested that a single molecule could be the "stores", the "erythropoietic" and the "inflammation" regulator of iron absorption and recycling [Cianetti et al., 2010; Fleming & sly, 2001; Nicolas et al., 2002), and that hepcidin acted principally or solely by binding to ferroportin, the only known cellular iron exporter, causing ferroportin to be phosphorylated, internalized, ubiquitylated, sorted (Nemeth et al., 2004) through the multivesicular body pathway and degraded in lysosomes (Ganz, 2005; Nemeth et al., 2004). Different stimuli can modulate hepcidin and act as positive or negative regulators. Four major regulatory pathways (erythroid, iron store, inflammatory and hypoxia-mediated regulation) that act through different signaling pathways to control the production of hepcidin are known (Cianetti et al., 2010). It is obvious that this complex network of interactions must be subjected to very close control in order to ensure that the iron erythropoietic demand is met and, in turn, adequate concentrations of iron in the circulation are always present (Cianetti et al., 2010; Piperno et al., 2009). Under normal conditions iron store and inflammatory regulation activate hepcidin transcription in the hepatocytes through the bone morphogenetic proteins (BMPs)/SMAD4 and signal transducer and activator of transcription-3 (STAT-3) pathways, respectively (Andrews, 2008; Piperno et al., 2009). The hemochromatosis protein HFE, transferrin receptor 2 (TfR2) and the membrane isoform of hemojuvelin (mHJV) are all positive modulators of hepcidin transcription and when defective, lead to hemochromatosis (HH) in humans (De Domenico et al., 2008; Piperno et al., 2009). Oppositely, hypoxia, anemia, increased erythropoiesis and reduced iron stores all negatively regulate hepcidin expression(Piperno et al., 2009). Emerging evidence suggests that erythropoiesis modulates hepcidin expression, with increased erythropoietic activity suppressing the action of hepcidin (Dallalio et al., 2006; Dunn et al., 2007; Kattamis et al., 2006; Pak et al., 2006; Vokurka et al., 2006). This in turn facilitates export of iron from the reticuloendothelial system and enterocytes, increasing the availability of iron for erythropoiesis (Dunn et al., 2007; Pak et al., 2006). Anemia and hypoxia also suppress hepcidin expression, although recent experiments indicate that functional erythropoiesis is required (Dunn et al., 2007; Pak et al., 2006; Vokurka et al., 2006) for these conditions to regulate hepcidin expression. Finally it is evident that erythropoiesis and iron metabolism are extremely intertwined in that alteration of one of the two may have a major impact on the second (Gardenghi et al., 2007; El Rassi et al., 2008; Rivella, 2009; Rund & Rachmilewitz, 2005; Weatherall & Clegg. 2001; Weatherall, 2001). That's the reason why thalassemia intermedia and thalassemia major are the best studied human models of hepcidin modulation by ineffective erythropoiesis. Beta-thalassemias are caused by mutations in the beta-globin gene resulting in reduced or absent beta-chain synthesis (for exhaustive reviews see Wetherall, 1998; Olivieri, 1999; Cao & Galanello, 2010; Ginzburg & Rivella, 2011). A relative excess of α-globin chain synthesis leads to increased erythroid precursor apoptosis, causing ineffective erythropoiesis which together with extramedullary expansion, splenomegalia and shortened red blood cells survival result in anemia (Huihui & Ginzburg, 2010). Patients either homozygous or compound heterozygous for mutation in the β-globin gene present with a broad range of clinical severity due to genotypically different mutations, combination inheritance with hemoglobinopathies, and additional modifying factors (Ginzburg & Rivella, 2011; Huihui & Ginzburg, 2010). Individuals with thalassemia major require regular red blood cell (RBC) transfusions to ameliorate anemia and suppress extramedullary erythropoiesis. Patients with beta-thalassemia intermedia show a milder clinical picture with more beta-globin chains synthesis and require only intermittent transfusions (Huihui & Ginzburg, 2010). Patients with beta-thalassemia have increased intestinal iron absorption which, in addition to transfusion dependence, contributes to iron overload (Huihui & Ginzburg, 2010). Progressive iron overload is the most salient and ultimately fatal complication of beta-thalassemia. Iron deposition occurs in visceral organs (mainly in the heart, liver and endocrine glands), causing tissue damage and ultimately organ dysfunction and failure (Fig.2). Both transfusional iron overload and excess gastrointestinal absorption are contributory. Paradoxically, excess gastrointestinal iron absorption persists despite massive increases in total body iron load (Fleming & Sly, 2001; Gardenghi et al., 2007; Rivella, 2009)(Fig.3). However, little is known about the relationship among ineffective erythropoiesis, the role of iron-regulatory genes, and tissue iron distribution in beta-thalassemia. If iron were a dominant regulator, patients with beta-thalassemia should express very high levels of hepcidin in serum; in contrast, the levels are very low, suggesting that the ineffective erythropoiesis alone is able to suppress the synthesis of hepcidin in spite of the presence of a severe iron overload (Cianetti et al, 2010; Piperno et al., 2009). Furthermore, serum from patients with thalassemia inhibited hepcidin mRNA expression in the HepG2 cell line, which suggested the presence of a humoral factor that down-regulates hepcidin (Weizer-Stern et al., 2006). The nature of the erythropoietic regulator of hepcidin is still uncharacterized, but may include one or more proteins during active erythropoiesis. Recent observations in thalassemia patients has suggested that one of these regulators could be the cytokine growth differentiation factor-15 (GDF15) (Piperno et al., 2009; Tanno et al., 2007). GDF15 is a divergent member of the transforming growth factor-beta superfamily that is secreted by erythroid precursors and other tissues. It has been identified as an oxygen-regulated transcript responding to hypoxia and as a molecule involved in hepcidin regulation (Cianetti et al., 2010; Bottner et al., 1999; De Caestecker, 2004; Tanno et al., 2007). Serum from thalassemia patients suppressed hepcidin mRNA expression in primary human hepatocytes and depletion of GDF15 reversed the hepcidin suppression (Piperno et al., 2009; Tanno et al., 2007). It was suggested that GDF15 overexpression arising from an expanded erythroid compartment contributed to iron overload in thalassemia syndromes by inhibiting hepcidin expression, possibly by antagonizing the BMP pathway. Without going into a detailed analysis of the GDF15 regulation mechanisms, we would like to recall the results obtained recently, that are in our view important to start reflecting on the existence of alternative ways that regulate hepcidin production (Cianetti et al., 2010). Recently a very interesting study demonstrated that expression of both GDF15 mRNA and protein was strongly and specifically responsive to intracellular iron depletion in a number of human cell lines and in vivo in humans (Lakhal et al., 2009; Cianetti et al., 2010). This up-regulation is independent of IRP1, IRP2 and the HIF pathway suggesting the involvement of a novel iron-regulatory pathway (Lakhal et al., 2009). This study showed that GDF15 was induced by over-expression of wild type ferroportin (Lakhal et al., 2009). This observation is very intriguing because it connects the iron-mediated regulation of GDF15 concentration to patho-physiological levels of iron: despite systemic iron overload, ineffective erythropoiesis and associated iron-fluxes in beta-thalassemia might generate an iron deficiency signal in a relevant molecular or cellular context and consequent stimulation of GDF15 expression in a particular erythroid compartment (Cianetti et al., 2010; Lakhal et al., 2009). Recent literatures provided at least two more molecules potentially involved in the regulation of hepcidin by erythropoiesis, i.e. the human twisted gastrulation factor (TWSG1) (Tanno et al., 2009) and the Oncostatin M (OsM) (Chung et al., 2010; Kanda et al., 2009). In contrast to GDF15, the highest-level expression of TWSG1 was detected at early stages of erythroblast differentiation before hemoglobinization of the cells (Tanno et al.,2009). In human cells, TWSG1 suppressed hepcidin through a BMP-dependent mechanism (Tanno et al., 2009). In vivo studies on thalassemic mice showed that TWSG1 expression was significantly increased in the spleen, bone marrow and liver. So it was proposed that TWSG1 might act with GDF15 to dysregulate iron homeostasis in beta-thalassemia (Tanno et al., 2009). In contrast to GDF15 and TWSG1, recent observations have showed that OsM could induce hepcidin expression in human hepatoma cell lines mainly through the JAK/STAT pathways (Kanda et al., 2009). Finally, results obtained by HuH7 hepatoma cells cocultured with primary human erythroblasts or erythroleukemic UT7 cells presented a 20- to 35-fold increase of hepcidin expression and identified OsM as responsible for increased levels of hepcidin (Chung et al., 2010). Furthermore, this study described the biological involvement of OsM in iron metabolism "in vivo" through direct transcriptional regulation of hepcidin gene expression and suggested a new OsM-hepcidin axis that might be critical in the development of hypoferremia in inflammation (Chung et al., 2010).

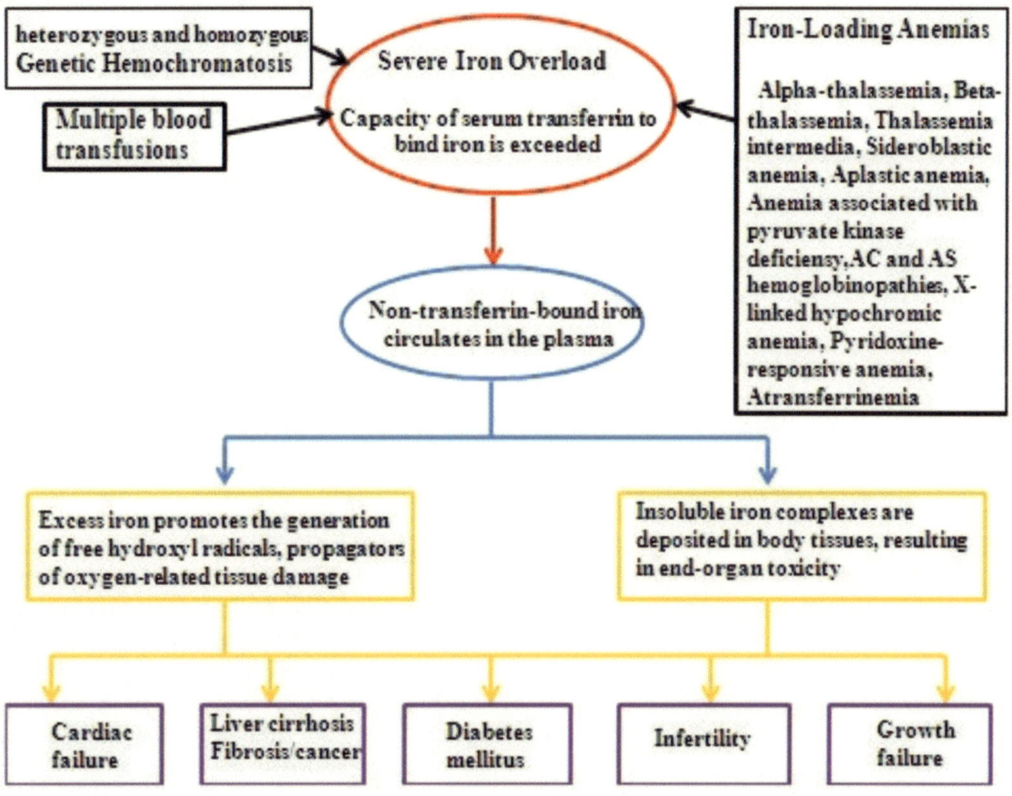

Fig. 2. **A summary of the causes of iron overload.** A schematic representation of the main causes of severe iron overload and its most important clinical manifestations.

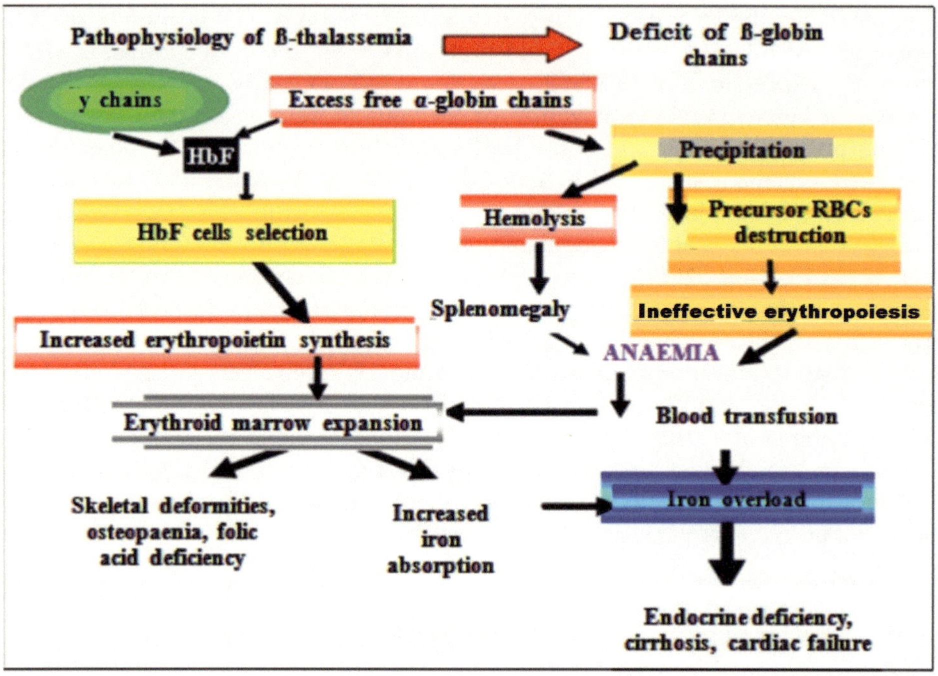

Fig. 3. **Pathophysiology of beta-thalassemia and corresponding clinical manifestations.** A summary of the effects of excess production of free alpha-globin chains. Excess unbound alpha-globin chains and their degradation products precipitate in red-cell precursors, causing defective maturation and ineffective erythropoiesis.

9. Ferroportin and erythroid cells

We reported for the first time the expression of FPN1 mRNA and protein in normal human erythroid cells at all stages of differentiation (Cianetti et al., 2005). The presence of an iron exporter was very surprising because the erythroid cells need to incorporate very high amounts of iron to support the continued synthesis of heme and hemoglobin (Cianetti et al., 2010). The IRE element in the 5′-UTR of FPN1 mRNA was demonstrated to be functional in erythroid cells and able to mediate translational modulation by cellular iron levels (Cianetti et al., 2005). Nonetheless, FPN1 protein expression appeared to maintain a constant level during different steps of erythroid differentiation and after iron treatments (Cianetti et al., 2005). A solution to this problem could be to use an upstream alternative promoters to produce mRNA species in which the 5′-UTR IRE could be spliced out or made non-functional (Cianetti et al., 2010). We described for the first time the existence of two alternative FPN1 transcripts (*variant II* and *III*), other than the IRE-containing canonical one (*variant I*), that did not contain the IRE element in their 5′-UT region, did not respond to iron treatments and together accounted for more than half of total FPN1 mRNA present in erythroid cells (Cianetti et al., 2005; Cianetti et al., 2010). These transcripts arise from the usage of alternative upstream promoters and differential splicing of 5'-UTR sequences. Interestingly, these transcripts were expressed mainly during the middle steps (4-11 days) of in vitro erythroid differentiation, corresponding to the maturation from late erythroid progenitors to polychromatophilic erythroblasts (Cianetti et al., 2005) (Fig.1). At these stages of erythroid differentiation TfR1, the receptor responsible for iron import in erythroid cells, is strongly and increasingly expressed (Sposi et al., 2000). Therefore, the non-IRE (*variant II* and *III*) FPN1 transcripts were expressed when erythroid progenitor/precursor cells need to accumulate iron into the cells (Cianetti et al.,2005). It was speculated that expression of the non-IRE FPN1 transcripts could produce a constant level of the transporter, unresponsive to the very high iron levels present in maturing erythroid cell. In contrast, IRE-containing FPN1 transcripts were mainly expressed in undifferentiated erythroid progenitors and in mature terminal erythroblasts, suggesting a possible role at these particular stages of erythroid differentiation (Cianetti et al., 2005; Cianetti et al., 2010). The existence of multiple FPN1 alternative transcripts indicated a complex regulation of the FPN1 gene in erythroid cells and the possibility that the control of FPN1 expression by iron conditions in different cell types might be complex. So in erythroid cells the regulation of FPN1 mRNA translation through the 5'-UTR IRE mechanism might be silenced because in this cell type a high level of iron uptake is needed to accumulate high amounts of iron required for optimal heme synthesis (Cianetti et al., 2005). A solution for this problem might be the utilization of an upstream alternative promoter to produce mRNA species in which the 5'-UTR IRE might be spliced out or made non functional (Cianetti et al., 2005; Cianetti et al., 2010). The alternative FPN1 transcripts are differentially expressed during erythroid differentiation, in particular indicating a sequential and specific activation pathway, with an apparently mutual exclusion between *variant I* IRE and *variant II/III* not containing the IRE transcripts (Cianetti et al., 2005) (Fig.1). These observations suggest that erythroid precursor cells need FPN1 transcript without a IRE to evade translational control by IRP-IRE system in order to export iron during the critical period when cells are committed to proliferate and differentiate (Cianetti et al., 2010). Once the precursor erythroid cells begin to produce hemoglobin, FPN1 without a IRE diminishes and FPN1 with a IRE predominates allowing erythroid cells to limit iron export through the IRP-IRE system and synthesize heme without developing microcytic anemia (Cianetti et al., 2010) (Fig.1).

10. New potential therapeutic opportunities

It is increasingly evident that the iron metabolism, heme and cellular erythropoiesis are inextricably linked, because iron metabolism (Andrews, 2005; Nemeth, 2008) and cellular heme (for exhaustive review see Tsiftsoglou et al., 2006) are two of the most relevant key regulators of erythropoiesis (Cianetti et al., 2010). The complex regulation of erythropoiesis suggests the existence of several molecular targets that could be exploited therapeutically for treatment of RBC disorders like thalassemias and anemias (Tsiftsoglou et al., 2009). We must differentiate between primary iron overload, and iron overload that accompanies ineffective erythropoiesis: in the latter case the administration of hepcidin might be considered as a new potential therapeutic approach to reduce iron overload in thalassemias and other forms of anemia associated with ineffective erythropoiesis (Cianetti et al., 2010; Tsiftsoglou et al., 2009). The reduced number or the absence of mature erythroid cells in beta-thalassemia patients is still very difficult to understand, and it has become one of the paradoxes among the most difficult to resolve : when the body has greater need for red blood cells instead it responds by decreasing their production (Rivella,2009). The most probable hypothesis to explain this phenomenon might rely on the existence of intrinsic and extrinsic mechanisms that would affect the process of differentiation: for example in cells where the synthesis of beta-globin gene is defective to the point that they ensure a stoichiometric between alpha and beta globin chains, a security mechanism can block the intrinsic maturation or, alternatively, an amount of heme in excess can be an extrinsic signal to prevent the differentiation that would lead to clusters of alpha globin chains production of reactive oxygen species (ROS) too toxic to survive (Cianetti et al, 2010; Rivella, 2009). There is much experimental evidence that oxidative stress may limit the process of differentiation. All this of course worsens the anemic outline (Rivella, 2009). So the contribution of these mechanisms to ineffective erythropoiesis might be different in each patient according to level of beta-globin synthesis and other extrinsic factors such as iron overload (Rivella,2009). At this point the question arises: is there a meeting point between different signaling pathways, although activated by different signals? Recent discoveries indicate that there is a potential for therapeutic intervention in beta-thalassemia by means of manipulating iron metabolism (Mabaera et al., 2008; Rivella, 2009; Rund & Rachmilewitz, 2005). A recent study suggested a link between EpoR/Jak/Stat signaling and iron metabolism, showing that in mice that completely lack Stat5 activity the cell surface levels of TfR1 on erythroid cells were decreased more than 2-fold (Kerenyi et al., 2008). Another study suggested a direct involvement of Epo in hepcidin regulation through the transcriptional factor C/EBP alpha (Pinto et al., 2008). In addition a link has been shown between Jak 2 and FPN1: Jak2 phosphorylates FPN1 following binding of this protein to hepcidin (De Domenico et al., 2009). Phosphorylation of FPN1 then triggers its internalization and degradation (De domenico et al., 2009). Therefore Jak2 might represent one of the major links at the interface between erythropoiesis and iron metabolism suggesting that use of Jak2 inhibitors, antioxidant, and analog of the hepcidin might be used to reduce ineffective erythropoiesis and abnormal iron absorption (Cianetti et al., 2010; Rivella, 2009). Administration of synthetic hepcidin or of agents that increase its expression, may be beneficial in controlling absorption of this metal (Piperno et al., 2009). Hepcidin agonists or stimulators of hepcidin production are being developed for the treatment or prevention of iron overload in hepcidin deficiency states, including hereditary hemochromatosis and beta-thalassemia (Ganz, 2011). In the mouse model of beta-thalassemia, transgenic hepcidin therapy improved iron overload as well as erythropoiesis suggesting that hepcidin deficiency or iron overload may adversely impact erythropoiesis in this disease (Ganz.2011). Hepcidin antagonists and inhibitors of hepcidin production may find utility in the treatment of iron-restricted anemias, alone or in combination with erythropoiesis-stimulating agents (Ganz,2011). Also GDF15 could be another potential therapeutic target for beta-thalassemia syndromes (Tanno et al., 2007). A major goal of hemoglobinopathy research is to develop treatments that correct the underlying molecular defects responsible for sickle cell disease and beta-thalassemia (Mabaera et al., 2008). One approach to achieving this goal is the pharmacologic induction of fetal hemoglobin (HbF). Although many of the events controlling the activity of the beta-globin locus are known, the details of those regulating normal human hemoglobin switching and reactivation of HbF in adult hematopoietic cells remain to be elucidated (Cianetti et al., 2010). If the molecular events in hemoglobin switching or gamma-globin gene reactivation were better understood and HbF could be fully reactivated in adult cells, the insights obtained might lead to a cure for these disorders (Cianetti et al., 2010). Agents that increase human HbF in patients may work at one or more levels: for example, hydroxyurea and 5-azacytidine kill dividing cells preferentially and may increase gamma-globin expression indirectly through this effect [for complete reviews see Mabaera et al., 2008; Bank, 2006). Butyrate may work both by histone deacetylase (HDAC) inhibition and by increasing gamma-globin translation on ribosomes (Bank, 2006; Mabaera et al., 2008). The Stem Cell Factor (SCF) induced an "in vitro" expansion of effective erythropoiesis and a reactivation of gamma-globin synthesis up to fetal levels, paving the way to its potential use in the therapeutic treatment of this disease (Gabbianelli et al., 2008). Recently it was reported the ability of thalidomide to increase gamma-globin gene expression and the proportion of HbF-containing cells in a human in vitro erythroid differentiation system (Aerbajinai et al., 2007) showing that thalidomide induced production of ROS that in turn caused p38 MAPK phosphorylation and globally increased histone H4 acetylation (Aerbajinai et al., 2007; Mabaera et al., 2008). All these experiments present a body of evidence that suggests an important role for intracellular signaling in HbF induction (Cianetti et al., 2010). However, the mechanisms of action of these agents are not yet defined and their role in beta-thalassemia therapy is still being explored in light of its acceptable toxicity profiles adding to their promise as therapeutic agents (Ginzburg & Rivella, 2011). Key genes controlling fetal/adult globin switching have been identified (e.g. BCL11 and cMYB) and may ultimately serve as direct targets for small molecules that would increase HbF levels in this patients (Bauer & Orkin, 2011; Ginzburg & Rivella, 2011; Wilber et al., 2011). Finally recent publications have demonstrated the importance of what has been termed the "integrated stress response" pathway in erythroid cells that is also activated from a variety of stress stimuli, including viral infection, NO, heat shock, ROS, endoplasmic reticulum stress, ultraviolet irradiation, proteosome inhibition, inadequate nutrients and, in erythroid cells, limiting amounts of heme (Chen, 2007; Cianetti et al., 2010; Mabaera et al., 2008 Wek et al., 2006).

11. Conclusion

Our understanding of the pathogenesis of iron-restricted anemias and iron-overload has been revolutionized by discovery of hepcidin and its role in iron homeostasis stimulating the development of new diagnostic and therapeutic modalities for these disorders. Further work is required to understand the mechanisms of hepcidin regulation by iron and erythroid activity and to understand the structure, the transport function and the complex regulation of the hepcidin receptor ferroportin. In conclusion we are increasingly convinced of the importance to study the molecular mechanisms of iron homeostasis dysregulation in thalassemia and in particular the GDF15-BMP-Hepcidin-Ferroportin regulatory way in order to understanding its contribute to iron overload.

12. References

Abboud S. & Haile DJ. (2000). A novel mammalian iron-regulated protein involved in intracellular iron metabolism. *J Biol Chem*, vol. 275, pp.19908-19912

Aerbajinai W., Zhu J., Gao Z., Chin K., & Rodgers GP. (2007). Thalidomide induces gamma-globin gene expression through increased reactive oxygen species-mediated p38 MAPK signaling and histone H4 acetylation in adult erythropoiesis. *Blood*, vol. 110, no. 8, pp. 2864-2871

Andrews N.C., (2000). Iron homeostasis: insights from genetics and animal models. *Nature Reviews Genetics*, vol. 1, no. 3, pp. 208-217

Andrews N.C. (2008). Forging a field: the golden age of iron biology. *Blood*, vol. 112, pp. 219-230

Andrews N.C. (2009). Genes determining blood cell traits. *Nat. Genet*, vol. 41, pp. 1161-1162

Babitt JL., Huang FW., Wrighting DM., Xia Y., Sidis Y., Samad TA., Campagna JA., Chung RT., Schneyer AL., Woolf CJ., Andrews NC., & Lin HY. (2006). Bone morphogenetic protein signaling by hemojuvelin regulates hepcidin expression. *Nature Genetics*, vol. 38, no. 5, pp. 531-539

Bali P.K., Zak O., & Aisen PA. (1991). New role for the transferrin receptor in the release of iron from transferrin. *Biochemistry*, vol. 30, pp. 324-328

Bank A. (2006). Regulation of human fetal hemoglobin: new players, new complexities. *Blood*, vol. 107, no. 2, pp. 435-443

Bauer DE., & Orkin S.H. (2011). Update on fetal hemoglobin gene regulation in hemoglobinopathies. *Curr opin Pediatr*, vol. 23(1), pp. 1-8

Becker EM., Greer JM., Ponka P., & Richardson DR. (2002). Erythroid differentiation and protoporphyrin IX down-regulate frataxin expression in Friend cells: characterization of frataxin expression compared to molecules involved in iron metabolism and hemoglobinization. *Blood*,vol. 99, pp. 3813-3822

Berardi AC., Wang A., Abraham J., and Scadden DT., (1995). Basic fibroblast growth factor mediates its effects on committed myeloid progenitors by direct action and has no effect on hematopoietic stem cells. *Blood*, vol. 86, no. 6, pp. 2123-2129,

Bernstein I.D., Andrews R.G., & Zsebo K.M. (1991) Recombinant human stem cell factor enhances the formation of colonies by CD34+ and CD34+lin- cells, and the generation of colony-forming cell progeny from CD34+lin- cells cultured with interleukin-3, granulocyte colony-stimulating factor, or granulocyte-macrofage colony-stimulating factor. *Blood*, vol. 77, no. 11, pp. 2316-2321

Böttner M., Laaff M., Schechinger B., Rappold G., Unsicker K., & Suter-Crazzolara C. (1999).

Characterization of the rat, mouse, and human genes of growth/differentiation factor-15/macrophage inhibiting cytokine-1 (GDF-15/MIC-1). *Gene*, vol. 237, no. 1, pp. 105-111

Canonne-Hergaux F., Zhang AS., Ponka P., Gros P. (2001). Characterization of the iron transporterDMT1 (NRAMP2/DCT1) in red blood cells of normal and anemic mk/mk mice. *Blood*, vol. 98, pp. 3823-3830

Cao A., & Galanello R. (2010). Beta-thalassemia. *Genet Med.*, vol. 12(2), pp. 61-76

Chen JJ. (2007). Regulation of protein synthesis by the heme-regulated eIF2alpha kinase: relevance to anemias. *Blood*, vol. 109, no. 7, pp. 2693-2699

Chung B., Verdier F., Matak P., Deschemin JC., Mayeux P., & Vaulont S. (2010). Oncostatin M is a potent inducer of hepcidin, the iron regulatory hormone. *The FASEB Journal*, vol. 24, no. 6, pp. 2093-2103

Cianetti L., Segnalini P., Calzolari A., Morsilli O., Felicetti F., Ramoni C., Gabbianelli M., Testa U., & **Sposi NM**. (2005). Expression of alternative transcripts of ferroportin-1 during human erythroid differentiation. *Haematologica*, vol.90, n.12, pp 1595-1606.

Cianetti L., Gabbianelli M., & Sposi N.M. (2010) Ferroportin and erythroid cells: an update. *Advance in Hematology*, vol.2010, Article ID 404173, 12 page

Cooperman SS., Meyron-Holtz EG., Olivierre-Wilson H., Ghosh MC., McConnell JP., Rouault TA. (2005). Microcytic anemia, erythropoieticprotoporphyria, and neurodegeneration in mice with targeted deletion of iron-regulatory protein 2. Blood, vol.106, pp. 1084-1091.

Dallalio G., Law E., & Means RT jr. (2006). Hepcidin inhibits in vitro erythroid colony formation at reduced erythropoietin concentrations. *Blood*, vol. 107, no. 7, pp. 2702-2704

De Caestecker M. (2004) The transforming growth factor-beta superfamily of receptors. *Cytokine and Growth Factor Reviews*, vol. 15, no. 1, pp. 1-11

De Domenico D., McVey Ward., & J. Kaplan. (2008) Regulation of iron acquisition and storage: consequences for iron-linked disorders. *Nature Reviews. Molecular Cell Biology*, vol. 9, no. 1, pp. 72-81

De Domenico I., Lo E., Ward DM., & Kaplan J. (2009) Hepcidin-induced internalization of ferroportin requires binding and cooperative interaction with Jak2. *Proceedings of the National Academy of Sciences of the United States of America*, vol. 106, no. 10, pp. 3800-3805

Demetri G. D., & Griffin JD. (1991). Granulocyte colony-stimulating factor and its receptor. *Blood*, vol. 78, no. 11, pp. 2791-2808

Domen J., & Weissman IL. (1999). Self-renewal, differentiation or death: regulation and manipulation of hematopoietic stem cell fate. *Molecular Medicine Today*, vol. 5, no. 5, pp. 201-208

Drysdale J., Arosio P., Invernizzi R., Cazzola M., Volz A., Corsi B., Biasiotto G., & Levi S. (2002). Mitochondrial ferritin : a new player in iron metabolism. *Blood Cells Mol Dis*, vol. 29, pp. 376-383

Donovan A., Brownlie A., Zhou Y., Shepard J., Pratt SJ., Moynihan J., Paw BH., Drejer A., Barut B., Zapata A., Law TC., Brugnara C., Lux SE., Pinkus GS., Pinkus JL., Kingsley PD., Palis J., Fleming MD., Andrews NC., & Zon LI. (2000). Positional cloning of zebrafish ferroportin 1 identifies a conserved vertebrate iron exporter. *Nature*, vol. 403, pp. 776-81

Drakesmith H., Schimanski LM., Ormerod E., Merryweather-Clarke AT., Viprekasit V., Edwards JP., Sweetland E., Bastin JM., Cowley D., Chinthammitr Y., Robson KJH., Townsend ARM. (2005). Resistance to hepcidin is conferred by hemochromatosis-associated mutations of ferroportin. *Blood*. Vol. 106, pp. 1092-1097

Dunn LL., Rahmanto JS., & Richardson DR. (2007). Iron uptake and metabolism in the new millennium. *Trends in Cell Biology*, vol. 17, no. 2, pp. 93-100

Du X., She E., Gelbart T., Truksa J., Lee P., Xia Y., Khovananth K., Mudd S., Mann N., Moresco E.M., Beutler E., & Beutler B. (2008). The serine protease TMPRSS6 is required to sense iron deficiency. *Science*, vol. 320, pp. 1088-1092

Emerson S.G., Thomas S., Ferrara JL., & Greenstein JL. (1989). Developmental regulation of erythropoiesis by hematopoietic growth factors: analysis on populations of BFU-E from bone marrow, peripheral blood, and fetal liver. *Blood*, vol. 74, no. 1, pp. 49-55

Fleming RE., & Sly WS. (2001). Hepcidin: a putative iron-regulatory hormone relevant to hereditary hemochromatosis and the anemia of chronic disease. *Proceedings of the National Academy of Sciences of the United States of America*, vol. 98, no. 15, pp. 8160-8162

Fried W. (1995). Erythropoietin. *Annual Review of Nutrition*, vol. 15, pp. 353-377

Fujita H., & Sassa S. (1989). The rapid and decremental change in haem oxygenase mRNA during erythroid differentiation of murine erythroleukaemia cells. *Br J Haematol*, vol. 73, pp. 557-560

Furuyama K., Kaneko K., & Vargas PD. (2007). Heme as a magnificent molecule with multiple missions: Heme determines its own fate and governs cellular homeostasis. *Tohoku J Exp Med*, vol. 213, pp. 1-16

Gabbianelli M., Sargiacomo M., Pelosi E., Testa U., Isacchi G., & Peschle C. (1990). Pure human hematopoietic progenitors: permissive action of basic fibroblast growth factor. *Science*, vol. 249, no. 4976, pp. 1561-1564

Gabbianelli M., Pelosi E., Montesoro E., Valtieri M., Luchetti L., Samoggia P., Vitelli L., Barbieri T., Testa U., & Peschle C. (1995). Multi-level effects of flt3 ligand on human hematopoiesis: expansion of putative stem cells and proliferation of granulomonocytic progenitors/monocytic precursors. *Blood*, vol. 86, no. 5 , pp. 1661-1670

Gabbianelli M., Morsilli O., Massa A., Pasquini L., Cianciulli P., Testa U., & Peschle C. (2008). Effective erythropoiesis and HbF reactivation induced by kit ligand in beta-thalassemia. *Blood*, vol. 111, no. 1, pp. 421-429

Gardenghi S., Marongiu MF., Ramos P., Guy E., Breda L., Chadburn A., Liu Y., Amariglio N., Rechavi G., Rachmilewitz EA., Breuer W., Cabantchik ZI., Wrighting DM., Andrews NC., de Sousa M., Giardina PJ., Grady RW., & Rivella S. (2007). Ineffective erythropoiesis in beta-thalassemia is characterized by increased iron absorption mediated by down-regulation of hepcidin and up-regulation of ferroportin. *Blood*, vol. 109, no. 11, pp. 5027-5035

Galy B., Ferring D., Minana B., Bell O., Janser HG., Muckenthaler M., Schümann K., Hentze MW. (2005). Altered body iron distribution and microcytosis in mice deficient in iron regulatory protein 2 (IRP2). *Blood*, vol. 106, pp. 2580-2589

Ganz T. (2005). Cellular iron: ferroportin is the only way out. *Cell Metabolism*, vol. 1, no. 3, pp. 155-157

Ganz T., & Nemeth E. (2006). Regulation of iron acquisition and iron distribution in mammals. *Biochimica et Biophysica Acta*, vol. 1763, no. 7, pp. 690-699

Ginzburg Y., & Rivella S. (2011). β-thalassemia: a model for elucidating the dynamic regulation of ineffective erythropoiesis and iron metabolism. *Blood*, vol.118, no. 16, pp. 4321-4330

Golde DW. (1991). The stem cell. *Scientific American*, vol. 265, no. 6, pp. 86-93

Grover CB. Jr. (1994). "Hematopoiesis" in *The molecular basic of blood*, Sander ed.

Gunshin H, Allerson CR, Polycarpou-Schwarz M., Rofts A., Rogers JT., Kishi F., Hentze MW., Rouault TA., Andrews NC., & Hediger MA. (2001). Iron-dependent regulation of the divalent metal ion transporter. *FEBS* Lett, vol. 509, pp. 309-316

Guo B., Brown FM., Philips JD., Yu Y., & Leibold EA. (1995). Characterization and expression of iron regulatory protein 2 (IRP2). Presence of multiple IRP2 transcripts regulated by intracellular iron level. *J. Biol. Chem*, vol. 270, pp. 16529–16535

Haile DJ., Rouault TA., Tang CK., Chin J., Harford JB., & Klausner RD. (1992). Reciprocal control of RNA-binding and aconitase activity in the regulation of the iron responsive element binding protein: role of the iron-sulfur cluster. *Proc. Natl Acad. Sci. USA*, vol. **89**, pp. 7536-7540

Henderson BR., Seiser C., & Kühn LC. (1993). Characterization of a second RNA-binding protein in rodents with specificity for iron responsive elements. *J. Biol. Chem.*, vol. 268, pp. 27327–27334

Hentze MW., Muckenthaler MU., & Andrews NC. (2004). Balancing acts: molecular control of mammalian iron metabolism. Cell, vol. 117, pp. 285-297

Horton MA. (1983). Expression of transferrin receptors during erythroid maturation. *Exp. Cell Res.*, vol. 144, pp. 361–366

Hubert N., & Hentze MW. (2002). Previously uncharacterized isoforms of divalent metal transporter (DMT)-1: Implications for regulation and cellular function. *Proc Natl Acad Sci* USA , vol. 99, pp. 12345-12350

Huihui L., & Ginzburg YZ. (2010). Crosstalk between iron metabolism and erythropoiesis. *Advances in Hematology*, vol. 2010, Article ID 605435, 12 pages

Iacopetta BJ., Morgan EH., & Yeoh GC. (1982) Transferrin receptors and iron uptake during erythroid cell development. *Biochim. Biophys. Acta*, vol. 687, pp. 204–210

Ingley E., Tilbrook PA., & Klinken SP. (2004). New insights into the regulation of erythroid cells. *IUMBMB Life*, vol. 56, no. 4, pp. 177-184

Ishikawa H., Kato M., Hori H., Kato M., Hori H., Ishimori K., Kirisako T., Tokunaga F., Iwai K. (2005). Involvement of heme regulatory motif in heme-mediated ubiquitination and degradation of IRP2. Mol *Cell*, vol. 19, pp. 171-181

Jonker JW., Buitelaar M., Wagenaar E., Van Der Valk MA., Scheffer GL., Scheper RJ., Plosch T., Kuipers F., Elferink RP., Rosing H., Beijnen JH., & Schinkel AH. (2002). The breast cancer resistance protein protects against a major chlorophyll-derived dietary phototoxin and protoporphyria. *Proc. Natl. Acad. Sci.* U.S.A, vol. 99, pp. 15649-15654

Kanda J., Uchiyama T., Tomosugi N., Higuchi M., Uchiyama T., & Kawabata H. (2009). Oncostatin M and leukemia inhibitory factor increase hepcidin expression in hepatoma cell lines. *International Journal of Hematology*, vol. 90, no. 5, pp. 545-552

Karthikeyan G., Lewis LK., & Resnick MA. (2002). The mithochondrial protein frataxin prevents nuclear damage. *Human Molecular Genetics*, vol. 11, no. 11, pp. 1351-1362

Kattamis A., Papassotiriou I., Palaiologou D., Apostolakou F., Galani A., Ladis V., Sakellaropoulos N., & Papanikolaou G. (2006). The effects of erythropoietic activity and iron burden on hepcidin expression in patients with thalassemia major. *Haematologica*, vol. 91, no. 6, pp. 809-812

Kaushanky K., Lok S., Holly RD., Broudy VC., Lin N., Bailey MC., Forstrom JW., Buddle MM., Oort PJ., Hagen FS., Roth GJ., Papayannopoulou T., & Foster DC. (1994). Promotion of megakaryocyte progenitor expansion and differentiation by the c-Mpl ligand thrombopoietin. *Nature*, vol. 369, no. 6481, pp. 568-571

Keel SB., Doty RT., Yang Z., Quigley JG., Chen J., Knoblaugh S., Kingsley PD., De Domenico I., Vaughn MB., Kaplan J., Palis J., & Abkowitz JL. (2008). A heme export protein is required for red blood cell differentiation and iron homeostasis. *Science*, vol. 319, pp. 825-828

Kerenyi MA., Grebien F., Gehart H., Schifrer M., Artaker M., Kovacic B., Beug H., Moriggi R., & Müllner EW. (2008). Stat5 regulates cellular iron uptake of erythroid cells via IRP-2 and TfR1. *Blood*, vol. 112, no. 9, pp. 3878-3888

Klausner RD., Rouault TA., & Harford JB. (1993). Regulating the fate of mRNA: the control of cellular iron metabolism. Cell, vol. **72**, pp. 19–28

Koury MJ., Sawyer ST., & Brandt SJ. (2002). New insights into erythropoiesis. *Current Opinion in Hematology*, vol. 9, no. 2, pp. 93-100

Krantz SB. (1991). Erythropoietin. *Blood*, vol. 77, no. 3, pp. 419-434

Lakhal S., Talbot NP., Crosby A., Stoepker C., Townsend AR., Robbins PA., Pugh CW., Ratcliffe PJ., & Mole DR. (2009). Regulation of growth differentiation factor 15 expression by intracellular iron. *Blood*, vol. 113, no. 7, pp. 1555-1563

Leary AG., Ikebuchi K., Hirai Y., Wong GG., Yang YC., Clark SC., & Ogawa M. (1988). Sinergism between interlukin-6 and interleukin-3 in supporting proliferation of human hematopoietic stem cells: comparison with interleukin-1 alpha. *Blood*, vol. 71, no. 6, pp. 1759-1763

Lee PL., & Beutler E. (2009). Regulation of hepcidin and iron-overload disease. *Annual Review of Pathology*, vol. 4, pp. 489-515

Levi S., Corsi B., Bosisio M., Invernizzi R., Volz A., Sanford D., Arosio P., Drysdale J. (2001). A human mitochondrial ferritin encoded by an intronless gene. *J Biol Chem*, vol. 276, pp. 24437-24440

Liu XB., Hill P., & Haile DJ. (2002). Role of the ferroportin iron-responsive element in iron and nitric oxide dependent gene regulation. *Blood Cells Mol Dis*, vol. 29, pp. 315-26

Loken M.R., Shah VO., Dattilio KL., & Civin CI. (1987). Flow cytometric analysis of human bone marrow: I. Normal erythroid development. *Blood*, vol. 69, no. 1, pp. 255-263

Lyman S.D., James L., Johnson L., Brasel K., De Vries P., Escobar SS., Downwy H., Splett RR., Beckmann MP., & McKenna HJ. (1994). Cloning of the human homologue of the murine flt3 ligand: a growth factor for early hematopoietic progenitor cells. *Blood*, vol. 83, no. 10, pp. 2795-2801

Lymboussaki A., Pignatti E., Montosi G., Garuti C., Haile DJ., Pietrangelo A. (2003). The role of the iron responsive element in the control of ferroportin/IREG1/MTP1 gene expression. *J. Hepatol.*, vol. 39, pp.710-715

Mabaera R., West RJ., Conine SJ., Macari ER., Boyd CD., Engman CA., Lowrey CH. (2008) A cell stress signaling model of fetal hemoglobin induction: what doesn't kill red blood cells may make them stronger. *Experimental Hematology*, vol.36, n.9, pp. 1057-1072

Martini LA., Tchack L., & Wood RJ. (2002). Iron treatment downregulates DMT1 and IREG1 mRNA expression in Caco-2 cells. *J Nutr*, vol. 132, pp. 693-696

Martin FM., Bydlon G., & Friedman JS. (2006). SOD2-deficiency sideroblastic anemia and red blood cell oxidative stress. *Antioxid Redox Signal*, vol. 8, pp. 1217-1225

Massagué J. (1998). TGF-beta signal transduction. *Annual Review of Biochemistry*, vol. 67, pp. 753-791

McEwen E., Kedershs N., Song B., Scheuner D., Gilks N., Han A., Chen JJ., Anderson P., & Kaufman RJ. (2005). Heme –regulated inhibitor kinase-mediated phosphorylation of eukaryotic translation initiation factor 2 inhibits translation, induces stress granule formation, and mediates survival upon arsenite exposure. *J Biol Chem*, vol. 280, pp. 16925-16933

McKie AT., Marciani P., Rolfs A., Brennan K., Wehr K., Barrow D., Miret S., Bomford A., Peters TJ., Farzaneh F., Hediger MA., Hentze MW., & Simpson RJ. (2000). A novel duodenal iron-regulated transporter, IREG1, implicated in the basolateral transfer of iron to the circulation. *Mol Cell*, vol. 5, pp. 299-309

McKie AT., & Barlow DJ. (2004). The SLC40 basolateral iron transporter family (IREG1/ferroportin/MTP1). Eur J Physiol, vol. 447, pp. 801-806

Metcalf D. (1989). The molecular control of cell division, differentiation committment and maturation in hemopoietic cells. *Nature*, vol. 339, no. 6219, pp. 27-30

Metcalf D. (1993). Hematopoietic regulators: redundancy or subtlety. *Blood*, vol. 82, no. 12, pp. 3515-3523

Millot S., De Falco L., & Beaumont C. (2009). Iron and erythropoiesis. *ESH Handbook Disorders of Iron Metabolism*, Cap.19, pp. 468-487

Mok H., Mendoza M., Prchal JT., Balogh P., & Schumacher A. (2004). Dysregulation of ferroportin 1 interferes with spleen organogenesis in polycythaemia mice. *Development*, vol. 131, pp. 4871-4881

Montosi G., Donovan A., Totaro A., Garuti C., Pignatti E., Cassanelli S., Trenor CC., Gasparini P., Andrews NC., & Pietrangelo A. (2001). Autosomal-dominant hemochromatosis is associated with a mutation in the ferroportin (SLC11A3) gene. *The Journal of Clinical Investigation*, vol. 108, pp. 619-623

Munoz M., Garcia-Erce JA., Remancha AF. (2011). Disorders of iron metabolism. Part II: iron deficiency and iron overload. *J Clin Pathol*, vol. 64, no. 4, pp. 287-296

Napier I., Ponka P., Richardson DR. (2005). Iron trafficking in the mitochondrion: Novel pathways revealed by disease. *Blood*, vol. 105, pp. 1867-1874

Nemeth E., Tuttle MS., Powelson J., Vaughn MB., Donovan A., Ward DM., Ganz T., & Kaplan J. (2004). Hepcidin regulates cellular iron efflux by binding to ferroportin and inducing its internalisation. *Science*, vol. 306, no. 5704, pp. 2090-2093

Nemeth E. (2008). Iron regulation and erythropoiesis. *Curr. Opin. Hematol.*, vol. 15, pp. 169-175

Nicolas G., Chauvet C., Viatte L., Danan JL., Bigard X., Devaux I., Beaumont C., Kahn A., and & Vaulont S. (2002). The gene encoding the iron regulatory peptide hepcidin is regulated by anemia, hypoxia, and inflammation. *The Journal of Clinical Investigation*, vol. 110, no. 7, pp. 1037-1044

Nunez MT., Glass J., Fischer S., Lavidor LM., Lenk EM., & Robinson SH. (1977). Transferrin receptors in developing murine erythroid cells. *Brit. J. Haematol.*, vol. 36, pp. 519–526

Ogawa M. (1993). Differentiation and proliferation of hematopoietic stem cells. *Blood*, vol. 81, no. 11, pp. 2844-2853

Ohgami RS., Campagna DR., Greer EL., Antiochos B., McDonald A., Chen J., Sharp JJ., Fujiwara Y., Barker JE., Fleming MD. (2005). Identification of a ferrireductase required for efficient transferrin-dependent iron uptake in erythroid cells. *Nat Genet*, vol. 37, pp. 1264-1269

Okumura N., Tsuji K., & Nakahata T. (1992). Changes in cell surface antigen expressions during proliferation and differentiation of human erythroid progenitors. *Blood*, vol. 80, no. 3, pp. 642-650

Olivieri NF. (1999). The beta-thalassemias. *N Engl J Med*, vol. 341, no. 2, pp. 99-109

Orkin SH. (1996). Development of the hematopoietic system. *Current Opinion in Genetics and Development*, vol. 6, no. 5, pp. 597-602

Orkin SH., & Zon LI. (2008). Hematopoiesis: an evolving paradigm for stem cell biology. *Cell*, vol. 132, no. 4, pp. 631-644

Pak M., Lopez MA., Gabayan V., Ganz T., & Rivera S. (2006). Suppression of hepcidin during anemia requires erythropoietic activity. *Blood*, vol. 108, no. 12, pp. 3730-3735

Palis J. (2008). Ontogeny of erythropoiesis. *Current Opinion in Hematology*, vol. 15, no. 3, pp. 155-161

Paradkar PN., Zumbrennen KB., Paw BH., Ward DM., Kaplan J. (2009). Regulation of mitochondrial iron import through differential turnover of mitoferrin1 and mitoferrin2. *Mol Cell Biol*, vol. 29, pp. 1007-1016

Pietrangelo A. (2002). Physiology of iron transport and the hemochromatosis gene. *American Journal of Physiology, Gastrointestinal and Liver Physiology*, vol. 282, no. 3, pp. G403-414

Pietrangelo A. (2004). Non-HFE Hemochromatosis. *Hepatology*, vol. 39, pp. 21-29

Pietrangelo A. (2004). The ferroportin disease. *Blood Cells, Molecules and Diseases*, vol. 32, pp. 131-138

Pietrangelo A. (2004). Hereditary Hemochromatosis–A new look at an old disease. *The New England Journal of Medicine*, vol. 350, pp. 2383-2397

Pinto JP., Ribeiro S., Pontes H., Thowfeequ S., Tosh D., Carvalho F., & Porto G. (2008). Erythropoietin mediates hepcidin expression in hepatocytes through EPOR signaling and regulation of C/EBP(alpha). *Blood*, vol. 111, no. 12, pp. 5727-5733

Piperno A., Mariani R., Trombini P., & Girelli D. (2009). Hepcidin modulation in human diseases: from research to clinic. *World Journal of Gastroenterology*, vol. 15, no. 5, pp. 538-551

Ponka P. (1997). Tissue-specific regulation of iron metabolism and heme synthesis: distinct control mechanisms in erythorid cells. *Blood*, vol. 89, no. 1, pp. 1-25

Ponka P., Beaumont C., Richardson DR. (1998). Function and regulation of transferrin and ferritin. *Semin Hematol*, vol. 35, pp. 35-54

Ponka P., Sheftel AD., Zhang AS. (2002). Iron targeting to mitochondria in erythroid cells. *Biochem Soc Trans.*, vol. 30, pp. 735-738

Puccio H., Simon D., Cossée M., Criqui-Filipe P., Tiziano F., Melki J., Hindelang C., Matyas R., Rustin P., Koenig M. (2001). Mouse models for Friedreich ataxia exhibit cardiomyopathy, sensory nerve defect and Fe-S enzyme deficiency followed by intramitochondrial iron deposits. *Nat. Genet.*, vol. 27, pp. 181-186

Quigley J.G., Yang Z., Worthington MT., Phillips JD., Sabo KM., Sabath DE., Berg CL., Sassa S., Wood BL., Abkowitz JL. (2004). Identification of a human heme exporter that is essential for erythropoiesis. *Cell*, vol. 118, pp. 757-766

Rassi FE., Cappellini MD., Inat A., & Taher A. (2008). Beta-thalassemia intermedia: an overview. *Pediatric Annals*, vol. 37, no. 5, pp. 322-328

Richardson DR., Ponka P., Vyoral D. (1996). Distribution of iron in reticulocytes after inhibition of heme synthesis with succinylacetone: examination of the intermediates involved in iron metabolism. *Blood*, vol. 87, pp. 3477-3488

Rivella S. (2009). Ineffective erythropoiesis and thalassemias. *Current Opinion in Hematology*, vol. 16, no. 3, pp. 187-194

Rund D., & Rachmilewitz E. (2005). Beta-thalassemia. *New England Journal of Medicine*, vol. 353, no. 11, pp. 1135-1146

Schaible UE., & Kaufmann SH. (2004). Iron and microbial infection. *Nature Rev. Microbiol.*, vol. 2, pp. 946-953

Schimanski LM., Drakesmith H., Merryweather-Clarke A., Viprakasit V., Edwards JP., Sweetland E., Bastin JM., Cowley D., Chinthammitr Y., Robson KJH., Townsend ARM. (2005). In vitro functional analysis of human ferroportin (FPN) and hemochromatosis-associated FPN mutations. *Blood*, vol. 105, pp. 4096-4102

Schranzhofer M., Schifrer M., Cabrera JA., Kopp S., Chiba P., Beug H., Müllner EW. (2006). Remodeling the regulation of iron metabolism during erythroid differentiation to ensure efficient heme biosynthesis. *Blood*, vol. 107, pp. 4159-4167

Shaw GC., Cope JJ., Li L., Corson K., Hersey C., Ackermann GE., Gwynn B., Lambert AJ., Wingert RA., Traver D., Trede NS., Barut BA., Zhou Y., Minet E., Donovan A., Brownlie A., Balzan R., Weiss MJ., Peters LL., Kaplan J., Zon LI., Paw BH. (2006). Mitoferrin is essential for erythroid iron assimilation. *Nature*, vol. 440, pp. 96-100

Sheftel AD., Zhang AS., Brown C., Shirihai OS., Ponka P. (2007). Direct interorganellar transfer of iron from endosome to mitochondrion. *Blood*, vol. 110, pp. 125-32

Sherr CJ. (1990). Colony-stimulating factor-1 receptor. *Blood*, vol. 75, no. 1 , pp. 1-12

Sipe DM., & Murphy RF. (1991). Binding to callular receptors results in increased iron release from transferrin at mildly acidic pH. J. *Biol. Chem.*, vol. 266, pp. 8002-8007

Shirihai OS., Gregory T., Yu C., Orkin SH., Weiss MJ. (2000). ABC-me: A novel mitochondrial transporter induced by GATA-1 during erythroid differentiation. *EMBO J*, vol. 19, pp. 2492-2502

Silvestri I., Pagani A., Nai A., De Domenico I., Kaplan J., & Camaschella C. (2008). The serine protease matriptase-2 (TMPRSS6) inhibits hepcidin activation by cleaving membrane hemojuvelin. *Cell Metabolism*, vol.8, n.6, pp. 502-511

Smith C. (2003). Hematopoietic stem cells and hematopoiesis. *Cancer Control*, vol. 10, no. 1, pp. 9-16

Sposi NM., Cianetti L., Tritarelli E., Pelosi E., Militi S., Barberi T., Gabbianelli M., Saulle E., Kühn L., Peschle C. & Testa U. (2000). Mechanisms of differential transferrin receptor expression in normal hematopoiesis. *Eur. J. Biochem.*, vol. 267, pp. 6762-6774

Stamatoyannopoulos G. (2005). Control of globin gene expression during development and erythroid differentiation. *Experimental Hematology*, vol. 33, no. 3, pp. 259-271

Tabuchi M., Tanaka N., Nishida-Kitayama J., Ohno H., Kishi F. (2002). Alternative splicing regulates the subcellular localization of divalent metal transporter 1 isoforms. *Mol Biol Cell*, vol. 13, pp. 4371-4387

Tamary H., Shalev H., Perez-Avraham G., Zoldan M., Lev Ii., Swinkels DW., Tanno T., & Miller JL. (2008). Elevated growth differentiation factor 15 expression in patients with congenital dyserythropoietic anemia type I. *Blood*, vol. 112, no. 13, pp. 5241-5244

Tanno T., Bhanu NV., Oneal PA., Goh SH., Staker P., Lee JT., Moroney JW., Reed CH., Luban NL., Wang RH., Eling TE., Childs R., Ganz T., Leitman SF., Fucharoen S., & Miller JL. (2007). High levels of GDF15 in thalassemia suppress expression of the iron regulatory protein hepcidin. *Nature Medicine*, vol. 13, no. 9, pp. 1096-1101

Tanno T., Porayette P., Sripichai O., Noh SJ., Byrnes C., Bhupatiraju A., Lee YT., Goodnough JB., Harandi O., Ganz T., Paulson RF., & Miller JL. (2009). Identification of TWSG1 as a second novel erythroid regulator of hepcidin expression in murine and human cells. *Blood*, vol. 114, no. 1, pp. 181-186

Taylor C.S., Willet B.J., Kabat D. (1999). A putative cell surface receptor for anemia-inducing feline leukemia virus subgroup C is a member of a transporter superfamily. *J Virol*, vol. 73, pp. 6500-6505

Testa U., Pelosi E., & Peschle C. (1993). The transferrin receptor. *Critical Reviews in Oncogenesis*, vol. 4, no. 3, pp. 241-276

Testa U.,Conti L., Sposi NM., Varano B., Tritarelli E., Malorni W., Samoggia P., Rainaldi G., Peschle C., & Belardelli F. (1995). IFN-beta selectively down-regulates transferrin receptor expression in human peripheral blood macrophages by a post-translational mechanism. *Journal of Immunology*, vol. 155, no. 1, pp. 427-435

Testa U. (2002). Recent developments in the understanding of iron metobolism. *The Haematology Journal*, vol. 3, no. 2, pp. 63-89

Thomson AM., Rogers JT., & Leedman PJ. (1999). Iron-regulatory protein, iron-responsive elements and ferritin mRNA translation. *Int. J. Biochem. Cell. Biol.*, vol. 31, pp. 1139-1152

Truksa J., Peng H., Lee P., & Beutler E. (2006). Bone morphogenetic proteins 2, 4, and 9 stmulate murine hepcidin 1 expression independently of Hfe, transferrin receptor 2 (Tfr2), and IL-6. *Proceedings of the National Academy of Sciences of the United States of America*, vol. 103, no. 27, pp. 10289-10293

Tsiftsoglou AS., Vizirianakis IS., & Strouboulis J. (2009). Erythropoiesis: model systems, molecular regulators, and developmental programs. *IUBMB Life*, vol. 61, no. 8, pp. 800-830

Tsiftsoglou AS., Tsamadou AI., & PapadopoulouLC. (2006). Heme as key regulator of major mammalian cellular functions: molecular, cellular, and pharmacological aspects. *Pharmacology and Therapeutics*, vol. 11, n. 2, pp. 327-345

Wang RH., Li C., Xu X., Zheng Y., Xiao C., Zerfas P., Cooperman S., Eckhaus M., Rouault T., Mishra L., & Deng CX. (2005). A role of SMAD4 in iron metabolism through the positive regulation of hepcidin expression. *Cell Metabolism*, vol. 2, no. 6, pp. 399-409

Weatherall DJ. (1998). Pathophysiology of thalassemia. *Baillieres Clin Haematol.*, vol. 11, no. 1, pp. 127-146

Weatherall DJ., & Clegg JB. (2001). The Thalassemia Syndromes. Weatherall DJ, Clegg JB, eds. *The thalassemia syndromes*, 4th ed. Oxford, United Kingdom: Blackwell Science, pp. 287-356

Weatherall DJ. (2001). Phenotype-genotype relationships in monogenic disease: lessons from the thalassaemias. *Nature Reviews. Genetics*, vol. 2, no. 4, pp. 245-255

Weissman IL. (2000). Stem cells: units of development, units of regeneration, and units in evolution. *Cell*, vol. 100, no. 1, pp. 157-168

Weizer-Stern O., Adamsky K., Amariglio N., Levin C., Koren A., Breuer W., Rachmilewitz E., Breda L., Rivella S., Cabantchik ZI., & Rechavi G. (2006). Downregulation of hepcidin and haemojuvelin expression in the hepatocyte cell-line HepG2 induced by thalassaemic sera. *British Journal of Haematology*, vol. 135, no. 1, pp. 129-138

Wek RC., Jiang HY., & Anthony TG. (2006). Coping with stress: eIF2 kinases and translational control. *Biochemical Society Transactions*, vol. 34(Pt1), pp. 7-11

Wilber A., Nienhuis AW., Persons DA. (2011). Transcriptional regulation of fetal to adult hemoglobin switching: new therapeutic opportunities. *Blood*, vol. 117, no. 15, pp. 3945-3953

Worwood M. (2005). Inherited iron loading: genetic testing in diagnosis and management. *Blood Reviews*, vol. 19, pp. 69-88

Vokurka M., Krijt J., Sulc K., & Necas E. (2006). Hepcidin mRNA levels in mouse liver respond to inhibition of erythropoiesis. *Physiological Research*, vol. 55, no. 6, pp. 667-674

Wrighting DM., & Andrews NC. (2006). Interleukin-6 induces hepcidin expression through STAT3. *Blood*, vol. 108, pp. 3204-3209

Yang F., Wang X., Haile DJ., Piantadosi CA., Ghio AJ. (2002). Iron increases expression of iron-export protein MTP1 in lung cells. Am *J Physiol Lung Cell Mol Physiol*, vol. 283, pp. 932-9

Zhang AS., Sheftel AD., Ponka P. (2005). Intracellular kinetics of iron in reticulocytes: evidence for endosome involvement in iron targeting to mitochondria. *Blood*, vol. 105, pp. 368-375

Zoller H., Koch RO., Theurl I., Obrist P., Pietrangelo A., Montosi G., Haile DJ., Vogel W., Weiss G. (2001). Expression of the duodenal iron transporters divalent-metal transporter 1 and ferroportin 1 in iron deficiency and iron overload. *Gastroenterology*, vol. 120, pp. 1412-9

Section 4

Iron Metabolism in Pathological States

4

Iron Deficiency in Hemodialysis Patients – Evaluation of a Combined Treatment with Iron Sucrose and Erythropoietin-Alpha: Predictors of Response, Efficacy and Safety

Martín Gutiérrez Martín[1], Maria Soledad Romero Colás[2], and José Antonio Moreno Chulilla[3]
[1]*Department of Medicine, University of Zaragoza, Investigation Group: Multifunctional Molecular Magnetic Materials, and INA (Institute of Nanocience of Aragon),*
[2]*Department of Medicine, University Hospital of Zaragoza,*
[3]*University Hospital of Zaragoza,*
Spain

1. Introduction

Chronic kidney disease is a public health problem and one of the outstanding causes of death in the industrialized world. The most serious condition is advanced chronic renal failure requiring replacement therapy by dialysis or kidney transplantation. In recent years the incidence is stabilizing but the prevalence is increasing probably due to the progressive aging of the population and increased comorbidity with other chronic disorders such as diabetes mellitus, hypertension and obesity (de Francisco et al. 2007). It is also a major cause of anemia in developing countries (Maiz, Abderrahim, and Zouaghi 2002) . The long-term survival and good quality of life of patients with chronic renal failure depends, among other factors, on hemoglobin, iron status and bone marrow response to erythropoiesis stimulating agents (ESA). Anemia is an almost constant complication of advanced renal failure which may contribute to worsen preexisting heart disease and, as a consequence, accelerate the progression of renal dysfunction (Kuwahara et al. 2011), (Silverberg et al. 2009). The administration of erythropoietin to patients with kidney and heart failure improves both processes, not only increasing hemoglobin but also by a direct effect of erythropoietin on cardiac function (Belonje, de Boer, and Voors 2008). In general, anemia is normocytic, normochromic and usually well tolerated until the advanced stages of kidney disease. It is usually a complication of stage 3 chronic kidney disease (KDOQI and National Kidney Foundation 2006). Its etiology is multifactorial: shortening of life span of erythrocytes, presence of inhibitors of erythropoiesis in plasma, inadequate production of endogenous erythropoietin (EPO) for the degree of anemia, blood loss, and iron and vitamin deficiency(Tsubakihara et al. 2010) (Belonje, de Boer, and Voors 2008), (Chamney et al. 2010). The outstanding cause is impaired secretion of erythropoietin due to renal disease, while other factors may contribute to its establishment, maintenance or aggravation.

The specific treatment of choice for anemia of chronic renal failure is recombinant human erythropoietin (rHuEPO), a drug considered a historic milestone since the time of its clinical use in 1986 (Winearls et al. 1986), and the major therapeutic advance in anemia of chronic renal failure. Erythropoietin remains vital in the treatment of anemia of renal failure, but in the coming years could be replaced by new erythropoiesis-stimulating agents under investigation (Schmid and Schiffl 2010). The use of erythropoietin led to a drastic reduction of transfusions and androgen therapy with the consequence of decreasing the complications of these treatments. Suitable doses of the drug, as well as the correction of other contributing factors to anemia, are necessary to maintain adequate levels of hemoglobin in the range of 11-12 g / dl (KDOQI 2007).

Iron is an essential factor to achieve and maintain effective erythropoiesis in patients with chronic renal failure treated with rHuEPO, due to frequent losses of blood in the hemodialyzer, overstimulation of erythropoiesis induced by erythropoietin and possible gastrointestinal bleeding. Moreover, the renal disease itself and chronic inflammation can sequester iron in the mononuclear phagocytic system preventing its use for erythropoiesis. These factors as a whole significantly increase the demand for iron. Capacity of intestinal iron absorption in these patients is not enough to maintain adequate levels of iron stores. On the other hand, the supply of iron improves response to rHuEPO and aids to lower its dose up to 30%. However, iron administration must be handled with caution, as an excess is not safe. The body has mechanisms to regulate iron absorption in the gastro-duodenal tract, but lacks a physiological mechanism to remove excess iron. Therefore treatment with intravenous iron should be monitored carefully.

Other causes of anemia in dialysis patients such as: hemolysis, aluminum intoxication, infection, chronic inflammation and hyperparathyroidism should not be overlooked; on the contrary the anemia of renal failure is not generally characterized by a lack of folic acid or vitamin B12 (Bravo, Galindo, and Bienchy 1994).

For all these reasons, patients need iron administration (usually intravenous) and regular monitoring of iron body stores. The diagnosis and treatment protocols should be optimized to adjust the cost, improve quality of life and prolong survival, as it has recently been reported that patients with hemoglobin above 12 g / dl have a higher survival rate than those with lower levels (Pollak et al. 2009).

The evaluation of anemia and iron status in chronic renal failure has peculiarities that make it different from other processes. Therefore we find it useful to include a brief description of the normal values in adults, the diagnosis of iron deficiency in general and the peculiarities of the diagnosis of iron status in patients with chronic renal failure. The World Health Organization specifies the normal range of hemoglobin and defines anemia as a hemoglobin decrease below the normal lower limit (Nutritional anaemias (Anonymous1968). Hematology analyzers measure the hemoglobin directly, with great precision and accuracy, while the hematocrit is a calculated value. Moreover hemoglobin remains constant from the extraction of blood until it is analyzed, while the hematocrit increases with time due to changes in erythrocyte volume (Tsubakihara et al. 2010). However some publications rely on hematocrit as an indicator of anemia, thus we consider both parameters. Red cell indices are very useful in the diagnosis of anemia whatever the etiology, and parameters of iron metabolism are essential for the diagnosis of iron deficiency anemia. Here we only state the normal range for adults of both sexes, excluding infants, children and pregnant women.

Below we present laboratory data useful for the study of iron deficiency anemia in general and the specific laboratory tests to evaluate iron status in chronic renal failure and hemodialysis patients.

1.1 Red blood cells: Normal values in adults

Hemoglobin: ♂: 14-17 g / dl; ♀: 12-14 g / dl
Hematocrit: ♂: 42-52% ♀: 36-46%
Red cell indices: mean corpuscular volume (MCV) 81-99 fl;
mean corpuscular hemoglobin (MCH), 27-31 pg; mean corpuscular hemoglobin concentration (MCHC) 34 ± 2 g/ dl
Reticulocytes: ♀: 0.4 to 2.4%, ♂: 0.6 to 2.6%; in absolute numbers: 40 - 100 x 10^9 / l

1.2 Assessment of normal iron status in adults

Serum iron: ♂ and ♀ postmenopausal 50-150 mg/dl; ♀ reproductive age 35-140 mg/ dl
Transferrin: 200-350 mg/dl
Transferrin saturation (serum iron x 100/ transferrin): 30%
Serum ferritin: ♂ and ♀ postmenopausal 30-400 ng/ml; ♀ reproductive age 15-150 ng/ml
Absence of iron stores in patients not on dialysis <10-15 ng/ml

Iron overload > 800 ng/ml. High levels of serum ferritin must be interpreted with caution in the clinical setting of tumors, inflammation and chronic conditions because ferritin may be elevated even if iron stores are normal or low. In these cases the soluble transferrin receptor is useful in estimating iron deposits. Normal levels of soluble transferrin receptor 0.8 to 1.8 ng /l.

1.3 Diagnosis of iron deficiency anemia

In patients without renal impairment, the diagnosis of iron deficiency anemia is based on the assessment of Hb (♂ <13 g/ dl and ♀ <12 g/ dl) and hematocrit (♂ <42% ♀ <36%) along with a decrease in mean corpuscular volume (MCV <80fl) mean corpuscular hemoglobin (MCH <25 pg) and mean corpuscular hemoglobin concentration (MCHC <32g/dl). The diagnosis of iron deficiency anemia also requires a reduction of serum iron below the following levels: (♂ and ♀ postmenopausal (<50 mg / dl) and ♀ reproductive age (<30 mg / dl), increased transferrin (> 360 mg / dl) decrease saturation of transferrin (<20%) and decreased serum ferritin (♂ and ♀ postmenopausal <30 ng / ml and ♀ reproductive age <15 ng / ml), all of them may be complemented by an increase in soluble transferrin receptor (> 2 ng /l).

1.4 Diagnosis of iron deficiency in chronic renal failure

In chronic kidney disease 60-80% of cases have absolute or functional deficiency of iron, especially in haemodialysed patients.

The European Best Practice Guidelines (EBPG) and the Kidney Disease Outcomes Quality Initiative (EBPG K / DOQI) have specified slightly different criteria for diagnosis of anemia in patients with chronic renal failure (Tsubakihara et al. 2010).

With respect to hemoglobin (Hb):

♂ Hb <13.5 g / dl (EBPG) and Hb <13.5 g / dl (K / DOQI)
♀ Hb <11.5 g / dl (EBPG) and Hb < 12.0 g / dl (K / DOQI)
> 70 years old Hb <12 g / dl (EBPG)

With respect to hematocrit, values differ by sex, race and age, decreasing values with increasing age, like hemoglobin. The reference values to define anemia by hematocrit in Japanese adult males are <40% and in adult women ♀ <35%(Tsubakihara et al. 2010)

If MCV is decreased or normal the most probable diagnosis is iron deficiency anemia, nevertheless other less frequent diagnoses must be ruled out such as: anemia of chronic disease, sideroblastic anemia, thalassemia, hemolytic anemia, aplastic anemia, myelodysplastic syndrome and pure red cell aplasia. The latter, though extremely rare has been associated with erythropoietin therapy, mainly if administered subcutaneously. On the contrary if the MCV is elevated macrocytic anemia should be considered due to deficiency of vitamin B12 and / or folic acid, liver disease, hypothyroidism, aplastic anemia, myelodysplastic syndrome or drugs that interfere with DNA synthesis.

The traditional parameters of iron metabolism, which are used for the diagnosis of iron deficiency in chronic kidney disease, are: serum iron <40 mg / dl, transferrin saturation < or = 20%, ferritin < or = 100 ng / ml and Hb <11 g / dl.(KDOQI and National Kidney Foundation 2006).

1.5 New red cell indices and iron status markers – Advantages over traditional markers

The anemia of chronic renal failure is complex and multifactorial, hence the analysis of individual parameters is neither accurate nor does it provide a predictive value to determine which patients will respond to therapy. This has led in recent years to the publication of numerous studies to find new laboratory tests that can identify patients with absolute or functional iron deficiency, in order to individualize and improve treatment. These parameters as well as others not related to the diagnosis of anemia have also been used to try to predict response to treatment with iron and erythropoietin.

Serum ferritin is not a good index for estimating iron deposits in the course of chronic kidney disease ((Kalantar-Zadeh, Kalantar-Zadeh, and Lee 2006). However on the other hands serum ferritin is useful for monitoring iron therapy in chronic kidney disease ((Nakanishi et al. 2010). To overcome drawbacks of ferritin as an estimator of iron stores several authors have studied the usefulness of soluble transferrin receptor with discrepant results.(Chang et al. 2007) have found a good correlation between the increase in soluble transferrin receptor and decreased iron stores. However (Gupta, Uppal, and Pawar 2009, 96-100) have not found any utility in transferrin soluble receptor as a marker of iron deficiency in patients with renal failure. In this context (Chen, Hung, and Tarng 2006a) studied the *TfR-F index* calculated by the ratio of transferrin receptor and the logarithm of serum ferritin, concluding that it is more sensitive than transferrin receptor to assess iron stores and may guide the IV iron therapy in hemodialysis patients better.

For over a decade reticulocyte parameters have been used to monitor erythropoiesis in various diseases, among which are patients with chronic renal failure and anemia (Remacha et al. 1997). (Agarwal, Davis, and Smith 2008) show that the fraction of immature reticulocytes behaves as an indicator of response in the anemia of chronic renal failure. (C.H. Fourcade, L. Jary, and and H. Belaouni 1999) have studied the reticulocyte profile under both regenerative and hypo regenerative bone marrow conditions. (Maconi et al. 2009) have made comparative studies of reticulocyte and erythrocyte parameters in the clinical setting of patients with anemia. (Brugnara, Schiller, and Moran 2006) have shown the usefulness of hemoglobin content of reticulocytes and red cells: Ret-He and RBC-He (Sysmex XE 2100) and CH and CHr (Bayer ADVIA 2120), in the identification of different stages of iron deficiency in hemodialysis patients. The correlation of both parameters is good and the performance of Ret-He is good for absolute iron deficiency, with an AUC of 0.913 a sensitivity of 93.3%, and a specificity of 83.2%. The diagnostic performance of Ret-He is less favorable for funcional iron deficiency, as the AUC is low (0.657).

Others such as (Kalantar-Zadeh et al. 2009), have studied iron metabolism markers and parameters of renal osteodystrophy looking for predictors of response to erythropoiesis-stimulating agents in hemodialysis patients and found that in the long term, low iron stores in patients with hyperparathyroidism and high bone marrow turnover are associated with hypo-responsiveness to ESA.

The sensitivity and specificity of some other parameters such as transferrin saturation, serum ferritin, hypochromic red cells (% Hypo), reticulocyte hemoglobin content (CHr) and soluble transferrin receptor (sTfR) have been published by (Tsubakihara et al. 2010). According these authors the most sensitive parameters to detect functional iron deficiency are serum ferritin and hypochromic red blood cells while the CHr is more specific. On the other hand CHr is the most sensitive parameter to detect iron overload, whereas ferritin (> 800ng/mL) and hypochromic red blood (<10%) cells are more specific (Tsubakihara et al. 2010).

In a multicenter study with participation of 9 hospitals in Europe, (Zini et al 2006) studied the utility of a new analytical parameter, low density hemoglobin, (LDH% Beckman-Coulter), compared with HCM, in hemodialysis patients with functional iron deficiency and concluded that they are useful parameters. The percentage of hypochromic red cells (%Hypo) has been incorporated to National Kidney Foundation KDOQI guidelines for monitoring recombinant human erythropoietin therapy. (Urrechaga 2010) (Urrechaga 2008) find a good correlation between (% Hypo) and low-density hemoglobin (LDH%), Both behave as good markers of iron deficiency in different types of anemia (anemia of kidney disease, iron deficiency anemia, anemia of chronic disease and beta thalassemia) and are equivalent. LDH% is a parameter calculated by a mathematical function based on mean cell hemoglobin concentration (MCHC) (Urrechaga 2010)

The anemia of chronic renal failure is also a chronic disease anemia, and therefore parameters such as IL6, TNF-alfa and other proteins such as neopterin, hepcidin and hemojuvelin should be evaluated. In this context (van der Putten et al. 2010 recently set out the clinical role of changes in hepcidin levels and response to treatment with EPO in patients with inflammation and renal and cardiac damage. Previously (Zaritsky et al. 2009) propose hepcidin as a new biomarker of iron status in chronic kidney disease. Moreover, pro-hepcidin has been proposed as a useful parameter in the evaluation of iron status in chronic kidney disease (Barrios, Espinoza, and Baron 2010; Arabul et al. 2009; Shinzato et al. 2008)

2. Objectives

This trial evaluates a treatment protocol for patients with anemia of chronic kidney disease on hemodialysis

It has two objectives:

a. To find new predictors of response
b. To evaluate a combined treatment regimen with EPO and iron in terms of safety, stability and efficacy.

Although planned in advance, this work meets the recommendation of Coyne (Coyne 2010) (2010) which specifies: "rather than focus on individual products, we should perform trials comparing anemia management strategies to assess safety, efficacy, and cost".

Hematological parameters	Hb	Coulter LH750®
	RBC, WBC	Coulter LH750®
	HCT, MCV, MCH, MRV, MCHC, MPV, MSCV	Coulter LH750®
	RET %, RET#, HLR%, HLR#	Coulter LH750®
	IRF	Coulter LH750®
	NE %, NE#	Coulter LH750®
Iron metabolism	Iron	COBAS-Integra 400 Roche® Diagnostic
	Transferrin	COBAS-Integra 400 Roche® Diagnostic
	TSAT	COBAS-Integra 400 Roche® Diagnostic
	Ferritin	COBAS-Integra 400 Roche® Diagnostic
	TfR-F index, sTfR	Roche® Diagnostic
	RBC Ferritin,	COBAS-Integra 400 Roche® Diagnostic
	EPO	Access 2 Beckman Coulter
	ESR	Alifax Beckman Coulter
Inflammation	Fibrinogen	ACL TOP IL
	CRP	High-sensitivity nephelometry. Beckman
	IL6	Access 2 Beckman Coulter
Vitamins	Vit B12, Folate, RBC Folate	Access 2 Beckman Coulter
Platelets	Plt	Coulter LH750®
	PPV	Coulter LH750®
	PDW	Coulter LH750®
Liver	ALT, GGT, AT III	Roche® Diagnostic
Calculated parameters	RPI	calculated : (RET% x HCT)/45
	RSf®	calculated : $\sqrt{MCV \cdot MRV}$ /1000
	Maf®	calculated : Hb x MCV/100
	VHDWf®	(MCV x Hgb)/(RDW x 10)

Table 1. Column 2 shows the panel of laboratory tests. These are grouped by category in column 1. Column 3 shows the instrumentation used. The tests were done with reagents supplied by the manufacturers of the devices, strictly following the operating instructions

manual. (CRP= C- reactive protein, EPO= Erythropoietin, ESR = Erythrocyte Sedimentation rate) Hb=Hemoglobin, HCT =Hematocrit ,HLR#=High light scatter reticulocytes (absolute), HLR%=High light scatter reticulocytes (relative to Hb), IRF=Immature reticulocyte fraction, Maf®=Microcytic anemia factor, IL6= Interleukin 6, MCH=Mean corpuscular Hemoglobin, MCHC=Mean corpuscular hemoglobin content, MCV=Mean corpuscular volume, MPV=Mean platelet volume, MRV=Mean reticulocyte volume, MSCV=Variance of MCV measurement, NE#=Neutrophils count (absolute), NE%=Neutrophils %, RBC=Red blood cell count, Plt= Platelets count, PPV=Platelet Packed Volume, RET#=Reticulocytes count (absolute), RET% = Reticulocytes %, RBC Folate= Intra-Red Blood Cells Folate), RPI= Reticulocyte production index , sTfR=soluble Transferrin Receptor, TSAT= Transferrin saturation, RBC Ferritin = Intra-Red Blood Cell Ferritin, TfR-F index =Transferrin Receptor-Ferritin Index (Soluble Transferrin Receptor/log Ferritin), VHDWf= Volumen Hemoglobin Distriburion Wide factor, WBC=White Blood Cells count.

To achieve these goals we used the laboratory data recommended in the 2006 KDOQI guide in order to evaluate anemia and iron status: *"Complete blood count (CBC) including red blood cell indices (mean corpuscular hemoglobin [MCH], mean corpuscular volume [MCV], mean corpuscular hemoglobin concentration [MCHC]), white blood cell count, differential and platelet count, absolute reticulocyte count, serum ferritin to assess iron stores and serum ferritin and the transferrin saturation (TSAT) or content of Hb in reticulocytes (CHr) to assess adequacy of iron for erythropoiesis"*; as well as other parameters that we feel could be useful in predicting response, according to publications mentioned above (see table 1)

3. Materials, patients and methods

3.1 Study groups and therapy

This is a prospective, open, nonrandomized trial. Forty-two patients from the dialysis department of the "Hospital Clinico Universitario de Zaragoza" (Spain) have been included. Patients were treated by hemodialysis (HD), EPO and Iron. Patients were not transfused during the study.

All patients gave informed consent. We analyzed the parameters specified in Table 1, monthly for 6 months.

In addition hemoglobin, reticulocyte and iron status were evaluated at the 7th month to assess response to therapy received during the sixth month.

3.2 EPO doses

3.2.1 Initial

- Pre-dialysis, 40 U / kg once a week
- Dialysis: 40 U / kg three times a week

3.2.2 Adjustment

- Evaluate four weeks later. If Hb increase exceeds 5%: do not change dose, otherwise increase 20 U / kg.

- Reassess every 4 weeks. Increase 20 U if the rise in hemoglobin is less than 5%
- Maximum 200 U / kg.
- Do not abruptly discontinue administration of erythropoietin, unless there is life threatening risk.

The maintenance phase begins when the target is reached (hemoglobin 12g/dl)

3.2.3 Maintenance

If the hemoglobin is 12 g / dl or greater decrease the dose of erythropoietin as follows:

- If the last dose was greater than 80 u / kg, reduced by half.
- If the last dose was less than 80 U / kg, left as maintenance 30 U / kg.

3.3 Iron therapy

3.3.1 Pre-dialysis

Iron (oral ferrous sulfate) is given to all patients with chronic renal failure non dialyzed with hemoglobin less than 11 g / dl or ferritin below 100 ng / mL and transferrin saturation below 20%.

Patients with an inadequate response to oral iron or gastrointestinal intolerance have been treated with 200 mg of Intravenous iron sucrose before starting the dialysis program.

3.3.2 Dialysis

All patients on dialysis included in this assay were treated with iron sucrose: 100 mg of iron sucrose in 100 cc saline in slowly perfusion at the end of each hemodialysis session (three times per week)

3.3.3 Target

Ferritin levels between 200 – 400 ng/ml and transferrin saturation > 20%

3.3.4 Adjustment of iron dose

As shown in table 2

Conditions	Adjustment of iron doses
If ferritin < 200 ng /ml	100 mg weekly
If ferritin 200-350 ng / ml	100 mg every 15 days
If ferritin 350 – 500 ng / ml	100 mg monthly.
If ferritin > 500 ng /ml	Stop iron therapy
If TfSat > 50%	Stop iron therapy regardless of serum ferritin

Table 2. Schedule for dose adjustment of Iron

With the exception of 7 patients, 6 laboratory panels per patient (one panel per month) are available. Of the 7 patients with missing data 3 died and 4 were transplanted. None of the deaths were related to the treatment with iron or erythropoietin. The laboratory data of these patients until death or transplantation were included in the statistical analysis.

Hemoglobin and iron status were also analyzed one month after the last (6th) panel in order to classify patients as responders or non-responders. Finally 224 laboratory panels were analyzed.

4. Definitions and criteria of response

Most authors only use hemoglobin as a criterion of response. This is correct when evaluating a long period of time, but for short periods the response may have started before there was an increase in hemoglobin. Therefore we have chosen a target compound in which the main data is the increase or maintenance hemoglobin, but giving the option to evaluate earlier data of erythropoiesis (reticulocytes and sTfR (Soluble transferrin receptor)) and the rise in hemoglobin over two months, instead of evaluating only the change in hemoglobin from one month to the next.

4.1 Criteria

Response was assumed if one of the following four conditions was fulfilled.

1. Increase of Hb ≥ 0.5 g/dl in the next control and/or increase of Hb for the following two controls > 0.8 g/dL, under condition that both changes are positive.
2. Achieve or maintain minimum levels of hemoglobin of 11 g/dl in women and 12 g/dl in men with the following two conditions:
3. Hb increase
4. Ret# >50 x 10^9/L
5. Increase of sTfR > 20%, provided that Hb also increases
6. Increase of Ret#>40 x 10^9/L provided that Hb also increases.

As can be seen to increase or maintain hemoglobin at normal levels is a prerequisite. However, we reduce the quantitative criteria for hemoglobin if the increase in reticulocytes or soluble transferrin receptor suggests an early recovery. Others consider, like us, the increase of reticulocytes as one of the criteria of response to erythropoietin (Brugnara, 2003)

4.2 Definition and classification of iron deficiency status

Applying the criteria of (Ng et al. 2009, c247-52) patients were divided into 4 groups, whose definitions and frequencies are as follows:

- Group 1. Absolute Iron deficiency. (Ferritin < 100ng/ml and Transferrin Saturation < 20%): 5
- Group 2. Functional Iron deficiency. (Ferritin ≥ 100ng/ml and Transferrin Saturation < 20%): 33
- Group 3. Ferritin < 100ng/ml and Transferrin Saturation ≥ 20%: 9
- Group 4. Iron repletion (Ferritin > 100ng/ml and Transferrin Saturation ≥ 20%): 198

To avoid confusion between functional iron deficiency and iron deficiency, hereinafter the latter will be referred to as absolute iron deficiency.

5. Statistical analyses

5.1 Directed at objective A

All statistical analyses were performed with SPSS.

All parameters were tested regarding departures from normal distribution by KS-test (Kolmogorov-Smirnov). In case of normal distributed parameters, group-wise means and standard deviations were calculated. In case of non-normality log transformation or description by non-parametric approaches (median, rank-correlation) were used to avoid biases related to not normally distributed parameters. All comparisons were performed by U-test. For parameters with significant group-wise differences the area under ROC curve (AUC) was calculated.

A correlation matrix (Pearson-correlation, rank-Spearman correlation) of all parameters was calculated and evaluated by factor analysis in order to gain information about relationship between the parameters and to reach a reduction of dimensions (variables) in subsequent statistical analysis (Härdle and Simar 2003) Parameters that were found associated using the statistical program were regarded as a parameter-class.

Bonferroni correction was used to avoid false positive results of significance due to multiple testing. The number of components N_C resulting from factor analysis was used for correction. Starting from a significance level of $\alpha=0.05$, $\alpha_{comp}=0.05/N_C$ was used for group-wise comparisons.

In order to calculate models describing dependence of binary outcome variable (response) on parameter values, logistic regression was performed. Parameters c_i determined in the model can be used in equations of the following type (n-dimensional model for logistic regression), where p_{resp} is probability of response, X_i is value of blood parameter and c_i is coefficient for blood parameter X_i within the model:

$$p_{resp} = \frac{1}{1+\exp(-(c_0 + c_1 X_1 + .. + c_n X_n))} \tag{1}$$

In practice, ranges of probability of response between 0 (prediction of no response) and 1 (prediction of response) can be calculated by putting all parameter values X_i into the formula.

Resulting models were evaluated by ROC analysis and calculating AUC, as mentioned above. Furthermore, practical issues like robustness of parameters and ability of a simple data management (e.g. avoiding usage of mean differences) were considered.

In addition cases were separated according to iron status classification and compared by univariate two-factor ANOVA (factors: iron status group, response) with post-hoc-comparisons

5.2 Statistical analyses directed to objective B

The descriptive statistics were carried out as follows.

The first step was to study the evolution of hemoglobin each month using parametric (Student) and nonparametric (comparing the overall monthly evolution of hemoglobin by the Kruskall-Wallis test) methods followed by bivariate comparisons of each month with the next(Mann-Whitney). Although hemoglobin fits a normal distribution we also used nonparametric tests to avoid false positive results due to sample size. In this section we choose hemoglobin as the dependent variable, not including any other criteria of response. This is because the purpose of this section to compare the parameters with hemoglobin, the therapeutic target that really determines the quality of life of patients.

In a second step we use multiple linear regression to obtain a mathematical model that relates the levels of hemoglobin with selected parameters.

The graphic presentation of hemoglobin evolution over time has been made by Box Plot to display the median, interquartile distribution, outliers and overlapping. We have also represented the means on a bar graph with confidence interval of 95%.

Finally we applied the same statistical model to the parameters that quantify the iron status: serum iron, transferrin, transferrin saturation, ferritin and soluble transferrin receptor. This statistical treatment is aimed to check whether iron treatment regimen is optimal, or requires changes.

6. Results

6.1 Descriptive statistics and groups

6.1.1 Demography

42 patients; gender F: 15, M: 27; age: median: 73 years (range: 22 - 88)

6.1.2 Responses

79 responses, 97 non responses, 88 not available (no EPO therapy, transplanted, death or missing data. (Table 3).

		Transferrin Saturation	
		< 20%	>20%
Ferritin ng/ml	<100	Group 1(ID) 5 (2%)	Group 3 9 (3.7%)
	>100	Group 2 (FID) 33 (13.5%)	Group 4 (IR) 198 (80.8%)

Table 3. Distribution of cases according to groups defined by Young and Chun (2009) (see text)

6.1.3 Iron status

Applying the criteria of Young and Chun (2009) frequencies of the four groups of iron status are:

- Group 1. - Absolute Iron deficiency (ID) (Ferritin < 100ng/ml and Transferrin Saturation < 20%): 5
- Group 2. - Functional Iron deficiency (FID) (Ferritin ≥ 100ng/ml and Transferrin Saturation < 20%): 33

- Group 3. - Ferritin < 100ng/ml and Transferrin Saturation ≥ 20% (Iron status is not well defined in this group). Transferrin saturation is enough for erythropoiesis, but iron stores may be low: 9
- Group 4. - Iron repletion (IR) (Ferritin > 100ng/ml and Transferrin Saturation ≥ 20%): 198

6.1.4 Descriptive statistics of all parameters

The descriptive statistics and comparison with normal distribution is shown in table 4.

	N	Mean	SD	Median	Minimum	Maximum	Comparison with normal distribution (Kolmogorov-Smirnov)
HLR (%)	189	0.825	0.36	0.836	0.062	2.24	n.s.
HLR# (n/mm³)	189	28.7	12.5	28.6	1.88	66.7	n.s.
RPI	189	1.55	0.534	1.59	0.12	3.14	n.s.
RET (%)	192	2.08	0.735	2.13	0.149	5.05	n.s.
RET# (n/mm³)	192	72.1	24.5	73.2	9.15	150	n.s.
IRF	189	0.387	0.0757	0.393	0.16	0.56	n.s.
Hb (g/dL)	224	11.1	1.44	11.1	7.18	14.8	n.s.
HCT (%)	192	34	4.33	33.9	21.7	45	n.s.
RBC 10³ / mm³)	195	3490	444	3470	2130	4690	n.s.
Maf	224	10.8	1.6	11	6.54	14.7	n.s.
RSf	189	0.11	0.00692	0.11	0.09	0.13	n.s.
MCV (fL)	224	97.3	4.93	97.6	83.8	113	n.s.
MSCV (fL)	189	95.9	6.04	95.5	83.5	116	n.s.
MRV (fL)	189	124	11	124	96.3	165	n.s.
MCH (g/L)	195	31.8	1.83	32.1	26.8	35.8	n.s.
EPO (IU/L)	238	21.3	39.6	12	1.75	465	$p<0.00001$
sTfRFindex	221	0.755	0.247	0.724	0.282	2.02	n.s.
sTfR (mg/L)	222	1.82	0.498	1.8	0.8	3.2	$p=0.046$
Fibrinogen (mg/dl)	222	521	121	518	246	993	n.s.
ESR (mm/ first hour)	222	43.2	28.2	35.5	1	142	$p=0.0038$
CRP (mg/L)	223	1.73	4.78	0.64	0	38.6	$p<0.00001$
IL6 (ng/L)	238	10.5	15.3	6.43	0.6	160	$p<0.00001$
Ferritin (ng/ml)	223	376	275	326	24.3	2290	$p<0.00001$
Plt (103/mm³)	192	213	56	216	92.5	368	n.s.
PPV (%)	192	0.178	0.0412	0.175	0.0713	0.288	n.s.
TfSat (%)	223	33.2	12.3	32.2	9.8	82.8	n.s.
Iron (μg/dL)	223	56.7	22.4	53.5	9.87	198	n.s.
MCHC (g/dl)	192	32.6	0.723	32.6	31	34.8	n.s.
MPV (fl)	191	8.46	1.07	8.34	6.13	11.4	n.s.

RDW (%)	192	15.8	1.47	15.7	13.2	20.9	n.s.
@NE	192	66.8	8.09	66.6	46.6	83.9	n.s.
NE#	192	5	1.61	4.79	1.16	9.74	n.s.
WBC (103/ mm^3)	192	7.33	2.2	7.46	0	14.9	n.s.
VitB12 (pg/ml)	224	534	218	484	180	1180	p=0.025
RBC Folate	223	723	796	421	107	3670	p<0.00001
PDW	192	16.7	0.554	16.6	15.6	18.5	n.s.
ALT (U/L)	222	14.8	12.2	12	1	73	p<0.00001
GGt (U/L)	222	31.5	38.8	17	4	211	p<0.00001
RBCFerritin (ng/ml of RBC)	224	731	345	638	223	2160	p=0.00023
Transferrin mg/dl	223	175	35.7	169	73.8	351	n.s.
ATIII (% of normal control)	220	101	16.9	101	62	149	n.s.

Table 4. Descriptive statistics and Kolmogorov-Smirnoff test (n.s. = not significant difference from normal distribution)

All parameters are normally distributed, with the exceptions of Ferritin, EPO, ESR, CRP, IL6, Vit B12, RBC, Folate, RBC ferritin, ALT and GGT. In all of these differences with the normal distribution are avoided by logarithmic transformation.

6.1.5 Factorial analysis

The coefficients given in Table 5 refer to the association of each parameter to one of the classes determined by factor analysis. The row-wise maximum relates each parameter to one of the 12 classes. Some of the parameters contribute to several components. As an example, Maf, which is a product of MCV and Hb, is associated to class 3 (contains Hb) as well as class 2 (contains MCV). In a similar manner, WBC is not only associated to Plt and Pct, but also to neutrophil-linked parameters NE# and NE%.

(See Table 5)

		Component											
		1	2	3	4	5	6	7	8	9	10	11	12
1	HLR %	0.97											
	HLR #	0.97											
	RPI	0.94											
	RET #	0.94											
	RET %	0.93											
	IRF	0.65		0.35									
2	Hb		0.97										
	HCT		0.97										
	RBC		0.92										
	Maf		0.88	0.40									

	VHDW		0.75						-0.37				
3	RSf			0.95									
	MCV			0.90									
	MRV			0.84									
	MSCV			0.84									
	MCH			0.81					-0.47				
4	EPO (log)				0.81								
	TfR-F index				0.51			-0.50				-0.42	
	sTfR				0.42			-0.38				-0.46	
5	Fibrinogen					0.83							
	ESR (log)		-0.33			0.78							
	CRP (log)					0.74							
	IL6 (log)					0.59						0.43	
	Ferritin (log)				-0.39	0.43		0.40					-0.40
6	Plt						0.94						
	PPV						0.88						
7	TfSat%							0.84					
	Iron							0.73					
8	MCHC								-0.79				
	MPV						-0.33		0.60				
	RDW				0.41				0.55				
9	NE #						0.35			0.80			
	NE %									0.75			
	WBC						0.40			0.63			
10	Vit. B12 (log)										0.77		
	RBC Folate (log)										0.75		
	PDW						-0.45				-0.57		
11	ALT (log)											0.78	
	GGT (log)											0.66	
	RBC Ferr. log)								-0.35			0.49	-0.35
12	Transferrin												0.84
	ATIII										0.37		0.53

Table 5. Factor analysis and correlation matrix.

Parameters with column maximum-wise (HLR% in case of class 1, Hb in class 2, Rsf® in class 3 and so on) are representative of class in the best manner.

6.1.6 Functional description of classes

It is worth noting that each of the classes (selected by factor analysis) contain a group of parameters that have a common physiological or pathological role.

- Class 1 is associated with erythropoietic activity: reticulocytes and reticulocyte indices
- Class 2 is related to parameters that provide information about the absence, presence or severity of anemia
- Class 3 is related to red cell indices and their derivatives obtained by mathematical formulas. They report on the type of anemia.
- Class 4 is associated with stimulation of erythropoiesis
- Class 5 is associated with chronic inflammatory disease
- Class 6 reports on platelets
- Class 7 is associated with iron status
- Class 8 is associated with microcytosis and anisocytosis.
- Class 9 reports on neutrophils.
- Class 10 reports on vitamin deficiency.
- Class 11 reports on liver disease.
- Class 12 reports of acute phase reactants not included in class 5.

6.1.7 Weekly erythropoietin dose and response to treatment

(See table 6)

			Response		Total	
EPO doses			No response	Response		Significance
	2000	Count	3	2	5	n.s.
		%	3.1%	2.5%	2.8%	
	3000	Count	3	2	5	n.s.
		%	3.1%	2.5%	2.8%	
	4000	Count	10	4	14	n.s.
		%	10.3%	5.1%	8.0%	
	6000	Count	14	11	25	n.s.
		%	14.4%	13.9%	14.2%	
	8000	Count	20	18	38	n.s.
		%	20.6%	22.8%	21.6%	
	12000	Count	18	15	33	n.s.
		%	18.6%	19.0%	18.8%	
	16000	Count	29	27	56	n.s.
		%	29.9%	34.2%	31.8%	
Total		Count	97	79	176	n.s.
		%	100.0%	100.0%	100.0%	

Table 6. No significant differences were found between the different doses of erythropoietin.

6.1.8 Univariate analysis of selected parameters comparing the groups of iron status and split by responders and no-responders

Table 7 shows statistical analyses of all parameters and their relations with the Iron Status classification and State of Response. In this analysis the iron status groups: ID, FID and IR are only taken into account. The 9 patients in group 3 have been excluded. ANOVA results have been compared with those of the Mann-Whitney test because the number of cases in each group is unbalanced. The Mann-Whitney, being nonparametric, is less affected by the imbalance. Parameters of the same class of those selected by factor analysis, behave similarly. Hb, RET# and sTfR show significant differences because they enter into the definition of response.

Parameters with column maximum are those that best represent their class as detailed above (material and methods).

Parameter	Iron Status	Response	Effect		Response via Mann Whitney U-Test
			Iron Status	Response status	
Rsf	**n.s.**	n.s.			
MCV	**n.s.**	n.s.			
MCH	**n.s.**	n.s.			
MSCV	n.s.	n.s.			
MRV	n.s.	n.s.			
HLR%	n.s.	n.s.			
HLR#	p=0.033	n.s.			
RET%	n.s.	n.s.			
RET#	n.s.	n.s.			
RPI	p=0.045	n.s.			
IRF	p=0.045	n.s.			
Hb	**p=0.000**	p=0.025	ID, FID < IR	Resp<nonresp	**p=0.0028**
HCt	**p=0.001**	p=0.029	ID < IR	Resp<nonresp	p=0.07
RBC	**p=0.002**	p=0.033	ID<IR	Resp<nonresp	**p=0.044**
Maf	**p=0.000**	p=0.039	ID < IR	Resp<nonresp	p=0.014
Plt	n.s.	n.s.			
PPV	n.s.	n.s.			
WBC	n.s.	n.s.			
TfRFindex	n.s.	n.s.			
sTfR	p=0.085	n.s.	ID<IR		
EPO	n.s.	p=0.016	FID: Resp<non resp IR: Resp>= non resp		**p=0.011**
ESR	n.s.	n.s.			
CRP	**p=0.000**	n.s.	FID > IR, ID		
IL6	**p=0.000**	n.s.	FID > IR,		
MCHC	n.s.	n.s.			**p=0.0007**
MPV	n.s.	n.s.			
RDW	p=0.031	n.s.	FID, ID <IR		

Ferritin	**p=0.000**	n.s.	trivial result	
Iron	**p=0.000**	n.s.	trivial result	
TSAT	**p=0.000**	n.s.	trivial result	
Vit. B12	n.s.	n.s.		
RBC Folate	n.s.	n.s.		
PDW	n.s.	n.s.		
ALT	n.s.	n.s.		
GGT	p=0.043	n.s.	ID, (FID) > IR	
RBC Ferr	n.s.	n.s.		
NE#	n.s.	n.s.	ID<IR	
NE%	n.s.	n.s.	ID<IR	
Transferrin	**p=0.000**	n.s.	trivial result	
AT III	n.s.	n.s.		

Table 7. Univariate two-factor ANOVA (Iron Status, Response) and Mann-Witney test. Significant differences for iron status are shown in column 3, for response status in column 4 and their effect in column 5. Parameters that enter into the definition of iron stages are logically associated with themselves; therefore we specify "trivial result".

6.1.9 Description of responses to therapy

Hereafter "case" means each result (6 per patient) for the referred parameter.

From 42 patients, 83 cases with EPO-treatment were considered as responses (38.6%). 132 cases (61.4%) were not responding. Among the responses, 40 (18.6% of 215) fulfilled 1 criterion of response, 36 cases (16.7%) 2 criteria, 5 cases (2.2%) 3 criteria and 2 cases (0.9%) 4 criteria. The distribution of responses according to the criteria is as follows:

- Criterion 1. - 63 cases. (Increase of Hb ≥ 0.5 g/dl in the next control and/or increased of Hb in the whole of the following two controls > 0.8 g/dL, under condition that both changes are positive)
- Criterion 2. - 48 cases (Achieve or maintain normal Hb for hemodialysis patients (male: 12 g/dl, female: 11 g/dl) under two conditions: Hb increase and Reticulocytes >50 x 10^9/L)
- Criterion 3. - 17 cases (Increase of sTfR > 20%, provided that Hb also increases)
- Criterion 4. -7 cases. (Increase of Ret#>40 x 10^9/L provided that Hb also increases)

6.1.10 Parameters predicting response

Table 8 shows the descriptive statistics and the response to combination therapy with iron and erythropoietin. We selected three variables (MCHC, EPO and Hb) with the highest levels of significance to determine their predictive value on response to therapy.

AUC of related ROC for these three parameters are respectively: 0.631 (95% CI: 0.54 - 0.70) for Hb, 0.612 (95% CI: 0.58 - 0.73) for EPO, and 0.662 (95% CI 0.57 – 0.73) for MCHC as shown in Figure 1, 2 and 3.

AUC of related ROC curves

	Non Response						Response						
	N	Mean	SD	Med	Min	Max	N	Mean	SD	Med	Min	Max	p
HLR %	78	0.795	0.372	0.803	0.117	2.24	66	0.897	0.332	0.895	0.256	1.57	0.076
HLR #	78	27.7	12.2	28.4	4.55	66.7	66	30.8	12.4	31.3	7.7	62	0.143
RPI	78	1.52	0.517	1.62	0.121	3.14	66	1.65	0.535	1.7	0.589	2.84	0.161
RET %	80	2.05	0.781	2.13	0.149	5.05	67	2.24	0.66	2.31	0.963	3.71	0.067
RET #	80	71.6	23.4	74.5	19.8	150	67	76.3	24.8	76.2	29	134	0.287
IRF	78	0.376	0.078	0.388	0.156	0.52	66	0.395	0.0622	0.396	0.225	0.52	0.226
Hb	**97**	**11.4**	**1.32**	**11.3**	**8.62**	**14.8**	**79**	**10.7**	**1.54**	**10.7**	**7.18**	**14.5**	**0.0028**
HCT	79	34.6	3.93	34.3	26.6	45	68	33.3	4.89	33	21.7	44.8	0.0752
RBC	**81**	**3540**	**385**	**3480**	**2750**	**4620**	**69**	**3410**	**502**	**3340**	**2130**	**4690**	**0.0442**
Maf	**97**	**11.1**	**1.51**	**11.3**	**7.86**	**14.4**	**79**	**10.4**	**1.69**	**10.5**	**6.54**	**13.8**	**0.0137**
VHDW	79	7.08	1.32	7.4	4.26	9.69	68	6.7	1.28	6.85	4.04	9.61	0.0505
RSf	78	0.11	0.006	0.11	0.0967	0.12	66	0.11	0.0076	0.11	0.094	0.134	0.744
VCM	97	97.4	4.63	97.5	83.8	109	79	97.4	5.11	98.1	85.8	109	0.891
MSCV	78	95.6	5.76	95.3	83.5	116	66	96.2	6.47	95.8	83.9	111	0.506
MRV	78	124	8.74	124	105	143	66	125	12.3	123	96.3	165	0.785
MCH	81	31.9	1.77	32.1	26.8	34.8	69	31.5	1.85	32	27.5	35.1	0.261
EPO	**97**	**11**	**11.9**	**8**	**1.8**	**78.6**	**79**	**18.4**	**27.6**	**10.1**	**1.1**	**200**	**0.0107**
TfR-F index	95	0.761	0.249	0.728	0.366	2.02	79	0.759	0.245	0.725	0.282	1.36	0.885
sTfR	95	1.85	0.495	1.8	1	3.2	79	1.82	0.512	1.8	0.8	3.1	0.752
Fibri-nogen	**96**	**539**	**128**	**526**	**284**	**993**	**79**	**498**	**110**	**487**	**264**	**836**	**0.0296**
ESR	97	44.2	29	35	8	125	78	40	27.9	32	3	142	0.309
CRP	97	1.89	5.5	0.69	0	38.6	79	1.33	2.93	0.64	0.11	24.3	0.552
IL-6	97	10.7	20.6	6.15	0.75	160	79	8.14	7.48	6.3	0.6	48.5	0.772
Ferritin	97	379	250	348	24.3	1940	79	344	211	320	33.2	1160	0.296
Plt	79	214	57	222	114	327	68	212	57.6	210	114	368	0.892
PPV	79	0.176	0.042	0.173	0.0919	0.27	68	0.178	0.0397	0.177	0.088	0.288	0.718
TfSat%	97	33.8	12.3	32.3	11.4	82.8	78	32.5	10.9	32.3	12.6	68.5	0.611
Iron	97	59.6	25.3	54.1	15.7	198	79	54.1	17.7	53.5	12.2	91.9	0.218
MCHC	**79**	**32.7**	**0.662**	**32.7**	**31.1**	**34.8**	**68**	**32.3**	**0.665**	**32.3**	**31**	**34**	**0.0007**
MPV	78	8.29	1.1	8.3	6.13	11.4	68	8.54	1.02	8.3	6.4	11	0.302
RDW	79	15.8	1.48	15.6	13.3	20.9	68	15.8	1.47	15.7	13.2	20.8	0.864
NE %	79	65.9	8.37	66.6	46.6	82.4	68	67.1	8.11	65.1	53.6	83.9	0.503
NE #	79	4.86	1.59	4.63	2.42	9.74	68	5	1.61	4.89	1.16	8.93	0.424
WBC	79	7.25	2.13	7.03	0	14.9	68	7.21	2.37	7.62	0	14.1	0.546
Vit B12	97	525	210	482	184	1160	79	527	199	498	191	1180	0.839
RBC Folate	96	691	804	318	107	3670	79	787	920	388	109	3500	0.38
PDW	79	16.7	0.612	16.7	15.6	18.5	68	16.6	0.52	16.6	15.6	17.9	0.516
ALT	96	13.5	9.99	12	1	56	79	15.8	13.5	13	1	73	0.22

GGt	96	30	38.5	16	4	201	79	33.1	39.1	19	5	210	0.286
RBC Ferr.	97	704	310	632	281	1950	79	698	309	583	230	2010	0.735
Transfer-rin	97	174	31.4	169	79.1	280	79	176	41.5	169	73.8	351	0.811
ATIII	95	102	15.6	103	68	149	78	103	19	104	65	149	0.724

Table 8. Descriptive statistics of all variables split by response o no response (from month to month). Significant differences have been highlighted.

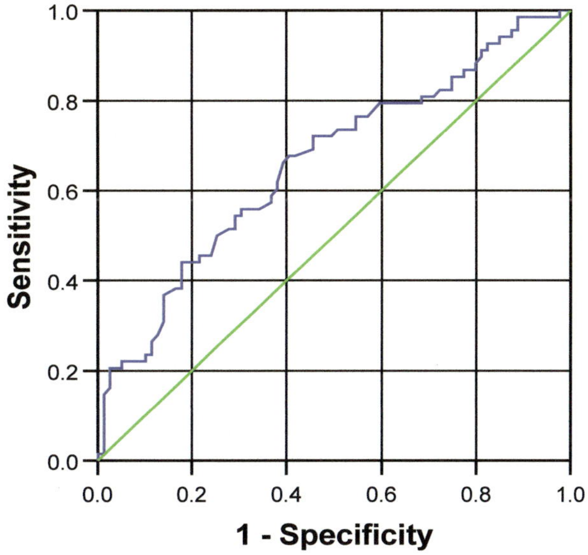

Fig. 1. MCHC AUC: 0.662 (0.573 – 0.75)

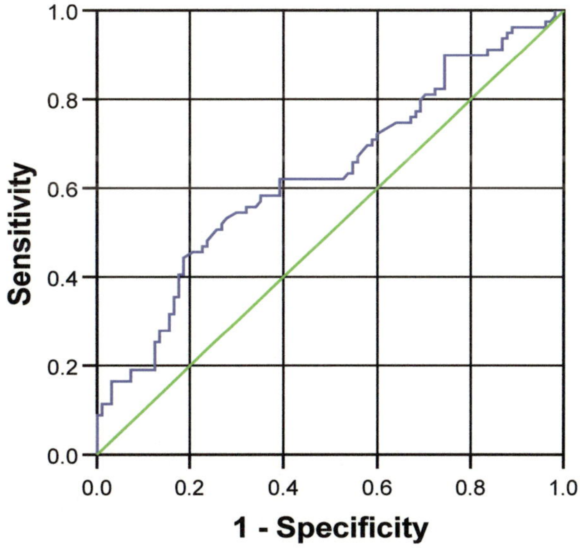

Fig. 2. HB AUC: 0.631 (0.548 – 0.714)

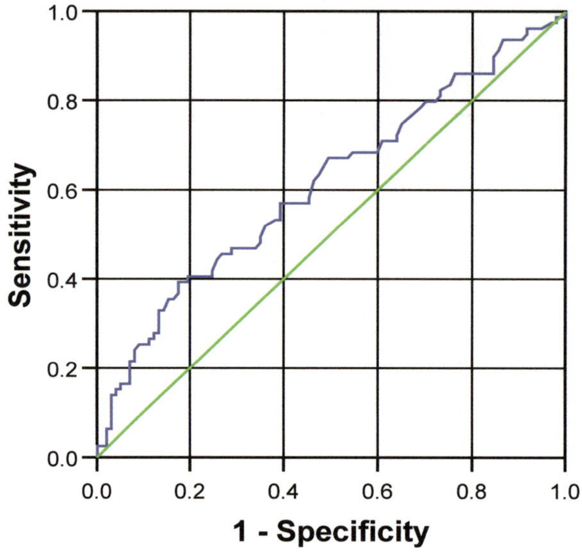

Fig. 3. EPO AUC: 0.612 (0.528 - 0.696)

6.1.11 ROC curves and AUC

The area under the curve of each of the three variables is too low to be practical in predicting response to treatment. So we tried to make a composite model with more prediction power.

6.1.12 Prediction model

Based on these results, several models to predict the response on the basis of parameters evaluated in this study have been calculated by logistic regression. The optimal model was chosen by achieving maximal AUC with a minimum of parameters and taking into account practical issues. The best three-parameter combination was RBC, EPO and MCHC (AUC=0.72). RBC, belonging to the same class as hemoglobin, slightly improves the AUC (+0.1). For this reason the model includes RBC, EPO and MCHC, instead of HB, EPO and MCHC. We could not find any other parameter able to increase the power of the predictive model. Figure 4 shows the ROC curve of this composite three parameter model. The AUC is 0.72 (%95 CI: 0.62 - 0.80). (Fig.4.)

The related formula is:

$$p_{resp} = \frac{1}{1 + exp(-(23.39 + 1.327 \cdot log(EPO) - 0.838 \cdot MCHC - 0.787 * \frac{RBC}{1000}))} \tag{2}$$

This model, being the best, has relative clinical utility because the AUC is not as high as would be desirable.

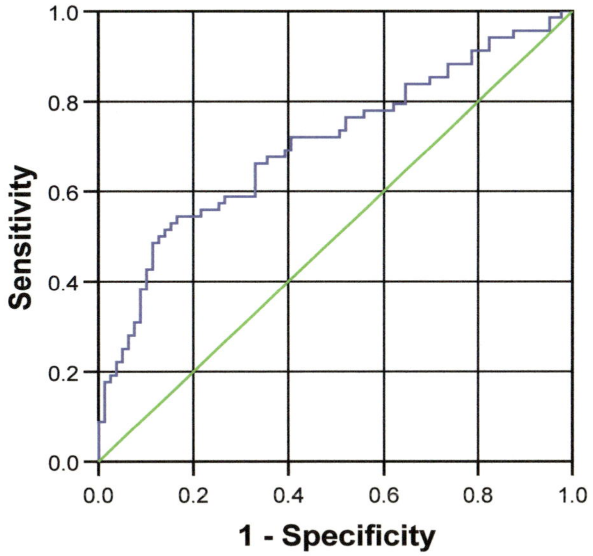

Fig. 4. ROC curve of the combination: RBC, EPO and MCHC (AUC: 0.72 (0.619 - 0.791)

7. Efficacy and safety

This section not only tries to verify the effectiveness and safety of treatment but also looks for correlations between hemoglobin and other variables. These correlations should not be interpreted as predictors of response, since hemoglobin is considered as a whole rather than month to month as in the previous section. Therefore we try to find a mathematical model to predict hemoglobin levels considering all the time of observation as a whole. For this purpose we have selected hemoglobin as a dependent variable. We have also selected explicative variables that measure the erythropoietic activity (reticulocytes and soluble transferrin receptor), indicators of iron status (serum iron, ferritin, transferrin and transferrin saturation), other nutritional factors (vitamin B12 and folic acid) and some indicators of acute or chronic inflammation (IL-6 and CRP) that can interfere with iron metabolism and erythropoiesis. (Table 9)

Statistical planning of this section is as follows:

- Descriptive statistics: means and frequencies
- Comparative evolution of hemoglobin in the 6 months: ANOVA and nonparametric
- Statistical comparison of patients with hemoglobin <11g/dl versus≥11g/dl: ANOVA, equality of variances and robust tests.
- Multiple linear regression stepwise forward (hemoglobin as dependent variable and all others as explicatory).
- Variables that did not fit the normal distribution have been replaced by their respective logarithms in parametric tests.

7.1 Descriptive statistics

Descriptive statistics are shown in table 9

	N	Min	Max	Mean	S.D.
EPO	245	1.75	465.12	23.5789	42.74901
IL-6	245	.60	375.39	15.3838	39.48357
CRP	243	.05	38.60	2.0386	4.86809
Hb	245	7.20	14,8	11.0665	1.54600
HCT	245	21.40	59.50	33.7563	4.62126
RETICULOCYTE	244	9.10	150.40	73.8156	24.98430
Fe	244	9.87	197.61	54.8609	22.59088
TRANSFERRIN	244	73.79	350.58	174.2232	34.89244
FERRITINE	244	33.20	2290.00	399.6719	292.31897
sTfR	244	.70	6.61	1.8598	.60920
B12	245	180.00	1455.00	541.3102	226.92288
FOLIC	245	1.60	200.00	27.5331	54.87474
FOLIC-INTRAE	244	85.50	3667.70	700.0311	770.10104
TSAT	244	8.54	87.09	31.9443	12.69501

Table 9. Descriptive statistics of variables used in this section

7.2 Hemoglobin stability

As shown in table 10, the means of hemoglobin vary from 10.9 to 11.3 during the six months follow-up period and remain always within the desired range. The minima of each month correspond to different patients, indicating at least a partial recovery of those who have held the minimum in any of the previous months. None of the patients exceeded 15 g / dl of hemoglobin as can be seen in the Box-Plot (Graph A1). This graph also shows the extreme values, which show only 6 out of a total of 245 samples. The evolution of individual patients who have had these outliers can be seen in Graph A-2.

MONTH	Mean (g/dl)	N	Standard deviation	Minimum	Maximum
1	10.9689	42	1.53798	7.2	14.3
2	11.1318	42	1.60113	7.2	14.2
3	10.9167	42	1.57231	7.2	14.9
4	10.9350	40	1.38408	7.4	14.6
5	11.1921	38	1.25383	8.2	13.5
6	11.2972	36	1.92628	8.1	14.8
Total	11.0665	245	1.54600	7.2	14.8

Table 10. Means of hemoglobin for each month during the six month follow-ups

7.3 Comparative statistics

7.3.1 Evolution of hemoglobin

Since hemoglobin fits normal distribution we compared the six month results globally using ANOVA with the result that no significant difference could be found ($F=0.394$, $p=0.853$).

To avoid possible errors due to sample size we have also used a nonparametric test (Kruskall-Wallis) with the same result: no significant difference (Chi square 1.473, p = 0.920). Median of hemoglobin and dispersion are represented as box plot on Fig. 5.

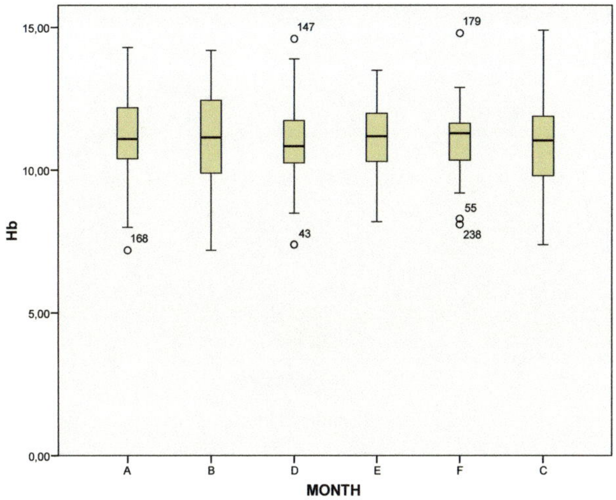

Fig. 5. Box-Plot of the evolution of Hb during the 6 months of dialysis. Outliers are identified with the sample number. Checking the table data we observe that all these extreme values come from different patients.

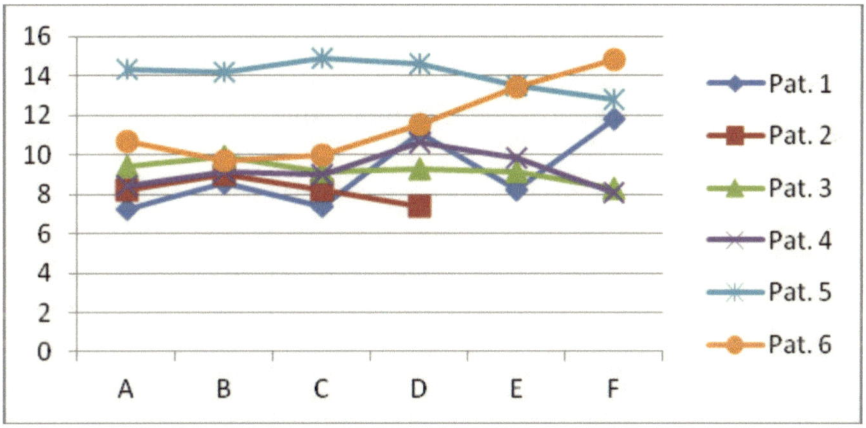

Fig. 6. Individual evolution of the six patients with extreme values. The vertical axis shows the values of hemoglobin (g / dl). The X axis shows the months of observation from A (first) to F (sixth). Patient 2 was excluded from the trial in the fourth month when the patient had a transplant. Patients 3 and 4 remained below 10g/dl of hemoglobin for most of the observation period. None of the patients exceeded 15 g/dl of hemoglobin.

Fig. 7 shows the mean hemoglobin concentration month by month and the error bars for 95% interval of confidence. The means remain in the range 10.9-11.3 g/dl. No significant differences with parametric methods (ANOVA, Student) and nonparametric (Kruskall - Wallis and Mann-Witney)

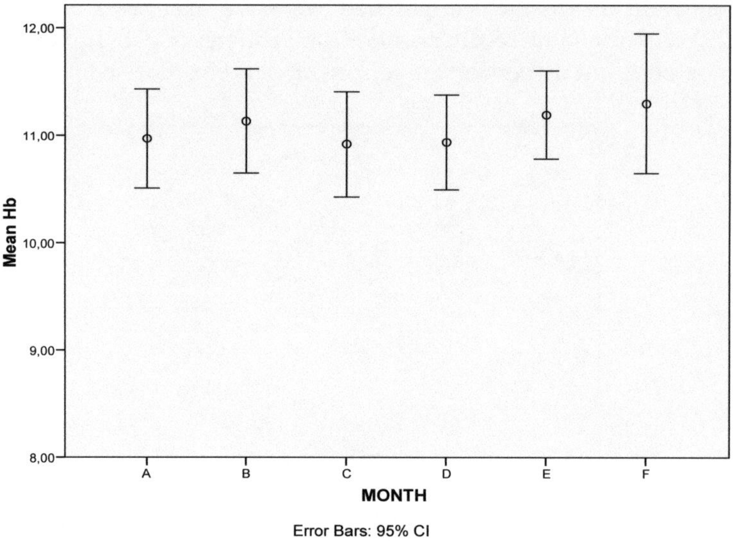

Fig. 7. Mean hemoglobin month by month. Error bars indicate confidence intervals of 95%

7.3.2 Patients with hemoglobin less than 11g/dl compared with those with hemoglobin ≥ 11g/dl

In this section we look for differences between the variables using a cutoff of 11 g/ dl of hemoglobin. Cases above and below this cutoff are almost balanced (n =117 (47.8%) <11g/dl) and n= 128 (52.2%≥ 11g/dl))

The homogenization of variances tested detected 5 variables with significant differences; therefore we applied robust tests to avoid false results due to bias. The table 11 shows the results.

	Statistic F	Sig.	Statistic Welch	Sig.
CRP	**4.629**	**.032**	**4.416**	**.037**
RET	1.597	.208	1.584	.209
Fe	**22.626**	**.000**	**23.323**	**.000**
TRANSF	.760	.384	.732	.393
FOLIC-INTRA	.441	.507	.435	.510
TSAT	**24.433**	**.000**	**24.665**	**.000**
Log EPO	**14.840**	**.000**	**14.479**	**.000**
Log IL-6	**9.970**	**.002**	**9.813**	**.002**
Log FERRITINE	.862	.354	.834	.362
Log sTfR	1.316	.252	1.296	.256
Log B12	.124	.725	.122	.727
Log FOLIC	.013	.908	.013	.909
SRTf/logFERR	.179	.672	.102	.751

Table 11. Homohenization of variances test using a hemoglobin cutoff of 11g/dl.

Table 12 shows the means and standard error of the variables split by an 11g/dl hemoglobin cut-off.

	Mean	Std. Error	Count	p (Welch)
EPO, Hb<11g/dl	32,316	5,245	117	
EPO, Hb>11	15,563	1,841	128	.000
iIL-6, Hb<11g/dl	21,233	4,972	117	
iIL-6, Hb>11	10,037	1,512	128	.002
RCP, Hb<11g/dl	2,742	,547	115	
RCP, Hb>11	1,406	,324	128	.037
Hb, Hb<11g/dl	9,850	,089	117	
Hb, Hb>11	12,178	,094	128	.000
RETIC, Hb<11g/dl	71,695	2,413	116	
RETIC, Hb>11	75,737	2,119	128	.209
Fe, Hb<11g/dl	47,936	1,661	116	
Fe, Hb>11	61,136	2,171	128	.000
TRANSFERRIN, Hb<11g/dl	176,270	3,843	116	
TRANSFERRIN, Hb>11	172,369	2,454	128	.393
FERRITINE, Hb<11g/dl	412,477	32,283	116	
FERRITINE, Hb>11	388,068	20,490	128	.362
sRTf, Hb<11Hb/dl	1,834	,065	116	
sRTf, Hb>11	1,883	,045	128	.256
B12, Hb<11g/dl	543,487	23,179	117	
B12, Hb>11	539,320	18,008	128	.727
FOLIC, Hb<11g/dl	30,862	5,583	117	
FOLIC, Hb>11	24,491	4,362	128	.909
FOLIC-INTRA, Hb<11g/dl	734,179	77,436	117	
FOLIC-INTRA, Hb>11	668,572	62,481	127	.510
sRTf:logF, Hb<11g/dl	,755	,028	116	
sRTf:logF, Hb>11	,761	,021	128	.751
TSAT, Hb<11g/dl	27,914	1,068	116	
TSAT, Hb>11	35,596	1,119	128	.000

Table 12. Means and standard error of the variables split by an 11g/dl hemoglobin cut-off.

7.3.3 Multiple linear regression

Since there is no significant difference in monthly hemoglobin we handle all the data together. The dependent variable is hemoglobin and the rest explicative. The hematocrit was excluded because it is obviously closely related to hemoglobin. For variables that do not fit the normal distribution we made a logarithmic transformation. The method used is forward stepwise multiple linear regression. In the resulting model only three variables remain: serum iron, log soluble transferrin receptor and log EPO. Note that the correlation coefficient of the latter is negative.

Model		Not standardized coefficients		Standardized coefficients	t	Sig.
Steps		B	Standard error	Beta	zero-order	Partial
1	(constant)	10.109	.251		40.321	.000
	Fe	.018	.004	.259	4.179	.000
2	(constant)	9.267	.334		27.765	.000
	Fe	.021	.004	.307	4.960	.000
	Log sRTf	2.672	.721	.229	3.705	.000
3	(constant) (Intercept)	10.396	.413		25.167	.000
	Fe	.018	.004	.261	4.301	.000
	Log sRTf	3.603	.728	.309	4.952	.000
	Log EPO	-1.053	.241	-.274	-4.363	.000

Dependent variable: Hb

Table 13. Forward step-wise multiple regression model. (Dependent variable hemoglobin)

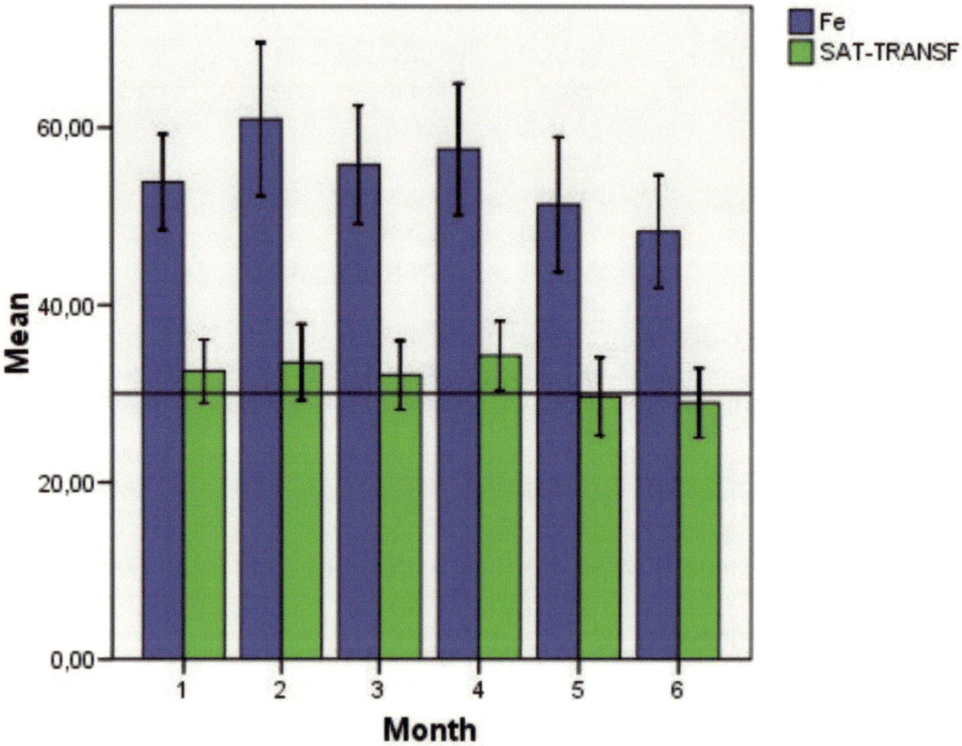

Fig. 8. Serum iron (mg/dl) and transferrin saturation (%) (TSAT). The central horizontal line plots the normal transferrin saturation of 30%. All means are above this line except for the sixth month. Nevertheless the latter is 28.6%, well above 20%. Error bars show the confidence interval 95%.

8. Iron, transferrin and saturation

Fig. 8. shows the serum iron and transferrin saturation for each of the six months of observation. The error bars show confidence intervals of 95%. All media, with their respective confidence intervals are in the field of 30% saturation of transferrin, enough for an adequate iron supply to erythroblasts. However, some individual values are below those desirable. Specifically, 33 cases (14.2%) have transferrin saturation less than 20%.

8.1 Ferritin

Descriptive statistic for ferritin split by months is shown in table 14.

	Mean	Std. Dev.	Std. Error	Count	Minimum	Maximum
FERRITIN. Total	399.672	292.319	18.714	244	33.200	2290.000
FERRITIN. A	425.107	325.013	48.450	45	39.900	1952.000
FERRITIN. B	378.284	249.318	37.586	44	33.200	1314.900
FERRITIN. C	416.134	247.962	38.725	41	42.600	1159.100
FERRITIN. D	376.029	317.108	50.139	40	49.400	1940.000
FERRITIN. E	371.563	219.388	35.589	38	40.000	972.400
FERRITIN. F	431.210	382.965	63.827	36	109.700	2290.000

Table 14. Evolution of ferritin during the observation period. Consecutive months are represented by A to F.

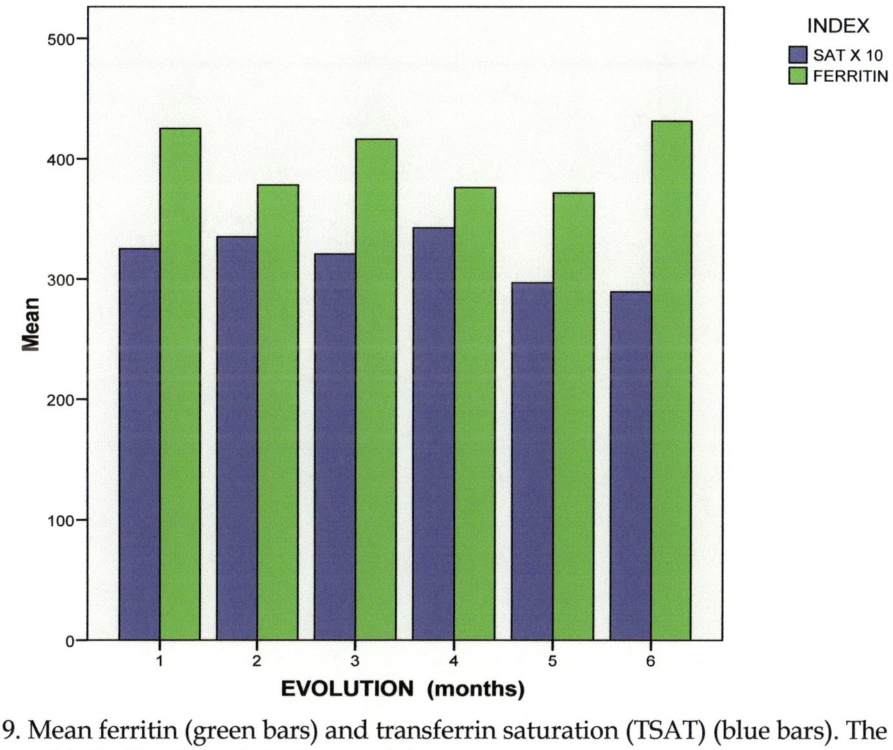

Fig. 9. Mean ferritin (green bars) and transferrin saturation (TSAT) (blue bars). The latter has been multiplied by 10 to fit in the graph better.

Mean ferritin is above 300 ng/ml in all cases. This does not necessarily mean that iron stores are adequate, as in renal failure and in other chronic diseases ferritin does not measure iron stores accurately. In 40 cases, the ferritin is less than 100 ng/ ml. In one case ferritin is above 2.000 ng/ dl and in six cases over 1.000. The standard deviation is high because ferritin does not fit a normal distribution.

8.2 Soluble transferrin receptor and soluble transferrin receptor/log ferritin index

Fig. 10. shows the evolution of soluble Transferrin Receptor

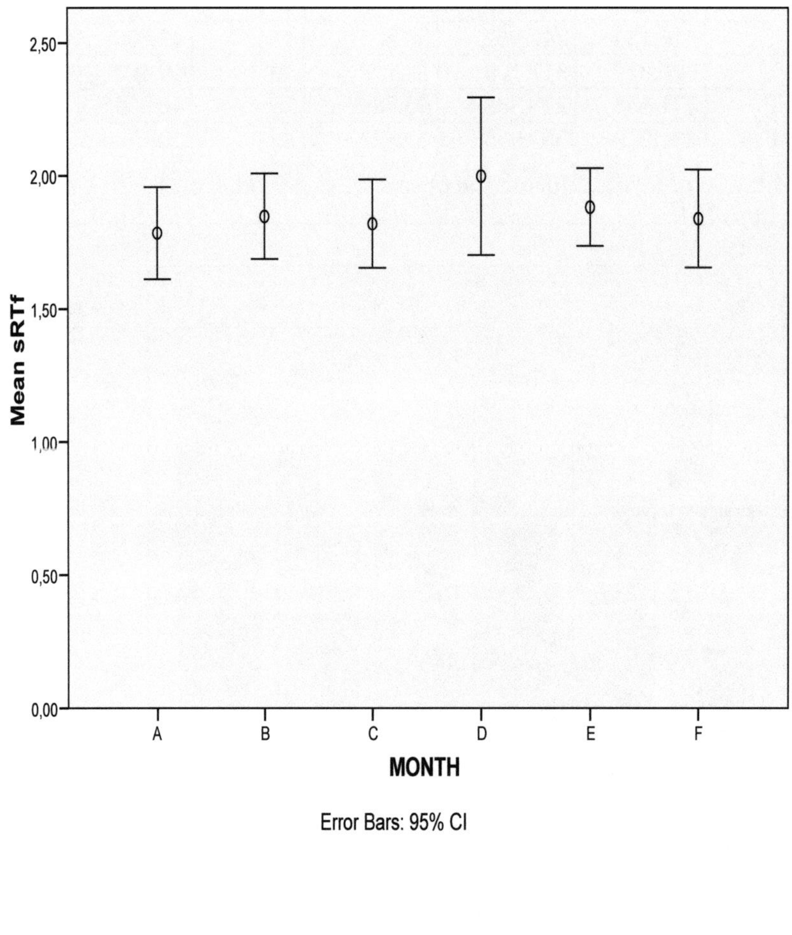

Fig. 10. Evolution of soluble Receptor of Transferrin

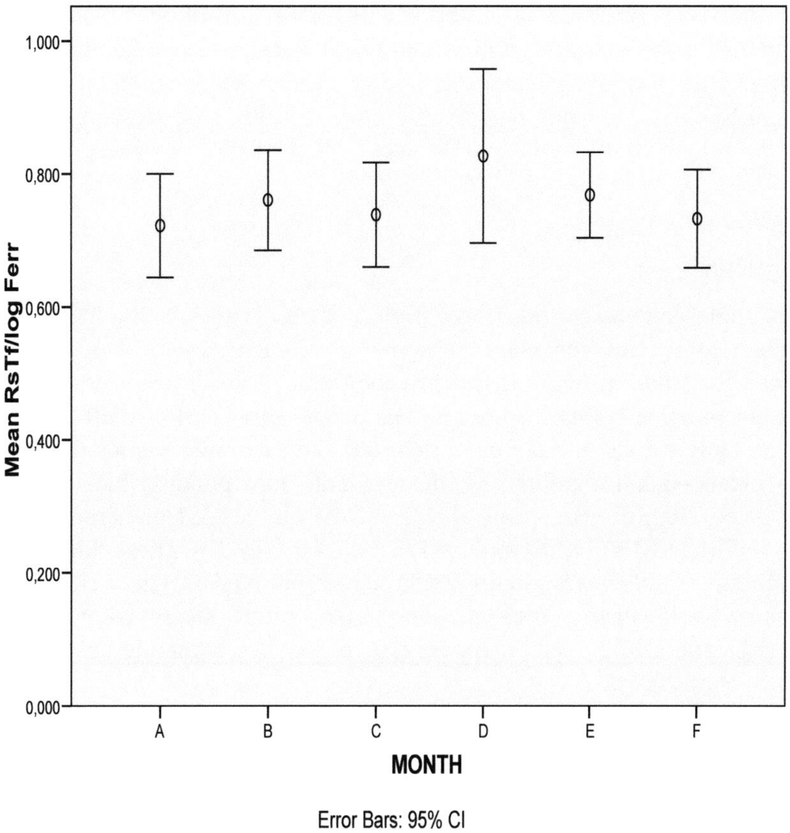

Fig. 11. Evolution of sTfR / Log Ferritin index.

9. Conclusions

9.1 Predictors of response to therapy

ANOVA shows significant differences between responders and non-responders for hemoglobin, hematocrit, red blood cells, erythropoietin, MCHC and Maf). Nevertheless only Hemoglobin (or red blood cells), EPO and MCHC were found to be the best predictors of response by multiple regression. However, the AUC of the ROC curves of each of these parameters separately is low and therefore its clinical utility is weak. The combination of red blood cells, erythropoietin and MCHC results in a mathematical model that significantly improves the predictive value of each of these variables, with an AUC of 0.72. (95% Confidence Interval: 0.62-0.80). The mathematical model is:

$$p_{resp} = \frac{1}{1+\exp(-(23.39+1.327\cdot\log(EPO)-0.838\cdot MCHC-0.787*\frac{RBC}{1000}))} \quad (3)$$

This model does not improve with the inclusion of additional variables and has the advantage that it only includes routine analytical data, without sophisticated tests. The statistical procedure that we have described (factorial analysis, data reduction, logistic regression and ROC curves) may be a useful tool for future studies with more patients and longer observation which may improve the accuracy of prediction of response.

9.2 Efficacy and safety

9.2.1 Hemoglobin

The mean hemoglobin level for the whole period of observation is X = 11.07g/dl; (SD 1.546; n = 245). When comparing the mean hemoglobin of each month, there are no significant differences and the small differences that are shown have no clinical significance. Therefore, the hemoglobin remains stable throughout the observation period with a mean within the desired range. Only six cases have been detected with extreme values (Box-Plot). None of the patients exceeded hemoglobin 15g/dl, and only two patients had hemoglobin levels persistently below 10g/dl. The cases above and below 11g/dl of hemoglobin are almost balanced (n =117 (47.8%) <11g/dl) and n= 128 (52.2%≥ 11g/dl)). These data confirm that this protocol maintains stable hemoglobin levels in the planned target. Achieved hemoglobin levels are somewhat lower than those recommended in the latest revision of K-DOKI clinical guidelines (KDOQI 2007), but conform to those recommended by others (Coyne 2010)(Akizawa et al. 2008).

When applying a cutoff of 11g/dl of hemoglobin there are significant differences above and below this value for the following parameters: C-reactive protein, serum iron, transferrin saturation, erythropoietin, and interleukin 6 (univariate analysis).

The stepwise multiple regression (with hemoglobin as the dependent variable), allowed us to develop a model in which, in the final step, only three parameters remain: serum iron, transferrin soluble receptor and erythropoietin (the latter with a negative beta coefficient). In this model the constant is 10.396 and the standardized beta coefficients: iron (0.261), log soluble transferrin receptor (0.309) and log erythropoietin (-0.274).

9.2.2 Iron

Means and standard deviations of the variables that establish the status of iron are as follows: serum iron 54.86 ± 22.59, transferrin 174.22 ± 34.89, transferrin saturation 31.94 % ± 12.70, ferritin 399.67 ± 292.31 and soluble transferrin receptor 1.86 ± 0.61. No significant differences were detected for these variables when comparing different months of observation.

Of these variables only the mean serum iron is significantly different (p <0.001) in cases with hemoglobin less than 11g/dl (x = 47.93) than in cases with more than 11g/dl hemoglobin (x = 61.14).

Although the mean transferrin saturation of each month is in the desired range, 33 cases (14.2%) had a transferrin saturation of less than 20%.

The mean index of transferrin soluble receptor / log ferritin is 0.7579 (above the 0.6 cut-off for iron deficiency) and the frequency distribution shows that 73.8% of the cases are above 0.6. These cases are likely to have iron deficiency, according to.(Chen, Hung, and Tarng 2006b)

Although the mean transferrin soluble receptor is 1.856 mg/L (less than 2 mg/L cut-off for iron deficiency), 37.2% had levels above 2 mg/L. These cases are likely to have iron deficiency, according to (Chang et al. 2007)

Therefore some patients have had iron deficiency at least once during the observation period in an amount ranging between 14.2% and 73.8%, depending on whether we use a less or more sensitive indicator.

Therefore, the iron dose should be increased slightly to maintain deposits and availability of iron in adequate quantity for normal erythropoiesis.

10. Discussion

Predictors of response reported so far are : albumin (Agarwal, Davis, and Smith 2008), clinical factors (Bamgbola, Kaskel, and Coco 2009) , (Bistrian and Carey 2000), protocol adherence(Chan et al. 2009), soluble receptor of transferrin (Chang et al. 2007; Chen, Hung, and Tarng 2006a), low iron stores (low ferritin and low transferrin saturation), malnutrition, hyperparathyroidism, and high-turnover bone disease (Kalantar-Zadeh et al. 2009).

In our model hypo-response to combination therapy with erythropoietin and iron occurs in patients with higher hemoglobin (11.4 in non-responders, versus 10.7 in responders), lower serum erythropoietin (11 in non-responders versus 18.4 in responders), higher MCHC (32.7 in non-responders versus 32.3 in responders). To our knowledge this is the first time that MCHC is included in a model to predict response to combination therapy with erythropoietin and iron in anemia in hemodialysis patients.

The difference in mean MCHC between responders and non-responders is marginal, but statistically significant.

It may seem odd that a higher level of hemoglobin is a predictor of no response, but can be explained by the fact that a level equal to or greater than 12g/dl hemoglobin involves a reduction of 50% of the dose of erythropoietin, according to our protocol. In a patient with chronic renal failure on hemodialysis serum erythropoietin level depends largely on that which is administered as a drug because the endogenous secretion is strongly suppressed. Of the three variables in the model, the serum erythropoietin is the most easily adjustable in the short term, since it can be achieved by increasing the dose. Although our protocol has been shown effective in maintaining a stable mean hemoglobin level of 11g/dl, it is insufficient to achieve the target of 12 g/ dl recommended in the latest revision of the K-DOKI guideline (KDOQI 2007). This trial had been designed before the amendment was published. Taking this into account it would be necessary to review the criteria for erythropoietin dose reduction conditioned by the level of hemoglobin. The importance of maintaining stable hemoglobin levels has been previously highlighted (Zaoui et al. 2011)

(Mathieu et al. 2008). The last authors describe a cohort of patients in Switzerland with stable hemoglobin levels, although slightly higher (mean hemoglobin 11.9 g/dl), than those presented in this paper.

Hemoglobin levels above 13g/dl, although recommended in some instances, have been associated with increased mortality. Recently, this increased mortality has been attributed to thrombocytosis induced by iron deficiency and therefore appropriate doses of intravenous iron could counteract the adverse effect of high doses of erythropoietin (Kalantar-Zadeh et al. 2009). However thrombocytosis associated with erythropoietin treatment to achieve high levels of hemoglobin can be attributed not only to iron deficiency but also to high doses of erythropoietin (Vaziri 2009).These data should be confirmed before raising the target hemoglobin level.

In the last decade hematological cell counters provide new erythrocyte and reticulocyte cell indices that are useful for the differential diagnosis of anemia. Some of these indices could be useful to establish the status of iron metabolism in the anemia of patients with advanced renal disease on hemodialysis and to predict response to treatment. If confirmed, the CBC would provide data that would spare more expensive laboratory tests. Unexpectedly, the best predictor in terms of this work is MCHC, an erythrocyte index of routine, instead of the most innovative. In general the red cell indices were used to assess the iron status rather than as predictors of response. Each author recommends the ones they have examined, but there is no consensus because the results are variable and generally not confirmed. Some of these indices are: reticulocyte hemoglobin equivalent (Ret He) (Brugnara, Schiller, and Moran 2006), serum soluble transferrin receptor (Chang et al. 2007), transferrin receptor-ferritin index (Chen, Hung, and Tarng 2006a), Soluble transferrin receptor and sTfR-F index (Choi 2008), soluble transferrin receptor and mean corpuscular hemoglobin (Choi 2007), as we have discussed in more detail in the introduction.

The serum iron is an infrequently used index of iron deficiency. In general, low serum iron is unreliable as a marker of iron deficiency because of the wide variation throughout the day. Transferrin saturation is generally preferred because in the case of iron deficiency, serum transferrin increases while serum iron decreased; but this is not the case in chronic renal failure in which both values decrease in parallel and thus the transferrin saturation shows little variation. In our patients the standard deviation of serum iron, expressed in percentage is 41%, while the same variation for transferrin is only 20%. Despite such a high dispersion, serum iron enters the multiple regression model, while transferrin saturation does not. Moreover serum iron is the only indicator of iron status with significant mean difference when applying a cutoff of 11g/dl hemoglobin. Therefore, although the serum iron is not a good indicator of iron status at the individual level, it may be useful in clinical trials.

Therefore we believe that serum iron should be taken into account in the case of anemia of chronic kidney disease.

It is not easy to compare our results with others because the treatment protocol and response criteria are different. Moreover there are no randomized clinical trials designed to look for safety of treatment with intravenous iron in the long term and it is unclear which of the two trends are correct: Increasing the dose of iron to save erythropoietin, or increasing the dose of erythropoietin to diminish the possible adverse effects of iron (Coyne 2010). The dilemma is important because high doses of erythropoietin also produce adverse effects. The most clear demonstration that increasing the number of patients treated with iron results in a decrease in erythropoietin dose in daily clinical practice (not only in clinical trials) are shown in the data published by (Hasegawa et al. 2011) . Although the balance between iron and erythropoietin therapy is still subject to discussion, it is clear that the combination therapy with both drugs reduce morbidity, mortality, hospital admissions and costs (Knight et al. 2010).

In the present trial initial iron dose is 100 mg three times a week intravenously at the end of dialysis. The initial dose of erythropoietin is 40 U / K (2,800 U for a person of average weight 70K) three times a week.

In a longitudinal study with data collected in Japan between 1999 and 2006 weekly doses of iron (160 mg / month) and erythropoietin (5531 U / week) are lower, but it must also be considered that the mean hemoglobin level was lower (10.4 g / dl)(Akizawa et al. 2008).

(Charytan et al. 2001) using a schedule similar to ours (iron sucrose injection administered as 1,000 mg in 10 divided doses by IV push) concludes that this therapy is safe and effective for the treatment of iron deficiency in patients with dialysis-associated anemia.

Iron Sucrose is the most widely iron used in patients with chronic kidney disease, but iron dextran of low molecular weight is equally effective (Atalay et al. 2011).

Several trials compare the costs and effectiveness of treatment of classical formulations of iron and erythropoietin with the new ones (some not yet approved for kidney patients) (Bhandari 2011)(Cuesta Grueso et al. 2010). Although the efficacy of these new drugs is similar to the former ones, there is no conclusive evidence to justify the increased cost of new formulations of iron and erythropoietin. In one study ferric carboxymaltose was effective in increasing the mean level of hemoglobin from 9.1 to 10.3 g / dl, but at the expense of 7.4% of serious adverse effects (Covic and Mircescu 2010). Of the new iron preparations only isomaltose iron at doses between 600 and 1,000 mg is cost effective compared with iron dextran (Bhandari 2011).

A comparative study was carried out: one branch with intravenous iron sucrose and the other with oral iron succinate. Both showed a positive response but the first one demonstrated better results. Although erythropoietin dose was lower in the intravenous iron branch, the total cost of both drugs together was higher. Gastrointestinal adverse events were higher in the oral branch (Li and Wang 2008).

Several reports have found that the detection and early treatment of anemia of chronic kidney disease with erythropoiesis-stimulating agents improves the quality of life, including cognitive and physical performances: memory, sustain attention, energy level, work capacity, aerobic capacity, and immune function (Fishbane 2010).

The alternative to transfusions most often used in patients with anemia of chronic kidney disease is erythropoietin and intravenous iron. Combination therapy is even more important in patients with anemia and cardio renal disease (Silverberg et al. 2009; Silverberg 2011; Silverberg 2010; Silverberg et al. 2010).

More than 90 % of end renal disease patients maintained on dialysis respond to traditional recombinant human erythropoietin (rHU EPO) or to EPO analogues (biosimilars, biogenerics) (Schmid and Schiffl 2010).

The therapeutic dose of EPO are higher than normal endogenous rates of EPO production in healthy subjects, and the amount of IV-iron given may be greater than the amount needed for normal erythropoiesis. This increase in erythropoietin and iron needs may be due to chronic inflammation and vitamin C deficiency, present in many patients with chronic kidney disease (Handelman 2007). The comparison between clinical trials is difficult not only for the selection of patients and the different doses of erythropoietin and iron, but also for the management of chronic inflammation and replacement of folic acid and vitamins B12 and C, data that are not always specified.

The doses of erythropoietin should be considered together with hemoglobin levels and resistance to treatment and comorbidities. In patients with chronic renal failure, without mention of heart disease, adverse effects are associated with low levels of hemoglobin (<9.5 g/ dl) despite high doses of erythropoietin (Bradbury et al. 2009), or with therapeutic targets of high hemoglobin levels (13.5 to 15 g / dl)(Belonje, de Boer, and Voors 2008) . In patients with simultaneous kidney and heart failure, erythropoietin improves cardiac function, even if it fails to raise the level of hemoglobin (Belonje, de Boer, and Voors 2008) (Pappas et al. 2008). To understand the role of erythropoietin it should be noted that its physiological effects are beyond the stimulation of erythropoiesis (Diskin et al. 2008).

Darbepoetin is as effective as epoetin alpha, but at a higher cost (Cuesta Grueso et al. 2010).

A possible way to save costs would be to give biosimilar erythropoietin rather than original. A clinical trial has demonstrated the equivalence of Eprex with GerEpo (biogeneric) in the short term, but the short duration of the trial (12 weeks) did not provide any conclusions about safety (Goh et al. 2007).

The current status of new anti-anemic drugs, including their indications and license in Europe and USA can be found in (Macdougall and Ashenden 2009). New intravenous iron preparations seem promising (Ferumoxytol), as well as erythropoietin with prolonged effect (CERA) and peptides that stimulate erythropoiesis by a mechanism different from erythropoietin (Hematide). Clinical trials are needed to establish the usefulness of these new drugs in patients with chronic kidney disease.

11. References

Nutritional anaemias. report of a WHO scientific group. 1968. *World Health Organization Technical Report Series* 405 : 5-37.

Agarwal, R., Davis J. L., and Smith L.. 2008. Serum albumin is strongly associated with erythropoietin sensitivity in hemodialysis patients. *Clinical Journal of the American Society of Nephrology : CJASN* 3 (1) (Jan): 98-104.

Akizawa, T., Pisoni R. L., Akiba T., Saito A., Fukuhara S.,. Asano Y, Hasegawa T., Port F. K., and Kurokawa K.. 2008. Japanese haemodialysis anaemia management practices and outcomes (1999-2006): Results from the DOPPS. *Nephrology, Dialysis,*

Transplantation : Official Publication of the European Dialysis and Transplant Association - European Renal Association 23 (11) (Nov): 3643-53.

Arabul, M., Gullulu M., Yilmaz Y., Eren M. A., Baran B., Gul C. B., Kocamaz G., and Dilek K.. 2009. Influence of erythropoietin therapy on serum prohepcidin levels in dialysis patients. *Medical Science Monitor: International Medical Journal of Experimental and Clinical Research* 15 (11) (Nov): CR583-7.

Atalay, Huseyin, Yalcin Solak, Kadir Acar, Nilgun Govec, and Suleyman Turk. 2011. Safety profiles of total dose infusion of low-molecular-weight iron dextran and high-dose iron sucrose in renal patients. *Hemodialysis International* 15 (3) (JUL): 374-8.

Bamgbola, O. F., Kaskel F. J., and Coco M.. 2009. Analyses of age, gender and other risk factors of erythropoietin resistance in pediatric and adult dialysis cohorts. *Pediatric Nephrology (Berlin, Germany)* 24 (3) (Mar): 571-9.

Barrios, Y., Espinoza M., and Baron M. A.. 2010. Pro-hepcidin, its relation with indicators of iron metabolism and of inflammation in patients hemodialyzed treated or not with recombinant erythropoietin. *Nutricion Hospitalaria: Organo Oficial De La Sociedad Espanola De Nutricion Parenteral y Enteral* 25 (4) (Jul-Aug): 555-60.

Belonje, A. M., de Boer R. A., and Voors A. A. 2008. Recombinant human epo treatment: Beneficial in chronic kidney disease, chronic heart failure, or both? editorial to: "correction of anemia with erythropoietin in chronic kidney disease (stage 3 or 4): Effects on cardiac performance by pappas et al.". *Cardiovascular Drugs and Therapy / Sponsored by the International Society of Cardiovascular Pharmacotherapy* 22 (1) (Feb): 1-2.

Bhandari, S. 2011. A hospital-based cost minimization study of the potential financial impact on the UK health care system of introduction of iron isomaltoside 1000. *Therapeutics and Clinical Risk Management* 7 : 103-13.

Bistrian, B. R., and Carey L. A. 2000. Impact of inflammation on nutrition, iron status, and erythropoietin responsiveness in ESRD patients. *Nephrology Nursing Journal : Journal of the American Nephrology Nurses' Association* 27 (6) (Dec): 616-22.

Bradbury, B. D., Danese M. D., Gleeson M., and Critchlow C. W. 2009. Effect of epoetin alfa dose changes on hemoglobin and mortality in hemodialysis patients with hemoglobin levels persistently below 11 g/dL. *Clinical Journal of the American Society of Nephrology : CJASN* 4 (3) (Mar): 630-7.

Bravo, J. A., Galindo P., and M. M. and Osorio Bienchy J.M. 1994. Anemia, insuficiencia renal cronica y eritropoyetina. *Nefrologia : Publicacion Oficial De La Sociedad Espanola Nefrologia* XIV (6) (23-02-1994): 687,687-694.

Brugnara, C., Schiller B., and Moran J. 2006. Reticulocyte hemoglobin equivalent (ret he) and assessment of iron-deficient states. *Clinical and Laboratory Haematology* 28 (5) (Oct): 303-8.

C.H. Fourcade, Jary L., and and Belaouni H. 1999. Reticulocyte ananalysis provided by the coulter GEN.S: significance and interpretation in regenerative and nonregn rative hematologic conditions. *Laboratory Hematology* 5 : 153,153-158.

Chamney, M., Pugh-Clarke K., Kafkia T., and Wittwer I.. 2010. CE: Continuing education article: MANAGEMENT OF ANAEMIA IN CHRONIC KIDNEY DISEASE. *Journal of Renal Care* 36 (2) (Jun): 102-11.

Chan, K., Moran J., Hlatky M., andLafayette R. 2009. Protocol adherence and the ability to achieve target haemoglobin levels in haemodialysis patients. *Nephrology, Dialysis, Transplantation : Official Publication of the European Dialysis and Transplant Association - European Renal Association* 24 (6) (Jun): 1956-62.

Chang, J., Bird R., Clague A., and Carter A. 2007. Clinical utility of serum soluble transferrin receptor levels and comparison with bone marrow iron stores as an index for iron-deficient erythropoiesis in a heterogeneous group of patients. *Pathology* 39 (3) (Jun): 349-53.

Charytan, C., Levin N., Al-Saloum M., Hafeez T., Gagnon S., and Van Wyck D. B. 2001. Efficacy and safety of iron sucrose for iron deficiency in patients with dialysis-associated anemia: North american clinical trial. *American Journal of Kidney Diseases : The Official Journal of the National Kidney Foundation* 37 (2) (Feb): 300-7.

Chen, Y. C., Hung S. C., and Tarng D. C. 2006a. Association between transferrin receptor-ferritin index and conventional measures of iron responsiveness in hemodialysis patients. *American Journal of Kidney Diseases : The Official Journal of the National Kidney Foundation* 47 (6) (Jun): 1036-44.

———. 2006b. Association between transferrin receptor-ferritin index and conventional measures of iron responsiveness in hemodialysis patients. *American Journal of Kidney Diseases : The Official Journal of the National Kidney Foundation* 47 (6) (Jun): 1036-44.

Choi, J. W. 2008. Soluble transferrin receptor and sTfR-F index for assessing concurrent iron deficiency in patients with chronic renal failure. *Annals of Hematology* 87 (7) (Jul): 575-6.

———. 2007. Combination index of soluble transferrin receptor and mean corpuscular hemoglobin for evaluating iron deficiency in end-stage renal disease. *Annals of Hematology* 86 (1) (Jan): 75-7.

Covic, A., and Mircescu G. 2010. The safety and efficacy of intravenous ferric carboxymaltose in anaemic patients undergoing haemodialysis: A multi-centre, open-label, clinical study. *Nephrology, Dialysis, Transplantation : Official Publication of the European Dialysis and Transplant Association - European Renal Association* 25 (8) (Aug): 2722-30.

Coyne, Daniel W. 2010. It's time to compare anemia management strategies in hemodialysis. *Clinical Journal of the American Society of Nephrology* 5 (4) (APR): 740-2.

Cuesta Grueso, C., Poveda Andres J. L., Garcia Pellicer J., andRoma Sanchez E. 2010. Cost minimisation analysis for darbepoetin alpha vs. epoetin alpha in chronic kidney disease patients on haemodialysis. *Farmacia Hospitalaria : Organo Oficial De Expresion Cientifica De La Sociedad Espanola De Farmacia Hospitalaria* 34 (2) (Mar-Apr): 68-75.

de Francisco, A. L., De la Cruz J. J., Cases A., de la Figuera M., Egocheaga M. I., Gorriz J. I., Llisterri J. I., Marin R., and Martinez Castelao A. 2007. Prevalence of kidney insufficiency in primary care population in spain: EROCAP study. *Nefrologia : Publicacion Oficial De La Sociedad Espanola Nefrologia* 27 (3): 300-12.

Diskin, C. J., Stokes T. J., Dansby L. M., Radcliff L., and Carter T. B. 2008. Beyond anemia: The clinical impact of the physiologic effects of erythropoietin. *Seminars in Dialysis* 21 (5) (Sep-Oct): 447-54.

Fishbane, S. 2010. The role of erythropoiesis-stimulating agents in the treatment of anemia. *The American Journal of Managed Care* 16 Suppl Issues (Mar): S67-73.

Goh, B. L., Ong L. M., Sivanandam S., Lim T. O., Morad Z., and Biogeneric EPO Study Group. 2007. Randomized trial on the therapeutic equivalence between eprex and GerEPO in patients on haemodialysis. *Nephrology (Carlton, Vic.)* 12 (5) (Oct): 431-6.

Gupta, S., Uppal B., and Pawar B. 2009. Is soluble transferrin receptor a good marker of iron deficiency anemia in chronic kidney disease patients? *Indian Journal of Nephrology* 19 (3) (Jul): 96-100.

Handelman, G. J. 2007. Newer strategies for anemia prevention in hemodialysis. *The International Journal of Artificial Organs* 30 (11) (Nov): 1014-9.

Härdle, W., and Simar L.. 2003. *Applied multivariate statistical analysis*. Berlin: Springer-Verlag.

Hasegawa, T., Bragg-Gresham J. L., Pisoni R. L., Robinson B. M., Fukuhara S., Akiba T., Saito A., Kurokawa K., and Akizawa T. 2011. Changes in anemia management and hemoglobin levels following revision of a bundling policy to incorporate recombinant human erythropoietin. *Kidney International* 79 (3) (Feb): 340-6.

Kalantar-Zadeh, K., Kalantar-Zadeh K., and Lee G. H. 2006. The fascinating but deceptive ferritin: To measure it or not to measure it in chronic kidney disease? *Clinical Journal of the American Society of Nephrology : CJASN* 1 Suppl 1 (Sep): S9-18.

Kalantar-Zadeh, K., Lee G. H., Miller J. E., Streja E., Jing J., Robertson J. A., and Kovesdy C. P. 2009. Predictors of hyporesponsiveness to erythropoiesis-stimulating agents in hemodialysis patients. *American Journal of Kidney Diseases : The Official Journal of the National Kidney Foundation* 53 (5) (May): 823-34.

Kalantar-Zadeh, K., Streja E., Miller J. E., and Nissenson A. R. 2009. Intravenous iron versus erythropoiesis-stimulating agents: Friends or foes in treating chronic kidney disease anemia? *Advances in Chronic Kidney Disease* 16 (2) (Mar): 143-51.

KDOQI. 2007. KDOQI clinical practice guideline and clinical practice recommendations for anemia in chronic kidney disease: 2007 update of hemoglobin target. *American Journal of Kidney Diseases : The Official Journal of the National Kidney Foundation* 50 (3) (Sep): 471-530.

KDOQI, and National Kidney Foundation. 2006. KDOQI clinical practice guidelines and clinical practice recommendations for anemia in chronic kidney disease. *American Journal of Kidney Diseases : The Official Journal of the National Kidney Foundation* 47 (5 Suppl 3) (May): S11-145.

Knight, T. G., Ryan K., Schaefer C. P., 'Sylva L. D, and Durden E. D. 2010. Clinical and economic outcomes in medicare beneficiaries with stage 3 or stage 4 chronic kidney disease and anemia: The role of intravenous iron therapy. *Journal of Managed Care Pharmacy : JMCP* 16 (8) (Oct): 605-15.

Kuwahara, M., Iimori S., Kuyama T., Akita W., Mori Y., Asai T., Tsukamoto Y., et al. 2011. Effect of anemia on cardiac disorders in pre-dialysis patients immediately before starting hemodialysis. *Clinical and Experimental Nephrology* 15 (1) (Feb): 121-5.

Li, H., and Wang S. X. 2008. Intravenous iron sucrose in chinese hemodialysis patients with renal anemia. *Blood Purification* 26 (2): 151-6.

Macdougall, I. C., and Ashenden M. 2009. Current and upcoming erythropoiesis-stimulating agents, iron products, and other novel anemia medications. *Advances in Chronic Kidney Disease* 16 (2) (Mar): 117-30.

Maconi, M., Cavalca L., Danise P., Cardarelli F., and Brini M. 2009. Erythrocyte and reticulocyte indices in iron deficiency in chronic kidney disease: Comparison of two methods. *Scandinavian Journal of Clinical and Laboratory Investigation* 69 (3): 365-70.

Maiz, H. B., Abderrahim E., and Zouaghi K.. 2002. Anemia and end-stage renal disease in the developing world. *Artificial Organs* 26 (9) (Sep): 760-4.

Mathieu, C. M., Teta D., Lotscher N., Golshayan D., Gabutti L., Kiss D.,. Martin P. Y, and Burnier M. 2008. Optimal and continuous anaemia control in a cohort of dialysis patients in switzerland. *BMC Nephrology* 9 (Dec 11): 16.

Nakanishi, T., Kuragano T., Nanami M., Otaki Y., Nonoguchi H., and Hasuike Y. 2010. Importance of ferritin for optimizing anemia therapy in chronic kidney disease. *American Journal of Nephrology* 32 (5): 439-46.

Ng, H. Y., Chen H. C., Pan L. L., Tsai Y. C., Hsu K. T., Liao S. C., Chuang F. R., Chen J. B., and Lee C. T. 2009. Clinical interpretation of reticulocyte hemoglobin content, RET-Y, in chronic hemodialysis patients. *Nephron.Clinical Practice* 111 (4): c247-52.

Pappas, K. D., Gouva C. D., Katopodis K. P., Nikolopoulos P. M., Korantzopoulos P. G., Michalis L. K., Goudevenos J. A., and Siamopoulos K. C. 2008. Correction of anemia with erythropoietin in chronic kidney disease (stage 3 or 4): Effects on cardiac performance. *Cardiovascular Drugs and Therapy/ Sponsored by the International Society of Cardiovascular Pharmacotherapy* 22 (1) (Feb): 37-44.

Pollak, V. E., Lorch J. A., Shukla R., and Satwah S. 2009. The importance of iron in long-term survival of maintenance hemodialysis patients treated with epoetin-alfa and intravenous iron: Analysis of 9.5 years of prospectively collected data. *BMC Nephrology* 10 (Feb 26): 6.

Remacha, A. F., Oliver A., Yoldi F., Lendinez M., DeLuis J., Villegas A., A. Gonzalez, and F. Sanchez. 1997. Reticulocytes and their maturity fractions in anemia. proposal of a new reticulocyte production index. *Blood* 90 (10) (NOV 15): 2766-.

Schmid, H., and Schiffl H. 2010. Erythropoiesis stimulating agents and anaemia of end-stage renal disease. *Cardiovascular & Hematological Agents in Medicinal Chemistry* 8 (3) (Jul): 164-72.

Shinzato, T., Abe K., Furusu A., Harada T., Shinzato K., Miyazaki M., and Kohno S. 2008. Serum pro-hepcidin level and iron homeostasis in japanese dialysis patients with erythropoietin (EPO) - resistant anemia. *Medical Science Monitor:*

International Medical Journal of Experimental and Clinical Research 14 (9) (Sep): CR431-7.

Silverberg, D. S. 2010. The role of erythropoiesis stimulating agents and intravenous (IV) iron in the cardio renal anemia syndrome. *Heart Failure Reviews* (Sep 24).

Silverberg, D. S., Wexler D., Iaina A., and Schwartz D. 2010. Anaemia management in cardio renal disease. *Journal of Renal Care* 36 Suppl 1 (May): 86-96.

———. 2009. The correction of anemia in patients with the combination of chronic kidney disease and congestive heart failure may prevent progression of both conditions. *Clinical and Experimental Nephrology* 13 (2) (Apr): 101-6.

Silverberg, Donald S. 2011. The role of erythropoiesis stimulating agents and intravenous (IV) iron in the cardio renal anemia syndrome. *Heart Failure Reviews* 16 (6) (NOV): 609-14.

Tsubakihara, Y., Nishi S., Akiba T., Hirakata H., Iseki K., Kubota M.,. Kuriyama S, et al. 2010. 2008 japanese society for dialysis therapy: Guidelines for renal anemia in chronic kidney disease. *Therapeutic Apheresis and Dialysis : Official Peer-Reviewed Journal of the International Society for Apheresis, the Japanese Society for Apheresis, the Japanese Society for Dialysis Therapy* 14 (3) (Jun): 240-75.

Urrechaga, E. 2010. The new mature red cell parameter, low haemoglobin density of the beckman-coulter LH750: Clinical utility in the diagnosis of iron deficiency. *International Journal of Laboratory Hematology* 32 (1 Pt 1) (Feb): e144-50.

———. 2008. Discriminant value of % microcytic/% hypochromic ratio in the differential diagnosis of microcytic anemia. *Clinical Chemistry and Laboratory Medicine : CCLM / FESCC* 46 (12): 1752-8.

van der Putten, K., Jie K. E., van den Broek D., Kraaijenhagen R. J., Laarakkers C., Swinkels D. W., Braam B., andGaillard C. A. 2010. Hepcidin-25 is a marker of the response rather than resistance to exogenous erythropoietin in chronic kidney disease/chronic heart failure patients. *European Journal of Heart Failure* 12 (9) (Sep): 943-50.

Vaziri, N. D. 2009. Thrombocytosis in EPO-treated dialysis patients may be mediated by EPO rather than iron deficiency. *American Journal of Kidney Diseases : The Official Journal of the National Kidney Foundation* 53 (5) (May): 733-6.

Winearls, C. G., Oliver D. O., Pippard M. J., Reid C., Downing M. R., and Cotes P. M. 1986. Effect of human erythropoietin derived from recombinant DNA on the anaemia of patients maintained by chronic haemodialysis. *Lancet* 2 (8517) (Nov 22): 1175-8.

Zaoui, P., Deray G., Ortiz J. P., and Rostaing L. 2011. Stability of hemoglobin levels: An indispensible paradigm change in medical management. *Nephrologie & Therapeutique* 7 (1 Suppl 2) (Feb): H5-7.

Zaritsky, J., Young B., Wang H. J., Westerman M., Olbina G., Nemeth E., Ganz T., Rivera S., Nissenson A. R., and Salusky I. B. 2009. Hepcidin--a potential novel biomarker for iron status in chronic kidney disease. *Clinical Journal of the American Society of Nephrology : CJASN* 4 (6) (Jun): 1051-6.

Zini,G., Machin, S., Briggs C., Preloznik-Zupan,I., Juncal, J. Romero, S., Beerenhout, C., Garcia, M., Pintado-Cros, T., Junior, E., Reis, A., Solenthaler, M., Goetgheluck, Q.,

Simon, R., Qian, C., Hou Z. 2006. Multicenter evaluation of Coulter MCH and the new derived LDH% parameters versus CHR and %Hypo for the assessment of iron metabolism disturbances. *Laboratory Hematology 2006; 12(4): pages 184 – 185 (PC)*

5

Role of Hepcidin in Dysregulation of Iron Metabolism and Anemia of Chronic Diseases

Bhawna Singh, Sarika Arora,
SK Gupta and Alpana Saxena
*University of Delhi, GGSIP University,
India*

1. Introduction

Iron is an essential element and its correct balance is necessary for good health and normal cellular functioning [1]. Hepcidin is the iron-regulatory hormone of hepatic origin. It is a defensin-like low-molecular-weight peptide that plays an important role in iron metabolism. Hepcidin and its receptor ferroportin play most important role in controlling the dietary absorption and tissue distribution of iron. Recently discovered hepcidin molecule has been recognized as the main hormone behind the pathogenesis of anemia of chronic disease.

Maintenance of normal Iron homeostasis in body

Iron is an important trace element that is crucial for human life. Its main functions include structural component of oxygen transportation and storage molecules, and of many enzymes. The control of this indispensable but potentially toxic substance is an important aspect of human health and disease. Intestinal absorption of dietary iron is a very dynamic process where non haem ferric form of iron (Fe^{3+}) is reduced to ferrous form (Fe^{2+}) by ferric oxidoreductase "duodenal cytochrome B" (DcytB) for transport across apical brush border. Iron is absorbed through the transporter DMT1 (divalent metal transporter 1) also called Nramp2 (natural-resistance-associated macrophage protein 2) [2, 3] present in apical intestinal epithelial cells. DMT1 mediates transport of non-transferrin bound iron (NTBI) along with other divalent metals (Fe^{2+}, Zn^{2+}, Mn^{2+}). This is a proton dependant Fe^{2+} import, therefore conversion of Fe^{3+} to Fe^{2+} is necessary. The enterocytes either store the iron as ferritin which is accomplished by Fe^{3+} binding to apoferritin or move to the basolateral surface of the cell from where it is transported out by the iron exporter ferroportin, reoxidized by hephaestin which is homolog of serum multi-copper oxidase ceruloplasmin that oxidizes Fe^{2+} to Fe^{3+} and facilitates incorporation of iron into transferrin. Iron is then collected by transferrin for distribution to tissues [4].

Iron transporter, ferroportin is a 571 amino acid long protein that is present in basolateral membrane of enterocytes and macrophages and is involved in iron-recycling in senescent erythrocytes and reticuloendothelial macrophages. The export is linked to a ferrooxidase. Iron in RBCs is phagocytosed by macrophages during recycling of iron from senescent red cells, exits the macrophage via ferroportin, assisted by the ferroxidase ceruloplasmin. Macrophages also take up iron from transferrin, transport it across the endosomal membrane via Nramp2 (natural resistance-associated macrophage protein) or divalent metal transporter1 (DMT1), and incorporate it in ferroproteins, including the storage protein ferritin.

Role of hepcidin in iron metabolism

Iron is utilized in nearly all cells, large amount of it being present in erythrocytes with lesser amounts in myoglobin. Iron is critical to a number of synthetic and enzymatic processes with greater requirement during periods of growth. Body plans to conserve iron by recycling it from senescent erythrocytes and from other sources. To maintain the homeostatic balance, essential mechanisms prevent excessive iron absorption in the proximal small intestine and regulate the rate of iron release from macrophages [5].

Maintenance of correct iron balance is vital to health. In heme or non-heme proteins, iron is involved in vital activities and biochemical reactions. Cell and tissue proliferation and immunity are also affected by iron. However, the ability to produce free radicals makes free iron a toxic element (Fenton reaction) [1].

Fenton reaction: $Fe2^{+} + H_2O_2 \rightarrow Fe3^{+} + OH^{*} + OH$

Over past few years immense research has been done and led to identification of a number of new proteins involved in iron homeostasis, hepcidin being an important hormone involved. Hepcidin acts as a systemic iron-regulatory hormone as it controls iron transport from iron-exporting tissues into plasma [6]. Hepcidin inhibits the intestinal absorption [7, 8], macrophage release [9, 10] and placental passage [8] of iron. It provides a more functional view of iron metabolism and reveals the mechanisms affecting iron status in patients with chronic inflammation and anemia.

Hepatocytes evaluate body iron status and release or down-regulate hepcidin according to the iron status of the body, with main function of hepcidin being reduction in plasma iron concentration. Hepcidin mRNA moves with the body's iron levels, increasing as they increase and decreasing as they decrease [11]. Hepcidin regulates iron uptake constantly on a daily basis, to maintain sufficient iron stores for erythropoiesis [12], as well as its feedback mechanism to prevent iron overload.

Hepcidin inhibits the cellular efflux of iron by binding to, and inducing the internalization and degradation of, ferroportin, the exclusive iron exporter in iron-transporting cells [6, 13, 14]. Thus, on one hand hepcidin decreases iron release from the spleen macrophages into the plasma and on other hand, it decreases duodenal iron absorption by diminishing the effective number of iron exporters on the membrane of enterocytes.

Hepcidin excess or deficiency might be the causative factor of dysregulation of iron homeostasis in hereditary and acquired iron disorders. In ferroportin mutations it has been observed that iron accumulates mainly in macrophages and is often combined with anemia [15]. It has been observed that hepcidin synthesis is increased by iron loading and decreased by anemia and hypoxia [16]. Anemia and hypoxia are associated with a dramatic decrease in liver hepcidin gene expression, which may account for the increase in iron release from reticuloendothelial cells and increase in iron absorption frequently observed in these situations [12]. Several studies have proved that there is local production of hepcidin by macrophages [17], cardiomyocytes [18] and fat cells [19], suggesting that hepcidin is involved in different regulatory mechanisms to control iron imbalance. Apart from this, few studies have proposed that hepcidin might also directly inhibit erythroid-progenitor proliferation and survival [20]. These modifications of hepcidin gene expression further suggest a key role for hepcidin in iron homeostasis under various pathophysiological conditions, which may support the pharmaceutical use of hepcidin agonists and antagonists in various iron homeostasis disorders.

2. Hepcidin

2.1 A peptide hormone

Hepcidin is a small, antimicrobial peptide hormone with a sequence of 25 amino acids which is produced by liver in response to inflammatory stimuli & iron overload. Hepcidin was first discovered in human urine and serum and later the studies done on the mice models led to most of the information on its structure, function expression and regulation. Originally hepcidin was isolated from plasma ultrafiltrate [21] and was called liver-expressed antimicrobial peptide (LEAP-1). Later when it was isolated from human urine, it was renamed as hepatic antimicrobial peptide (HAMP). Currently known as 'hepcidin' because of its hepatic origin and bactericidal effect *in vitro* [7], this newly discovered peptide has been established to be regulated by inflammation, iron stores, [22] hypoxia and anemia [16].

Hepcidin is thought to be the primary regulator of iron homeostasis whose production is mainly controlled by the erythropoietic activity of the bone-marrow, the body iron stores, and presence of inflammation in the body. Hepcidin was discovered accidentally when its gene was knocked out in a group of mice and they were noticed to develop iron overload. On contrary when hepcidin was over expressed, mouse fetuses died in utero because they developed severe hypoferremia thus it indicates that hepcidin may be involved in maternal-fetal iron transport across placenta [23,24]. It is also proved to be a type II acute phase protein [25].

2.2 Overview of structure

Hepcidin exists as precursor protein, a full-length preprohepcidin which comprises of 84 amino acids (aa). Subsequent to the enzymatic cleavage at the C-terminus, 64 aa long pro-hepcidin peptide is exported from cytoplasm into the lumen of endoplasmic reticulum followed by removal of a 39 aa pro-region peptide by a furin-like proprotein convertase [21, 7]. The 25 amino acid form is the mature bioactive hepcidin.

Structural analysis of hepcidin by NMR spectroscopy has revealed that the mature hepcidin molecule exists as a simple hairpin structure with disulfide bridges linking the two arms in a ladder like configuration. There are four disulfide bonds present between the cysteine molecules in the mature hepcidin. The hairpin loop has an indistinct β-sheet structure steadied by four disulfide bonds between the two anti-parallel strands. An atypical feature is the presence of a cysteine bridge between two adjacent cysteines near the turn of the hairpin that might be acting as a vital domain in the activity of the molecule [26]. These specific disulfide bonds formed between adjacent cysteines are stressed and might have a greater chemical reactivity. Like other antimicrobial peptides, hepcidin displays spatial separation of its positively charged hydrophilic side chains from the hydrophobic ones, a characteristic of peptides that disrupt bacterial membranes.

The predominant form of hepcidin in human urine is 25 aa long (hepcidin-25), along with two peptides which are shorter at the amino terminus, hepcidin-22 and hepcidin-20 [7]. Both of these isoforms which are truncated at the N-terminus of hepcidin-25 are detectable in human serum and urine while 22 aa isoform has been identified only in urine [27] suggesting that it may be a urinary degradation product of hepcidin-25 [28]. Recent studies have shown that the iron regulating bioactivity is almost exclusively due to the 25 aa peptide, signifying that the five N-terminal amino acids are essential for this activity [29, 30]. The 25 aa form has been proved to have both antibacterial [7] and antifungal activities [21] making hepcidin a member of the family of cysteine rich, cationic, antimicrobial peptides (AMP) which includes the defensins and cathelicidins [14] and is responsible for providing first line of defense at mucosal barriers [7, 21].

2.3 Genetics of hepcidin

In humans, *HAMP* is the gene that encodes for hepcidin. Human hepcidin is encoded by a 0.4-kilobase (kb) mRNA generated from 3 exons of a 2.5-kb gene on chromosome 19q13.1. The development of severe iron overload by knocking out the gene in mice suggested that hepcidin is involved in iron metabolism [23]. Animal models of iron overload include mice deficient in Upstream factor 2 (*Usf2)* that do not express the antimicrobial peptide hepcidin [31]. Constitutive overexpression of hepcidin in *HAMP* transgenic mice leads to iron-deficient anemia [8]. These findings indicate a key role for hepcidin in regulation of iron absorption in mammals and make *HAMP* a functional candidate for association with juvenile hereditary hemochromatosis that is not linked to 1q.

2.4 Assay methods

Various techniques have been employed to measure hepcidin / prohepcidin. Commercially available ELISA, dot blot assay using non-commercially available antibodies for the semi-quantitative measurement of hepcidin in urine [25] and more advanced technologies such as surface-enhanced laser desorption/ionization time-of-flight mass spectrometry (SELDI-TOF MS) and liquid chromatography tandem mass spectrometry (LC/MS-MS) [32, 33,34] have taken the lead in hepcidin quantification.

Choice of right sample and a validated and reliable method is still being explored to assay levels of hepcidin. Hepcidin has been quantitated in serum as well as urine by various techniques although till date urinary hepcidin estimation has been more popular in most of the studies. Urinary secretion of hepcidin is under the control of glomerular filtration and tubular reabsorption and to some extent local production of hepcidin in renal tissue might also contribute towards the urinary hepcidin [35]. In spite of the fact that concentrations of urine and serum correlate with each other [36], the use of urine hepcidin measurements might be misleading.

2.5 Regulation of hepcidin and its effects

Hepcidin is homeostatically regulated by two factors- iron and erythropoietic activity. Hepcidin levels are regulated by a feedback mechanism: Iron- increased plasma and stored iron stimulate hepcidin production, which in turn blocks dietary iron absorption and further iron loading whereas hepcidin is suppressed in iron deficiency [37], allowing increased absorption of dietary iron and replenishment of iron stores. Thus the feedback loop between iron and hepcidin ensures that plasma iron concentration is tightly controlled. At the cellular level, hepcidin regulates iron by binding with ferroportin. When plasma hepcidin concentration is elevated, the rate of hepcidin-ferroportin binding and subsequent ferroportin internalization and degradation lead to a decreased release of iron into the plasma. Hepcidin transcription implicates numerous proteins through several molecular cascades. Major proteins involved are the bone morphogenetic protein (BMP), the haemochromatosis protein HFE, TfR2 (Tf receptor 2) and the BMP co-receptor HJV (haemojuvelin) and membrane-bound serine protease matriptase 2 (TMPRSS6). Second process regulating hepcidin production is the process which consumes most iron, erythropoiesis [38]. Increased erythropoietic activity suppresses hepcidin production which allows the release of stored iron from macrophages and hepatocytes, and increased iron absorption, all resulting in greater supply of iron for hemoglobin synthesis.

2.6 Role of hepcidin in inflammation

The discovery of hepcidin regulation by inflammatory mechanisms has greatly increased the understanding of anemia caused in chronic inflammatory diseases. During inflammation although iron stores tend to increase, but availability of iron from stored forms and absorption decreases. Increased iron stores and inflammation induce hepcidin production, whereas hypoxia, anemia, and increased erythropoiesis moderates hepcidin synthesis [6, 16, 39, 40]. The link between inflammation and production of hepcidin by liver is attributed to IL-6, produced at sites of inflammation [41]. IL-6 is believed to induce production by binding a transcription activator to the hepcidin promoter. Human hepatocytes increase hepcidin mRNA in the presence of IL-6 or lipopolysaccharide and in the presence of IL-6 produced by monocytes exposed to lipopolysaccharide [25].

Studies have confirmed that changes in hepcidin expression is not by direct transcriptional mechanism but hypoxia-inducible factor (HIF)-1 alpha may down regulate hepcidin or it may be mediated by haemojuvelin, which may be increased by the HIF-dependent induction of furin activity [42, 43]. In a recent study Nemeth et al have suggested that hepcidin is a type II acute-phase protein. Hepcidin peptide was observed to be 100 times higher in urine of patients suffering from chronic infections and severe inflammatory diseases in contrast to patients with less severe inflammatory disorders [25]. Nicolas et al observed in mice models that inflammation from injection of turpentine resulted in induction of hepcidin mRNA and decrease in serum iron by 6 times and 2 times respectively [16]. The hypoferremic response to turpentine-induced inflammation, a standard inflammatory stimulus, was absent in the USF2/hepcidin-deficient mice, indicating that this response is fully dependent on hepcidin. In another study by Shike et al it was seen that infection with the fish pathogen Streptococcus iniae amplified hepcidin mRNA expression 4500-fold in white bass liver [44].

Whereas IL-6 induces hepcidin mRNA other cytokines like IL-1 or tumor necrosis factor (TNF-) inhibit it [25]. Recent studies have proposed that inflammation may perpetuate the iron deficiency of obesity by hepcidin mediated inhibition of dietary iron absorption. Serum hepcidin has been found to be elevated in obese women despite iron depletion, suggesting that it is responding to inflammation rather than iron status. The source of excess hepcidin however was proposed to be liver and not adipose tissue. The iron deficiency of obesity is thus a condition of a true body iron deficit rather than maldistribution of iron due to inflammation [45].

2.7 Role of hepcidin in innate immunity

Role of iron in bacterial growth is well established. Iron is required for bacterial growth and trivial to modest increase in iron intake may diminish host resistance to infection [46]. Bacterial cells tend to develop various means [47] for acquiring iron in environments where very little free iron is available. Iron overload increases the susceptibility to intracellular and blood pathogens [48, 49]. In response to bacterial infections, the host has its own mechanisms of withholding iron from microbes. These include increasing the production of iron binding proteins, reducing dietary iron assimilation, increasing hepatic production of hemoglobin and hemin scavengers (haptoglobin and hemopexin, respectively), and the release of apolactoferrin from neutrophils to sequester iron at sites of bacterial invasion. Conditions under which the level of iron in serum is increased compromise these host defenses and thereby predispose the host to invasion from these iron-requiring microbes [50].

The amphipathic hepcidin contains a motif of numerous cationic residues, well recognized in antimicrobial peptides that bind to negatively charged phospholipids on the cytoplasmic membranes of many microbes (bacterial, parasitic, and fungal). It has been speculated that hepcidin might subsequently disrupt membrane function, penetrate cells in order to damage them, or excite an immune response through chemotactic properties. Operating downstream of potent cytokines and Toll-like receptors, hepcidin contains potential binding sites for transcription factors NF-κB, HNF3 and C/EBP in its regulatory region and is thus recruited by bacterial lipopolysaccharides and inflammation [21]

In addition to its direct importance in bacterial growth, excess iron plays a crucial role in impairment of the host immune system [51, 52]. Results from different animal models indicates that excessive iron may have profound effects on T-cell function, with increased $CD8^+$ counts at the expense of reduced $CD4^+$ cell counts and a reduced mitogenic response to standard antigens and impaired hypersensitivity responses. Thus it appears that Th1 responses (cellular immune responses) may be down regulated by excess iron.

Iron has a direct inhibitory effect on vital gamma interferon-mediated pathways in macrophages, such as NO formation (by inhibition of inducible NO synthase), TNF-α formation, major histocompatibility complex class II expression, and ICAM-1 expression [53, 54, 55]. As a consequence, gamma interferon pathways become ineffective at destroying intracellular pathogens in iron-overloaded macrophages. This has been shown to detrimentally affect the immune response to *Legionella, Listeria, Ehrlichia,* and some viruses, where NO is critical [56]. *The identification of NRAMP-1 (natural resistance-associated macrophage protein 1)—which both is involved with modulation of iron metabolism in macrophages and plays an important role in early-phase macrophage activation and therefore in host innate immunity also explains the critical relation between immune response and iron [57].

Significance of hepcidin as a mediator of innate immunity has been highlighted by Ganz in his research. It was observed that hepcidin concentration amplified about 100-fold in the urine samples of one of the urine donors who developed a systemic infection [58]. Also its composition was seen to resemble that of drosomycin, a 4-disulfide insect defensin synthesized in body of drosophila in response to infections. Hepcidin, by its regulatory action on iron metabolism may thus be expected to have an important role in immune regulation. Hepcidin, by inducing macrophage sequestration of iron, robs bacteria of this element. Hepcidin thus provides an uncongenial internal milieu for microbes that successfully enter the bloodstream. Microbes require iron for the production of the superoxide dismutase that protects them from host oxygen radicals [59, 60].

2.8 Role of hepcidin in anemia of chronic diseases

Anemia is frequently associated with a wide variety of chronic infections, inflammatory diseases and malignancies. Chronic diseases are characterized with disturbance in iron homeostasis leading to anemia, referred to as anemia of chronic diseases. Mild to moderate anemia that is usually normocytic, normochromic, later can turn into hypochromic and microcytic. Hepcidin is the underlying cause of anemia in such settings. Hepcidin mediated anemia i.e, Anemia of Chronic Diseases (ACD) has been referred by a variety of other names also like Anemia of Inflammation (AI) and anemia of cancer (in case of malignancy). Anemia in patients with chronic infections could not be explained in earlier times though Locke et al (1932) had observed that infection was associated with hypoferremia [61]. The expression of proteins involved in iron homeostasis is altered by cytokine action although its role in anemia of inflammation has not been ascertained [62]. It has been established that the inflammatory cytokine IL-6 stimulates synthesis of hepcidin which is responsible for most or all of the features of this disorder [58]. It is now seen as a key mediator of hypoferremia in inflammation [4, 16, 63].

3. Anemia of Chronic Disease (ACD)

Dysregulated iron metabolism occurs in chronic inflammatory diseases. The immune driven anemia due to inflammatory cytokines (IL-1β, TNFα, IFNγ) and impaired erythropoiesis leads to anemia of chronic disease (ACD) [64]. Therefore, patients suffering from chronic disorders like infection, cancer or an autoimmune disorder often develop ACD. ACD is probably the second most common anemia next to anemia due to iron deficiency [65, 66]. It has been proved that noninfectious diseases also lead to anemia as observed in chronic infections, thus formulating the term 'anemia of chronic disease'. Hepcidin plays an important role in pathogenesis of ACD as it redirects iron from intestinal absorption as well as deters its release from macrophages [67].

A newly identified gene, hemojuvelin is essential for iron homeostasis and is required for normal expression of hepcidin in hepatocytes [68]. The laboratory picture of ACD is typically characterized by normochromic or mild microcytic anemia with reduced serum iron concentrations and transferrin saturation and raised bone marrow iron stores and ferritin [69, 70]. The condition is marked by a low reticulocyte count indicating an underproduction of red cells. Transferrin concentrations are normal or slightly reduced and serum transferrin receptor (TfR) levels are slightly enhanced [69, 71, 72].

3.1 Anemia of inflammation

Anemia of inflammation is an intricate pattern of anemia encountered in critically ill patients. It is characterized by anemia with high ferritin levels and maintenance of iron stores in organs [73]. Role of hepcidin in development of anemia of inflammation has been explicated by Rivera et al. Stimulation of hepatocytes forms hepcidin, thus preventing absorption of iron due to internalization and destruction of ferroportin. Iron gets accumulated in the duodenal cells which are shed and recycling of iron is stopped as iron is trapped in macrophages. In other words anemia of inflammation can be defined as inappropriate preservation of iron in the milieu of anemia [73]. Nemeth et al have showed that hepcidin is imperatively linked to inflammatory cytokines [74] and increased production of hepcidin by hepatocytes is due to the action of IL-6. Hepcidin thus synthesized, negatively regulates intestinal iron absorption and macrophage iron release, thus leading to hypoferremia [74, 75]. This is consistent with clinical finding of hypoferremia soon after the onset of inflammation. Inflammation-induced hepcidin expression might account for iron sequestration within cells of the Reticulo-endothelial System (RES).Cytokines thus exert a pivotal role in the control of iron sequestration within cells of the RES. A direct inhibitory role for hepcidin on iron release by cells of the RES has been proposed but not proven [16]. A potential NF-κB-binding site has been identified in the promoter region of mouse hepcidin [11. Plasma ferritin is secreted from cells of the RES depending on the iron concentration within the cell. High ferritin levels in chronic inflammatory conditions result from the reduced uptake of iron into erythroid precursors, and may serve as an indicator of how much iron is being deposited within the RES [76].

3.2 Anemia of cancer

Anemia is a common occurrence in various malignant conditions. Anemia of cancer is referred to as anemia of inflammation when cause is not bleeding or bone marrow infiltration or chemotherapy. Tumor cells lead to the occurrence of anemia by either infiltrating into the bone marrow [64] or by destroying the erythroid progenitor cells by oxidant injury due to free radicals or by producing proinflammatory cytokines [65, 66]. Various neoplastic disorders like Hodgkin`s disease, lung and breast carcinoma are associated with anemia of cancer. As in chronic inflammatory disorders and infections, certain cancers release inflammatory cytokines. Role of hepcidin in pathogenesis of anemia by virtue of decreased iron release from macrophages and enterocytes as well as induction of its expression by IL-6 is well established [13, 74]. Hepcidin is up-regulated in multiple myeloma patients by both IL-6-dependent and IL-6-independent mechanisms and may play a role in the anemia of multiple myeloma [77]. Some recent reports indicate ectopic production of hepcidin by hepatic adenomas, where severe anemia of cancer was resolved after tumor resection [63, 78]. Besides invasion of cancer cells into bone marrow, the anemia of cancer worsens by chemotherapy and radiation that damage the bone marrow.

3.3 Human diseases related to altered hepcidin expression

In recent years anemia associated with various diseases has been specifically described in terms of hepcidin playing a key role in the pathogenesis. Hemochromatosis is one of the most important disease caused by iron dysregulation. Hemochromatosis is characterized by continued absorption of dietary iron despite adequate or raised iron stores, with the subsequent accumulation of iron in liver and other body tissues. Hereditary hemochromatosis (HH) is a condition resulting most commonly from mutation in HFE gene. Hemochromatosis protein (HFE) is an atypical major histocompability class I protein, located on chromosome 6 [79]. The hemochromatosis (HFE) gene related HH is characterized by an inappropriately increased iron absorption, which leads to iron accumulation in liver and pancreas. HFE emerges to be involved in the maintenance of body iron homeostasis. HFE controls and modulates hepcidin, though its exact role in assessing body iron is not very clear. Four main types of HH have been identified and remarkably, genes implicated encode for proteins involved in hepcidin synthesis and its interaction with ferroportin. Major mutation C282Y causes a conformational change of the HFE protein [80]. It is now well known that hepcidin controls iron homeostasis by diminishing cellular iron efflux by binding to the transmembrane iron exporter ferroportin on enterocytes and macrophages, thus disrupting the function of ferroportin and subsequently inducing its internalization [13, 81].

HFE is implicated in upstream modulation of the regulation of hepcidin expression as is suggested by incongruously low concentrations of hepcidin associated with mutations in HFE [77, 82]. Hepcidin concentrations in urine are negatively correlated with the severity of HH. It has been proposed that availability of hepcidin measurements in both urine and serum, may aid in strategic approach for the treatment [83].

A few other disorders associated with this type of anemia are thalassemia, Inflammatory Bowel Disease (IBD) like Crohn's disease and celiac disease, Chronic Kidney Disease (CKD), rheumatoid arthritis and atherosclerotic lesions like ischemic heart disease.

Iron overload due to blood transfusions or due to increased iron absorption lead to decrease in hepcidin. Murine models of human thalassemia, have also demonstrated decreased hepcidin mRNA expression [84]. On one hand the proinflammatory cytokines like IL-6 in particular have been observed to have a definitive role in pathogenesis anemias of IBD [85, 86] and rheumatoid arthritis [87]. IBD is characterized by interplay of inflammatory and cytotoxic mechanisms. On the other hand anemia of CKD is predominately driven by impaired erythropoietin production, its production being reduced by inflammation [88, 89] along with antiproliferative effects of accumulating uremic toxins [90]. Hepcidin production is affected by iron status of the body, presence of inflammation, anaemia, hypoxia and erythropoietin in CKD [91]. Also several studies have proposed protective effect of sustained iron depletion or mild iron deficiency against ischemic heart disease, referred to as "iron hypothesis" [92, 93, 94]. Increased retention of iron in macrophages by elevated hepcidin and reducing the mobilization of iron from macrophages within atherosclerotic plaque might aid in promoting the evolution of atherosclerotic plaque. Low levels of hepcidin might result in increased macrophage iron loads promoting uptake of lipids through stimulation of expression of the scavenger receptor-1 in macrophages [95]103] and causing lipid peroxidation, and evolution of foam cells. Interruption of iron acquisition and storage in plaque macrophages by iron restriction or iron chelation inhibit lesion initiation and progression [96, 97].

3.4 Future prospects of hepcidin

Application of hepcidin assay in urine as well as serum has paved way to various studies and its use hepcidin as a diagnostic and therapeutic tool. In the recent times knowledge on hepcidin, its role in physiological and clinic pathological states has grown tremendously. Molecular mechanisms of hepcidin activity amplified our understanding of the regulation of iron transport. In fact quantitative assays for serum and urinary hepcidin can lead to establish the role of hepcidin, as compared to common parameters, such as serum ferritin and transferring saturation [91].

Hepcidin analysis is being explored by researchers to establish its role with novel tools for differential diagnosis, therapeutic regimes and monitoring of disorders of iron metabolism in various disease conditions like hereditary hemochromatosis and anemia associated with chronic diseases. Role of hepcidin in the pathogenesis of anemia of CKD as well as its effect in resistance to erythropoeisis stimulating agents is well established [98]. The potential clinical benefits of hepcidin measurement are the improved assessment of functional iron status that can be used to assess erythropoietin response and efficacy of iron treatment in patients with chronic disease anemias. Since hepcidin inhibits intestinal iron absorption, need of oral or parentral iron supplementation can be in such patients can be reviewed by evaluation of hepcidin level. Possibility of exploiting hepcidin-lowering or enhancing agents may prove to be an effective strategy for curing the main consequences of hepcidinopathies, anemia or iron overload, respectively.

4. References

[1] Aisen P, Enns C, Wessling-Resnick M. Chemistry and biology of eukaryotic iron metabolism. Int J Biochem Cell Biol 2001; 33: 940-59.

[2] Fleming MD, Andrews NC. Mammalian iron transport: an unexpected link between metal homeostasis and host defense. J Lab Clin Med 1998; 132: 464-8.

[3] Fleming MD, Trenor CC III, Su MA, et al. Microcytic anaemia mice have a mutation in Nramp2, a candidate iron transporter gene. Nat Genet. 1997; 16: 383-6.

[4] Andrews NC. Metal transporters and disease. Curr Opin Chem Biol 2002; 6: 181-186.

[5] Andrews NC. Disorders of iron metabolism. N Engl J Med 1999; 341: 1986-95.

[6] Ganz T. Hepcidin and its role in regulating systemic iron metabolism. Hematology Am Soc Hematol Educ Program. 2006:507; 29-35.

[7] Park CH, Valore EV, Waring AJ, Ganz T. Hepcidin, a urinary antimicrobial peptide synthesized in the liver. J Biol Chem 2001; 276:7806-10.

[8] Nicolas G, Bennoubn M, Porteu A, Mativet S, Beaumont C, Grandchamp B, et al. Severe iron deficiency anemia in transgenic mice expressing liver hepcidin. PNAS 2002; 99: 4596-4601.

[9] Fleming RE, Sly WS. Hepcidin: a putative iron regulatory hormone relative to hereditary hemochromatosis and the anemia of chronic disease. Proc Natl Acad Sci USA 2001; 98:8160–2.

[10] Singh PK, Parsek MR, Greenberg EP, Welsh MJ. A component of innate immunity prevents bacterial biofilm development. Nature 2002; 417:552–5.

[11] Pigeon C, Llyin G, Courselaud B et al. A new mouse liver-specific gene, encoding a protein homologous to human antimicrobial peptide hepcidin, is over expressed during iron overload. J Biol Chem 2001; 276: 7811–9.
[12] Finch C. Regulators of iron balance in humans. Blood 1994; 84:1697–702.
[13] Nemeth E, Tuttle MS, Powelson J, Vaughn MB, Donovan A, Ward DM, Ganz T, Kaplan J. Hepcidin regulates cellular iron efflux by binding to ferroportin and inducing its internalization. Science 2004; 306: 2090–3.
[14] De Domenico I, Mc Vey Ward D, Kaplan J. Regulation of iron acquisition and storage: consequences for iron-linked disorders. Nat Rev Mol Cell Biol 2008; 9:72–81.
[15] Njajou OT, de Jong G, Berghuis B, Vaessen N, Snijders PJLM, Goossens JP, et al. Dominant hemochromatosis due to N144H mutation of SLC11A3: clinical and biological characteristics. Blood Cell Mol Dis 2002; 29:439-43.
[16] Nicolas G, Chauvet C, Viatte L, Danan JL, Bigard X, Devaux I, et al. The gene encoding the iron regulatory peptide hepcidin is regulated by anemia, hypoxia, and inflammation. J Clin Invest 2002; 110:1037-44.
[17] Peyssonnaux C, Zinkernagel AS, Datta V, Lauth X, Johnson RS, Nizet V. TLR4-dependent hepcidin expression by myeloid cells in response to bacterial pathogens. Blood 2006; 107:3727-32.
[18] Merle U, Fein E, Gehrke SG, Stremmel W, Kulaksiz H. The iron regulatory peptide hepcidin is expressed in the heart and regulated by hypoxia and inflammation. Endocrinology 2007; 148:2663-68.
[19] Bekri S, Gaul P, Anty R, Luciani N, Dahman M, Ramesh B, et al. Increased adipose tissue expression of hepcidin in severe obesity is independent from diabetes and NASH. Gastroenterol 2006; 131:788-96.
[20] Dallalio G, Law E, Means RT Jr. Hepcidin inhibits in vitro erythroid colony formation at reduced erythropoietin concentrations. Blood 2006; 107:2702–4.
[21] Krause A, Nietz S, Magert HJ, Schultz A, Forssmann WG, Schultz-Knappe P, et al. LEAP-1, a novel highly disulfide-bonded human peptide, exhibits antimicrobial activity. FEBS Lett 2000; 480:147-50.
[22] Pigeon C, Ilyin G, Courselaud B, Leroyer P, Turlin B, Brissot P, et al. A new mouse liver-specific gene, encoding a protein homologous to human antimicrobial peptide hepcidin, is over expressed during iron overload. J Biol Chem 2001; 276:7811-9.
[23] Nicolas G, Bennoun M, Devaux I, Beaumont C, Grandchamp B, Kahn A, Vaulont S. Lack of hepcidin gene expression and severe tissue iron overload in upstream stimulatory factor 2 (USF2) knockout mice. Proc Natl Acad Sci U S A. 2001; 98: 8780-5.
[24] Ganz T. Hepcidin in Iron Metabolism. Curr Opin Hematol 2004; 11: 251-4.
[25] Nemeth E, Valore EV, Territo M, et al. Hepcidin, a putative mediator of anemia of inflammation, is a type II acute-phase protein. Blood 2003; 101:2461–3.
[26] Hunter HN, Fulton DB, Ganz T, Vogel HJ. The solution structure of human hepcidin, a peptide hormone with antimicrobial activity that is involved in iron uptake and hereditary hemochromatosis. J Biol Chem 2002; 277:37597-603.

[27] Kemna EHJM, Tjalsma H, Podust VN, Swinkels DW. Mass spectrometry-based hepcidin measurements in serum and urine: analytical aspects and clinical implications. Clin Chem 2007; 53:620-8
[28] Ganz T. Hepcidin. A regulator of intestinal iron absorption and iron recycling by macrophages. Best Pract Res Clin Haematol 2005;18:171-82
[29] Rivera S, Nemeth E, Gabayan V, Lopez MA, Farshidi D, Ganz T. Synthetic hepcidin causes rapid dose-dependent hypoferremia and is concentrated in ferroportin-containing organs. Blood 2005; 106:2196-9.
[30] Nemeth E, Preza GC, Jung CL, Kaplan J, Waring AJ, Ganz T. The N-terminus of hepcidin is essential for its interaction with ferroportin: structure-function study. Blood 2006;107:328-33.
[31] Nicolas G, Bennoun M, Devaux I, Beaumont C, Kahn A, Vaulont S. Lack of hepcidin gene expression and severe tissue iron overload in upstream stimulatory factor 2 (USF2) knockout mice. PNAS 2001; 98: 8780-5.
[32] Murphy AT, Witcher DR, Luan P, et al. Quantitation of hepcidin from human and mouse serum using liquid chromatography tandem mass spectrometry. Blood (2007) 110:1048–1054.
[33] Murao N, Ishigai M, Yasuno H, Shimonaka Y, Aso Y. Simple and sensitive quantification of bioactive peptides in biological matrices using liquid chromatography/selected reaction monitoring mass spectrometry coupled with trichloroacetic acid clean-up. Rapid Commun Mass Spectrom 2007; 21:4033–8.
[34] Kemna E, Tjalsma H, Laarakkers C, Nemeth E, Willems H, Swinkels D. Novel urine hepcidin assay by mass spectrometry. Blood 2005;106:3268–70.
[35] Kulaksiz H, Theilig F, Bachmann S, Gehrke SG, Rost D, Janetzko A, Cetin Y, Stremmel W. The iron-regulatory peptide hormone hepcidin: expression and cellular localization in the mammalian kidney. J Endocrinol 2005; 184:361–70.
[36] Kemna EHJM, Tjalsma H, Podust VN, Swinkels DW. Mass spectrometry-based hepcidin measurements in serum and urine: analytical aspects and clinical implications. Clin Chem 2007; 53:620–28.
[37] Ganz T, Olbina G, Girelli D, Nemeth E, Westerman M. Immunoassay for human serum hepcidin. Blood 2008; 112: 4292–7.
[38] Pak M, Lopez MA, Gabayan V, Ganz T, Rivera S. Suppression of hepcidin during anemia requires erythropoietic activity. Blood 2006; 108: 3730–5.
[39] Nicolas G, Viatte L, Bennoun M, Beaumont C, Kahn A, Vaulont S. Hepcidin, a new iron regulatory peptide. Blood Cells Mol Dis 2002; 29:327–35.
[40] Kemna EHJM, Tjalsma H, Willems HL, Swinkels DW. Hepcidin: from discovery to differential diagnosis. Haematologica 2008; 93:90–7
[41] Erslev AJ. Anemia of chronic disease. In: Beutler E, Coller BS, Lichtman MA, Kipps TJ, Seligsohn U. Williams hematology. New York, NY: McGraw-Hill, 2001:481–6.
[42] Peyssonnaux C, Zinkernagel AS, Schuepbach RA, Rankin E, Vaulont S, Haase VH, Nizet V, Johnson RS.Regulation of iron homeostasis by the hypoxia-inducible transcription factors (HIFs). J Clin Invest 2007; 117:1926–32.
[43] Silvestri L, Pagani A, Camaschella C. Furin mediated release of soluble hemojuvelin: a new link between hypoxia and iron homeostasis. Blood 2008; 111:924–931

[44] Shike H, Lauth X, Westerman ME, Ostland VE, Carlberg JM, Van Olst JC et al. Bass hepcidin is a novel antimicrobial peptide induced by bacterial challenge. Eur J Biochem 2002; 269:2232-37.

[45] Tussing-Humphreys LM, Nemeth E, Fantuzzi G, Freels S, Guzman G, Holterman AL, et al. Elevated systemic hepcidin and iron depletion in obese premenopausal females. Obesity 2010; 18: 1449-56.

[46] Gangaidzo IT, Moyo VM, Mvundura E, Aggrey G, Murphree NL, Khumalo H et al. Association of pulmonary tuberculosis with increased dietary iron. J Infect Dis 2001;184: 936-9.

[47] Braun V, Killmann H. Bacterial solutions to the iron-supply problem. Trends Biochem Sci. 1999;24: 104-9.

[48] Collins HL. The role of iron in infections with intracellular bacteria. Immunol Lett. 2003; 85: 193-5.

[49] Jurado RL. Iron, infections, and anemia of inflammation. Clin Infect Dis. 1997; 25: 888-95.

[50] Marx JJ. Iron and infection: competition between host and microbes for a precious element. Best Pract Res Clin Haematol 2002; 15:411-26.

[51] Walker EM Jr, Walker SM. Effects of iron overload on the immune system.Ann. Clin Lab Sci 2000; 30: 354-65.

[52] Weiss G. Iron and immunity: a double-edged sword. Eur J Clin Investig 2002; 32(Suppl. 1): 70-8.

[53] Bogdan C. Nitric oxide and the regulation of gene expression. Trends Cell Biol 2001; 11: 66-75.

[54] Weiss G, Fuchs D, Hausen A, Reibnegger G, Werner ER, Werner-Felmayer G, et al. Iron modulates interferon-gamma effects in the human myelomonocytic cell line THP-1. Exp Hematol 1992; 20:605-10.

[55] Recalcati S, Pometta R, Levi S, Conte D, Cairo G. Response of monocyte iron regulatory protein activity to inflammation: abnormal behavior in genetic hemochromatosis. Blood 1998; 91: 2565-72.

[56] Weinberg ED. Modulation of intramacrophage iron metabolism during microbial cell invasion. Microbes Infect 2000; 2:85-9.

[57] Zwilling BS, Kuhn DE, Wikoff L, Brown D, Lafuse W. Role of iron in Nramp1-mediated inhibition of mycobacterial growth. Infect Immun 1999; 67:1386-92.

[58] Ganz T. Hepcidin, a key regulator of iron metabolism and mediator of anemia of inflammation. Blood 2003;102(3): 783-788

[59] Dey R, Datta SC Leishmanial glycosomes contain superoxide dismutase. Biochem J 1994; 301: 317–9.

[60] Zhang Y, Lathigra R, Garbe T, Catty D, Young D. Genetic analysis of superoxide dismutase, the 23 kilodalton antigen of mycobacterium tuberculosis. Mol Microbiol 1991; 5:381–91.

[61] Locke, A, Main, ER, Rosbach, DO. The copper and non-hemoglobinous iron contents of the blood serum in disease. J Clin Invest 1932; 11:527-42.

[62] Ludwiczek, S, Aigner, E, Theurl, I, Weiss, G. Cytokine-mediated regulation of iron transport in human monocytic cells. Blood 2003; 101:4148-54.

[63] Weinstein DA Loda MF, Wolfsdorf JI, Andrews NC. Inappropriate expression of hepcidin is associated with iron refractory anemia: implications for the anemia of chronic disease. Blood 2002; 100: 3776-81.

[64] Weiss G, Goodnough LT. Anemia of Chronic Disease. N Engl J Med 2005; 352(10): 1011-23.

[65] Weiss G. Pathogenesis and treatment of anaemia of chronic disease. Blood Rev 2002; 16:87-96.

[66] Means RT Jr. Recent developments in the anemia of chronic disease. Curr Hematol Rep 2003; 2:116-21.

[67] Laftah AH, Ramesh B, Simpson RJ, Solanky N, Bahram S, Schumann K, et al. Effect of hepcidin on intestinal iron absorption in mice. Blood 2004; 103: 3940-4.

[68] Papanikolaou G, Samuels ME, Ludwig EH, MacDonald ML, Franchini PL, Dubé MP et al. Mutations in HFE2 cause iron overload in chromosome 1q-linked juvenile hemochromatosis. Nat Genet 2004; 36:77- 82.

[69] Konjin A, Hershko C. The anaemia of inflammation and chronic disease, In Iron in Immunity, Cancer and Inflammation 1989; edited by Desousa M, Brock JH Chichester, Wiley and Sons pp 111−43.

[70] Cartwright GE. The anemia of chronic disorders. Semin Hematol 1966; 3: 351−68

[71] Means RT, Krantz SB. Progress in understanding the pathogenesis of the anemia of chronic disease. Blood 1992; 80: 1639−47.

[72] Kuiper-Kramer EP, Huisman CM, vanRaan J, vanEijk HG. Analytical and clinical implications of soluble transferrin receptor in serum. Eur J Clin Chem Clin Biochem 1996; 34: 645−9.

[73] Rivera S. Hepcidin is the principle mediator of anemia of inflammation. Presented at: annual meeting of the American College of Chest Physicians; October 31, 2005; Montreal, Quebec.

[74] Nemeth E, Rivera S, Gabayan V, Keller C, Taudorf S, Pedersen BK et al. IL-6 mediates hypoferremia of inflammation by inducing the synthesis of the iron regulatory hormone hepcidin. J Clin Invest 2004; 113:1271-6.

[75] Andrews NC. Anemia of inflammation: the cytokine-hepcidin link. J Clin Invest 2004; 113(9): 1251-3.

[76] Cavill I. Iron and erythropoietin in renal disease. Nephrol Dial Transplant 2002; 17 [Suppl 5]: 19–23.

[77] Bridle KR, Frazer DM, Wilkins SJ, Dixon JL, Purdie DM, Crawford DH, et al. Disrupted hepcidin regulation in HFE-associated haemochromatosis and the liver as a regulator of body iron homeostasis. Lancet 2003; 361:669-73.

[78] Chung AYF, Leo KW, Wong GC, Chuah KL, Ren JW, Lee CGL. Giant hepatocellular adenoma presenting with chronic iron deficiency anemia. Am J Gastroenterol 2006; 101: 2160–2.

[79] Simon M, Bourel M, Genetet B, Fauchet R. Idiopathic hemochromatosis: demonstration of recessive transmission and early detection by family HLA typing. N Engl J Med 1977; 297:1017-21.

[80] Lyon E, Frank EL. Hereditary hemochromatosis since discovery of the HFE gene. Clin Chem 2001; 47:1147-56.

[81] De Domenico I, Ward DM, Nemeth E, Vaughn MB, Musci G, Ganz T, et al. The molecular basis of ferroportin-linked hemochromatosis. Proc Natl Acad Sci U S A 2005; 102:8955-60.

[82] Nicolas G, Viatte L, Lou DQ, Bennoun M, Beaumont C, Kahn A, et al. Constitutive hepcidin expression prevents iron overload in a mouse model of hemochromatosis. Nat Genet 2003; 34:97-101.

[83] Swinkels DW, Janssen MCH, Bergmans J, Marx JJM. Hereditary Hemochromatosis: Genetic Complexity and New Diagnostic Approaches. Clin Chem 2006; 52: 950-68.

[84] Adamsky K, Weizer O, Amariglio N, Harmelin A, Rivella S, Rachmilewitz E et al. Decreased hepcidin mRNA expression in thalassemic mice. Br J Haematol 2004; 124: 123-24.

[85] Arnold J, Sangwaiya A, Bhatkal B, Geoghegan F, Busbridge M. Hepcidin and inflammatory bowel disease: dual role in host defence and iron homoeostasis. Eur J Gastroenterol Hepatol 2009 ; 21(4):425-9.

[86] Bergamaschi G, Sabatino A, Albertini R, Ardizzone S, Biancheri P, Bonetti E et al. Prevalence and pathogenesis of anemia in inflammatory bowel disease. Influence of anti-tumor necrosis factor- treatment. Haematologica 2010; 95: 199-205.

[87] Murakami M, Nishimoto N. The value of blocking IL-6 outside of rheumatoid arthritis: current perspective. Curr Opin Rheumatol 2011;23(3):273-7.

[88] Barany P, Divino Filho JC, Bergstrom J. High C-reactive protein is a strong predictor of resistance to erythropoietin in hemodialysis patients. Am J Kid Dis 1997; 29(4): 565–8.

[89] Cooper AC, Mikhail A, Lethbridge MW, Kemeny DM, MacDougall IC. Increased expression of erythropoiesis inhibiting cytokines (IFN-gamma, TNF-alpha, IL-10, and IL-13) by T cells in patients exhibiting a poor response to erythropoietin therapy. J Am Soc Nephrol 2003; 14(7):1776-84.

[90] Eschbach JW. Anemia management in chronic kidney disease: role of factors affecting epoetin responsiveness. J Am Soc Nephrol 2002; 13:1412-4.

[91] Swinkels DW, Wetzels JFM. Hepcidin: a new tool in the management of anaemia in patients with chronic kidney disease? Nephrol Dial Transplant 2008; 23(8): 2450-53.

[92] Sullivan JL. Iron and the sex difference in heart disease risk. Lancet 1981; 13; 1(8233):1293-4.

[93] Sullivan JL. The iron paradigm of ischemic heart disease. Am Heart J 1989; 117: 1177–88.

[94] Sullivan JL. Stored iron and vascular reactivity. Arterioscler Thromb Vasc Biol 2005; 25:1532–5.

[95] Kraml PJ, Klein RL, Huang Y, Nareika A, Lopes-Virella MF. Iron loading increases cholesterol accumulation and macrophage scavenger receptor I expression in THP-1 mononuclear phagocytes. Metabolism 2005; 54:453–9.

[96] Minqin R, Rajendran R, Pan N, Kwong-Huat TB, Ong WY, Watt F et al. The iron chelator desferrioxamine inhibits atherosclerotic lesion development and decreases

lesion iron concentrations in the cholesterol-fed rabbit. Free Radic Biol Med 2005; 38:1206–11.
[97] Lee TS, Shiao MS, Pan CC, Chau LY. Iron-deficient diet reduces atherosclerotic lesions in apoE-deficient mice. Circulation 1999; 99: 1222–29.
[98] Young B, Zaritsky J. Hepcidin for Clinicians. Clin J Am Soc Nephrol 2009; 4: 1384-87

Section 5

Iron Metabolism in Pathogens

6

Iron Metabolism in Pathogenic Trypanosomes

Bruno Manta, Luciana Fleitas and Marcelo Comini
Group Redox Biology of Trypanosomes,
Institut Pasteur de Montevideo,
Uruguay

1. Introduction

1.1 Unique features, evolution and life cycle of trypanosomes

Trypanosomatids comprise a large group of flagellated unicellular protists with free-living and parasitic lifestyles. Several members of this family are widely known for being vertebrate pathogens of biomedical and veterinary importance. They belong to the order *Kinetoplastida,* which together with the groups *Diplonemida* (deep-see organisms) and *Euglenida* (photosynthetizing organisms) form the phylum Euglenozoa (Simpson *et al.*, 2006; Roger & Simpson, 2009). Kinetoplastids represent one of the most ancient eukaryotic lineages that diverged after the acquisition of the mitochondrion and share unique biochemical and subcellular features including the nuclear and mitochondrial gene expression mechanism, the energy and thiol redox metabolism and the organization of the mitochondrial DNA, named kinetoplast, and the compartmentalization of the almost entire glycolytic pathway in a peroxisome-like organelle called the glycosome. Phylogenetic studies support the theory that hemoflagellate trypanosomes evolved from a free-living bodonid that subsequently became an insect parasite, which later gained capacity to adapt to mammalian hosts (Adl *et al.*, 2005, 2007; Hamilton *et al.*, 2004; Simpson *et al.*, 2002). An early split of the genus *Leishmania* from the trypanosome taxon together with the existence of two well-defined clades within the genus *Trypanosoma* (the "*brucei*" clade and the "*cruzi*" clade) are strong evidences that the different lineages of pathogenic trypanosomes have evolved independently. Although they share a common ancestor, trypanosomes from the "*brucei*" and "*cruzi*" clades evolved and are geographically confined to the African and New World (South-America and Oceania) continents, respectively. In contrast to members from the "*cruzi*" clade, several lines of evidence indicate that African trypanosomes co-evolved with their mammalian hosts and insect vectors (Hamilton *et al.*, 2007; Maslov *et al.*, 1996; Stevens *et al.*, 1998; Stevens *et al.*, 2001). Parasitic trypanosomes are naturally transmitted by arthropods, *e.g.* tsetse fly for *T. brucei*, kissing bug for *T. cruzi*, and sand fly for *Leishmania* spp. (Fig. 1). Occasionally, bats can also act as vector agents (Dávila & Silva, 2000) and, more recently, rats and ticks are discussed as potentially involved in transmission of *T. cruzi* and *Leishmania* parasites to mammals (Herrera & Urdaneta-Morales, 2001; Colombo et al, 2011; Dantas-Torres, 2011). The natural infectious cycle of these parasites is initiated when non-dividing infective trypanosomes (metacyclic stage) are mechanically introduced in the mammal *via* insect bites or by involuntary deposition of infected feces from insects in the mucosa or injured dermis of mammals. Depending on the trypanosomatid species, parasites can reside in the host dermis (*L. major*), infect mucosa (*L. brasilienzis* and *L. amazoniensis*) or internal tissues/organs (*T. cruzi, L. donovani* and *L. infantum*) or remain in the extracellular fluids (*i. e., T. brucei* ssp.). Inside the mammal hosts, parasites shuttle between proliferative and non-proliferative forms. Indeed, the non-proliferative stages play an important role in the perpetuation of the life cycle since they are pre-adapted to survive in the poikilothermic arthropod (Comini *et al.*, 2011). They are taken up during insect blood meal of an infected host and further differentiate to dividing forms. The transformation to the quiescent infective stages occurs in the gut (*T. cruzi*) or salivary glands (*T. brucei* and *Leishmania* spp.) of the invertebrate. Trypanosomes undergo important metabolic and morphological changes to adapt to the growth conditions imposed by the different hosts and environments (extracellular medium and cell tissues) they inhabit. Fine tuning of energy metabolism, organelle reorganization and dedicated nutrient uptake are some of the mechanisms the parasite exploits to survive in the human host, as will be discussed below.

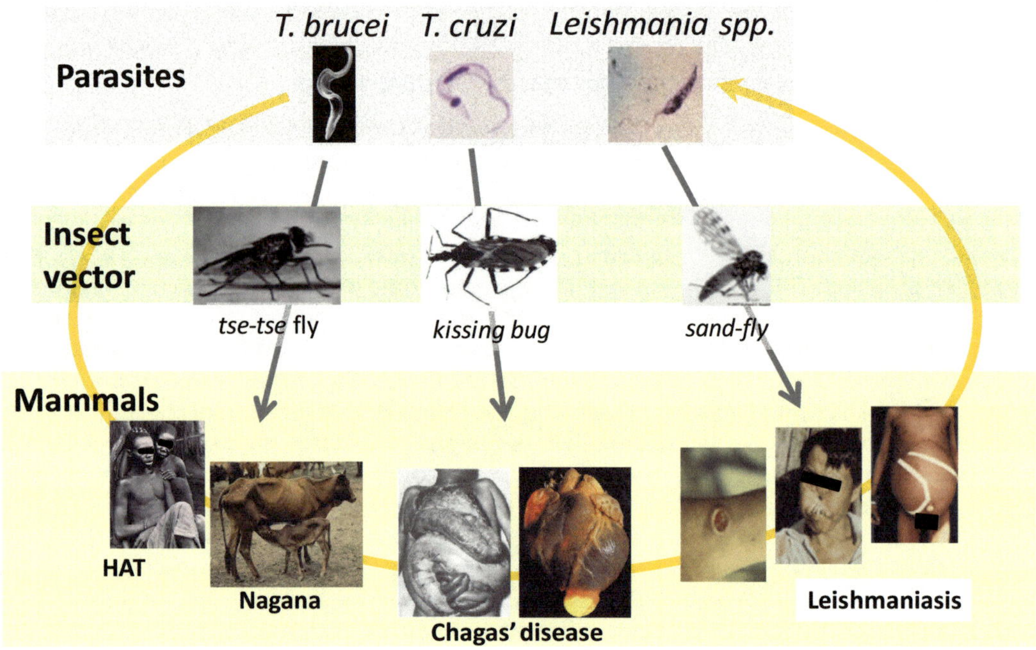

Fig. 1. Life cycle and diseases caused by trypanosomatids.
The genus *Trypanosoma* and *Leishmania* include species that are pathogenic for mammals. The natural cycle of these parasites involves their transmition by different but specific arthropods (insect vectors). Inside the host each species exhibit a peculiar tropism for different tissues, organs and systems resulting in different pathologies. For instance, *T. brucei* is an extracellar parasite that resides in the host´s bloodstream and cerebrospinal fluid; different strains of *T. cruzi* invade cardiomiocytes or nervous tissue from the digestive system; depending on the *Leishmania* species, the parasites invade the dermis, mucosa or internal organs (e. g., spleen). The diseases associated with infection are devastating and fatal if left untreated. Human pathogens from the "*brucei*" complex (*T. b. rodhesiense* and *T. b. gambiense*) cause sleeping sickness or human African trypanosomiasis (HAT; see section1); *T. b. brucei* produces nagana disease of cattle; *T. cruzi* is the ethiologic agent of Chagas disease in Latin-America; *L. infantum* and *L. donovani* produces visceral leishmaniasis, *L. major* and *L. amazonensis* causes cutaneous leishmaniasis, and *L. brasiliensis* is responsible for

a mucocutaneous infection. During their life cycle, the parasites undergo important biochemical and ultrastructural remodeling to adapt to the different hosts.The cycle is closed when insect feeds on infected mammals.

1.2 Trypanosomiasis: Disease, burden and treatment

Different members of the Trypanosomatida family are etiologic agents of highly disabling and often fatal diseases of humans and livestock (see Fig. 1). With respect to the parasites that are the major focus of this chapter, members from the *T. brucei* complex are transmitted by tsetse flies of the genus *Glossina* spp., which is found exclusively in equatorial Africa. The human pathogens *T. b. gambiense* and *T. b. rodhesiense* differ in their geographical distribution with the first subspecies being endemic of west and central regions while the last is mainly present in east and southern Africa (Barrett *et al.*, 2003).

HAT present two main clinical phases with compromise of the hematolymphatic system (acute phase) and the central nervous system (CNS, chronic phase). The *T. b. rhodesiense* infection develops rapidly as an acute disease that is characterized by a high parasite load, severe anemia and thrombocytopenia accompanied by hypertrophy of the reticuloendothelial system. If untreated, the pathology evolves to a pancarditis with congestive heart failure, pulmonary edema and physiological collapse (Barrett *et al.*, 2003). Due to this fast and lethal development, along with the limited sanitary conditions of endemic regions, HAT caused by *T. b. rhodesiense* is usually under-diagnosed explaining - at least partly - why 90% of the reported cases of African sleeping sickness are ascribed to *T. b. gambiense (*Birkholtz *et al.*, 2011). In contrast, HAT produced by *T. b. gambiense* displays a more discrete development without characteristic symptoms in the early phase, unless the patient develops a generalized lymphadenopathy, which hinders an accurate diagnosis. The second stage of HAT starts when the parasites invade internal organs, including the CNS. For *T. b. rhodesiense* and *T. b. gambiense* this phenomena can take place within few weeks and up to years upon infection, respectively. Invasion of the CNS by the parasite is typically accompanied by intense headache, sleeping disorders and mental dysfunction, leading to a comatose state and sudden death (Barrett *et al.*, 2003). The differential pathogenicity and clinical manifestations of both diseases have been formerly explained on the basis of mutual host-parasite adaptations that shaped pathogen virulence and host resistance during evolution (Fèvre *et al.*, 2006). However, the hypothesis of a co-evolutionary virulence attenuation of *T. b. gambiense* has recently been challenged by studies on phylogenetic relationships within the *T. brucei* taxon (Balmer *et al.*, 2011).

The World Health Organization (WHO) estimates that sixty million people are at risk of infection as a consequence of at least 300 separate active foci in 36 African countries (Jacobs *et al.*, 2011), most of them in rural areas of extreme poverty. Around 300,000 people are currently infected with trypanosomes and 48,000 of them dye per year (Cavalli & Bolognesi, 2009). The lack of local human and financial resources combined with the burden of conflicts in most of the endemic countries impedes to achieve full control of HAT (Cavalli & Bolognesi, 2009). However, after continued control programs spanning vector eradication, early diagnosis and treatment, and surveillance (Barrett *et al.*, 2003; Cavalli, 2009) the number of annual infections fell almost 5- to 7-fold in the last three decades[1]. Unfortunately, this progress is not

[1] http://www.who.int/mediacentre/factsheets/fs259/en/

accompanied by the development of new chemotherapeutic options (see below) and is endangered by the increasing drug resistance of the naturally circulating strains of *T. brucei* ssp. (Cavalli & Bolognesi, 2009; Delespaux & de Koning, 2007; Jacobs *et al.*, 2011; Matovu *et al.*, 2001). In addition to HAT, animal trypanosomiasis represents a major problem for the agricultural and nutritional development of endemic regions. About ten million square kilometers of arable land are infested by tsetse flies (Matovu *et al.*, 2001) capable of transmitting *T. b. brucei, T. congolense* and *T. vivax* (Nagana-disease) or *T. evansi* (Surra-disease) between domestic and wild (reservoirs) animals. For Africa, the total economic losses due to animal trypanosomiasis are estimated to be US$ 4.75 billion per year[2]. The recent detection of members from the "*brucei*" clade in countries from Asia, Central- and South-America should raise alarm considering the serious threat these pathogens entails for the well-developed agricultural economies of these regions (Luckins & Dwinger, 2004; Batista *et al.*, 2007, 2009; Da Silva *et al.*, 2011; Dávila & Silva, 2000; Mekata *et al.*, 2009).

Confronted with the lack of prospect for vaccine development against trypanosomiasis, chemotherapy remains as the only short- and mid-term therapeutic choice for these diseases. Nevertheless, the few drugs currently available against HAT (acute phase: pentamidine and suramine, chronic phase: melarsoprol and efluornithine[3]) are far from optimal: most of them were originally developed for veterinary use, lacking safety compliance, and present a limited efficacy against late-stage disease (Steverding, 2010). An additional drawback associated with the inappropriate use of these drugs lies on the emergence of resistance. Unfortunately, pharmaceutical companies are less prone to engage and invest in drug discovery and development against diseases that affect the world´s poorest people (Barrett *et al.*, 2003; Cavalli & Bolognesi, 2009; Matovu *et al.*, 2001). However, in the last years, scientists, policy-makers and non-profit institutions (WHO, TDR, Médecins Sans Frontieres, FioCruz Institute, **D**rugs for **N**eglected **D**isease **i**nitiative), together with a few pharmaceutical companies (Glaxo SmithKline®, Bayer®), have joined efforts to improve this situation. As mentioned above, trypanosomes present several unique biochemical and biological features that can be exploited for the development of specific therapies. These include several organelles (glycosomes, acidocalcisomes, kinetoplast) that are absent in the mammalian host, and metabolic pathways and cellular functions that differ significantly from host counterparts, namely carbohydrate metabolism, protein and lipid modification, thiol-redox metabolism, cell cycle, programmed cell death, etc. (Naula & Burchmore, 2003). Despite the obvious indispensability of iron for pathogenic trypanosomatids, the mechanisms and components comprising the uptake, storage and usage of this metal have been poorly investigated. In the next sections will be reviewed the state-of-the-art regarding iron-homeostasis and metabolism in African trypanosomes.

2. Iron acquisition and homeostasis

Owing the extracellular and parasitic lifestyle of African trypanosomes, it deems important to comment first on the mechanisms and components controlling iron homeostasis in the human host. Dietary ferric iron (Fe^{3+}) is reduced to its ferrous form (Fe^{2+}) by a ferrireductase

[2] Amounts in terms of agricultural Gross Domestic Product, data taken from:
http://www.fao.org/ag/againfo/programmes/en/paat/disease.html

[3] It must be noted that efluornithine is active only against *T. b. gambiense* but not *T. b. rodhesiense* (Cavalli & Bolognesi, 2009; Jacobs *et al.*, 2011; Matovu *et al.*, 2001).

present in the membrane of enterocytes, and then incorporated *via* a divalent metal transporter. Cytosolic iron is exported to the circulation from the basolateral membrane of enterocytes through ferroportin with the concomitant reoxidation to Fe^{3+} by the multicopper oxidase hephaestin (Kosman, 2010). Iron circulates in plasma bound to the glycoprotein transferrin (Tf), which is internalized by cells *via* a specific transferrin receptor (TfR1) in a clathrin-dependent mechanism. In the acidic environment of the endosome Tf, iron and TfR1 disassemble. Apo-Tf is released to circulation whereas TfR1 is recycled back to the membrane. Fe^{3+} is exported from the late endosomal vesicle through the concerted action of transporters and metalloreductases (Hentze *et al.*, 2010; Kurz *et al.*, 2011). How this "labile iron pool" (LIP, Hider & Kong, 2011; Kakhlon & Cabantchik, 2002) is trafficked within the cell remains poorly understood (Hentze *et al.*, 2010; Anderson & Vulpe, 2009; Atanasiu *et al.*, 2007; Hentze *et al.*, 2010; Subramanian *et al.*, 2011). Other major source of iron comprises the recycling of heme-iron from senescent erythrocytes, a task carried out by specialized macrophages of the reticuloendothelial system known as Kupffer cells (Anderson & Vulpe, 2009; Schultz *et al.*, 2010). The liver is both the major site for iron storage and also the central metabolic regulator. Induced by different stimuli -from iron availability to inflammatory stresses- (Zhang & Enns, 2009), hepatocytes produce and secrete a 25-aminoacid hormone, hepcidin (Atanasiu *et al.*, 2007), which regulates the levels of systemic iron by a negative-loop mechanism that involves ferroportin turnover. Intracellular iron homeostasis is regulated post-transcriptionally by the iron regulatory protein 1 (IRP1, see section 3.3.3.1). The vast majority of iron is dedicated to hemoglobin or myglobin synthesis, but also the biogenesis of iron-sulfur (Fe/S) proteins demands this metal. Both processes occur mostly in the mitochondria, representing the main subcellular compartment for iron utilization (Levi & Rovida, 2009). Iron is stored bound to ferritin heteropolymers, which can hold up to 4500 Fe^{3+} atoms (Andrews, 2010). Heme-iron is also essential in mammalian physiology (see section 4) but it poses an independent mechanism of absorption that remains mostly unsolved (Schultz *et al.*, 2010). As envisaged, iron homeostasis is tightly controlled at several levels -from absorption to mobilization and utilization- and in an interdependent manner in humans.

Iron is an essential element also for *T. brucei*, therefore the parasite has developed exceptional mechanisms to guarantee metal supply from a host that (un)intentionally limits metal availability in response to infection (see section 5). For example, iron-deficiency induced by ferritin upregulation and reduction of iron-transferrin saturation is a classical immune-based response mounted during the acute phase of the infection to limit parasite proliferation (Chisi *et al.*, 2004). Also the chronic stage is accompanied by a notorious iron deprivation (*e.g.* anemia, see section 5) but, in this case, its origin is a chronic inflammatory disorder involving macrophage hyperactivation along with iron accumulation within the reticuloendothelial system (Stijlemans *et al.*, 2008). In the bloodstream, trypanosomes acquire the metal[4] *via* a high affinity receptor-mediated endocytosis of iron-loaded Tf (see Fig. 2; Grab *et al.*, 1992, 1993; Steverding *et al.*, 1995). The trypanosomal Tf receptor (TfR) was identified as a heterodimeric complex of proteins encoded by the expression-site-associated-gene (ESAG) 6 and ESAG 7 (Salmon *et al.*, 1994; Steverding *et al.*, 1995). ESAG 6 and 7 are truncated forms of variable surface glycoproteins (VSG) that lack the C-terminal domain, and, in the case of ESAG 7, the glycophosphatidylinositol (GPI) anchor. Under normal growth

[4] The incorporation of heme-bound iron is discussed in section 4.

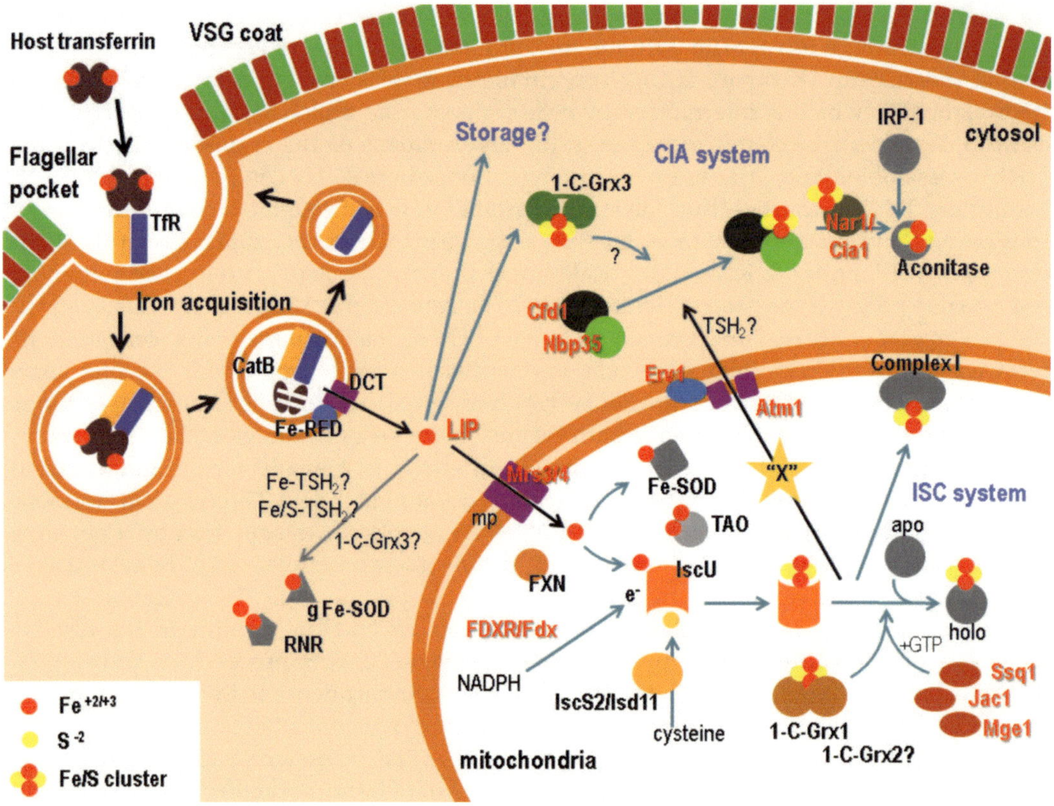

Fig. 2. Working model for iron acquisition and utilization in *Trypanosoma brucei*.
Iron is incorporated from the host bloodstream through receptor (TfR) mediated internalization of loaded transferrin (Tf, upper left) at the flagellar pocket. In the late endosomes, Tf is degraded by a cathepsin B-like protease (CatB) and iron is released to the cytosol through the concerted action of a ferric reductase (Fe-RED) and a divalent cation transporter (DCT). Once in the cytosol iron is complexed to low molecular mass ligands forming the labile iron pool (LIP, see section 2) that probably fuels the synthesis of iron-dependent enzymes like the glycosomal superoxide dismutase (gFe-SOD) or ribonucleotide reductase (RNR), and the biogenesis of cytosolic Fe/S clusters (CIA system, section 3.3.1). Mitochondrial Fe/S cluster biogenesis depends on iron imported in a membrane-potential dependent (mp) fashion at expenses of the inner membrane carriers Mrs3/4. Mitochondrial iron is either incorporated to iron-centered enzymes (*e.g.* Fe-SOD and trypanosomal alternative oxidase, TAO) or participates in Fe/S cluster biogenesis (ISC system, see section 3.3.1.2). Black letters refer to proteins that have been reported in *T. brucei* and red letters denote components of the iron- and Fe/S cluster metabolism not yet identified in trypanosomes but with essential functions in yeast or mammals. CIA proteins are depicted in green tones, ISC proteins in orange-brown tones, membrane transporters in purple and Fe or Fe/S cluster receiving proteins in grey. Fe and sulfur atoms are shown as red and yellow spheres, respectively. Scheme based in Lill & Mühlenhoff, 2008; Hentze *et al.*, 2010 and Taylor & Kelly, 2010.

conditions the TfR localizes at the flagellar pocket wherefrom bound-transferrin is internalized and proteolyticaly degraded in the endolysosome by a cathepsin-B like protease (O'Brien *et al.*, 2008; Mussmann *et al.*, 2003), which finally releases iron. The relevance of the endocytic pathway as the sole source of iron for the parasite was demonstrated using antibodies anti-TfR that inhibited growth of *T. brucei in vitro* (Grab *et al.*, 1992). Expression of TfR in the parasite is regulated by iron availability and post-transcriptional control that does not involve the IRE/IRP1 system typical for mammals (Fast *et al.*, 1999). Iron starvation induced by iron chelators or species-specific transferrins lead to a 3- to 10-fold upregulation in the expression of TfR with a concomitant redistribution of the receptor from the flagellar pocket to the entire parasite surface (Fast *et al.*, 1999; Mussmann *et al.*, 2004). This, together with the rapid recycling of TfR (Kabiri & Steverding, 2000) and gene-specific (in)activation events (van Luenen *et al.*, 2004) allows trypanosomes to efficiently compete for limiting substrate and withstand iron-deprivation until a new set of higher affinity TfR is expressed. For instance, sequence polymorphisms in ESAG 6 and 7 were proposed to determine the affinities of TfR for transferrins from different mammalian species (Bitter *et al.*, 1998) permitting for a rapid adaptation of the parasite to distinct hosts. It was also suggested that the TfR repertoire may allow the parasite to overcome anti-TfR antibody response by the host (Gerrits *et al.*, 2002). However, estimations and studies by Steverding (1998, 2003, 2006) disproved this hypothesis and supported the view that high affinity TfRs were evolutionary selected to enable the parasite to cope with the diversity of mammalian transferrins (Steverding, 2003, 2006).

In the aerobic and buffered milieu of the cytosol iron is never free, mostly because it can readily produce highly toxic oxygen species through Fenton chemistry (see section 3.2.2), but also because the ferric form tends to form insoluble hydroxides. The cellular labile or chelatable iron pool is defined as the intracellular pool of redox-active iron that is not associated with proteins. LIP comprises ~ 5 % of the total cellular iron and consist of Fe^{2+} and Fe^{3+} associated with a diverse population of low molecular mass ligands such as organic anions (phosphate, citrate, inositol phosphate, etc.), polypeptides such as glutathione (GSH) and/or components of membranes (phospholipids, etc; Kakhlon & Cabantchik, 2002). Whether this percentage represents the situation in trypanosomes is unknown. The nature of the ligand(s) can vary between cells and among different physiological states but recent reports support the notion that intracellular GSH (2-5 mM) is the most relevant low molecular mass complexing agent in most GSH-dependent organisms (Hider & Kong, 2011; Kumar *et al.*, 2011; Mühlenhoff *et al.*, 2010; Overath *et al.*, 1986). The nature of this LIP in trypanosomes was never assessed and it is worthy to speculate that trypanothione ($T(SH)_2$, see below), and not GSH, will be the relevant physiological ligand. Beyond that $T(SH)_2$ is the most abundant intracellular low molecular mass thiol in trypanosomes (Krauth-Siegel & Comini, 2008), our working model is supported by experimental evidences showing the formation of $T(SH)_2$-Fe and $T(SH)_2$-Fe/S complexes *in vitro* (Ceylan *et al.* 2010; Manta *et al.*, unpublished, Fig. 2) and by the extensive documentation showing that most thiol-dependent functions in these organisms evolved to use $T(SH)_2$ and not GSH as cofactor (reviewed in Irigoín *et al.*, 2008; Krauth-Siegel and Comini, 2008). How iron enters and exits the LIP and which are the proteins involved in this process remain as open questions. Recent studies propose a link between the LIP and Fe/S protein metabolism by means of a mechanism that involves Fe/S clusters as signalling molecule and cytosolic monothiol glutaredoxins as mediators (see section 3.2.1; Kumar *et al.*, 2011; Mühlenhoff *et al.*, 2010). In fact, the nature of monothiol glutaredoxins (*i.e.* iron-sulfur proteins that use GSH as ligand cofactor for Fe/S cluster assembly) make these proteins exceptional candidates for the integration of the cellular iron and Fe/S cluster status with thiol redox status, and as signal transducer regulating iron uptake and utilization (Mühlenhoff *et al.*, 2010; Rodriguez-Manzaneque *et al.*, 2002; Rouhier *et al.*, 2010; Ye *et al.*, 2010). Another important form of "low-molecular mass" iron species are the dinitrosyl iron complexes (DNIC, Bosworth *et al.*, 2009) formed between LIP and low molecular mass thiols when nitric oxide is present (Vanin, 2009). This point is addressed in the next section.

3. Cellular fates of Iron

Iron is an important redox or structural cofactor of several indispensable proteins of trypanosomes. For instance, DNA synthesis, protein translation, oxidant defense and cytochrome respiration are important cellular functions that involve the utilization of this metal (Taylor & Kelly, 2010).

In this section we will review the most relevant iron-related molecules and metabolic pathways of bloodstream *T. brucei*. Whenever possible, the components and mechanisms employed by the parasite to incorporate different forms of iron onto target molecules will be described. Taking advantage of the recent availability of genome sequencing data for the most representative species of *Trypanosoma* (Berriman *et al.*, 2005; El-Sayed *et al.*, 2005; Ivens *et al.*, 2005) and the current knowledge of the iron metabolism in model eukaryotes (Hentze *et al.*, 2010), we here provide a state-of-the-art view of iron metabolism in African trypanosomes.

3.1 Dinitrosyl iron complexes

Parasites circulating in host´s bloodstream or inside the phagolysosome of activated macrophages are exposed to reactive oxygen and nitrogen species. In both cases, the second messenger nitric oxide (•NO) is produced by endothelial or immune cells, which, if not neutralized rapidly, can lead to the formation of the highly reactive oxidant peroxynitrite (Girard *et al.*, 2005). The effect of •NO and derivatives was studied in *T. brucei* (Lu *et al.*, 2011; Steverding *et al.*, 2009; Vincendeau *et al.*, 1992) and *T. cruzi* (Piacenza *et al.*, 2007; Alvarez *et al.*, 2011 and see papers quoted in Irigoín *et al.*, 2008). A recent work by Bocedi *et al.* (2010) demonstrated the formation *in vitro* of a DNIC involving the parasite specific dithiol $T(SH)_2$. Based on the high intracellular concentration of $T(SH)_2$ the authors proposed that formation of this complex may play an important role in trapping •NO and, thus, preventing the formation of dangerous oxidants. This work raises the possibility for a new potential link between iron and low-molecular mass thiols in trypanosomes.

3.2 Mononuclear iron proteins

Mononuclear iron proteins can be classified according to their biological function, by Fe centre type, by type and number of prosthetic centres, and by sequence similarity. The iron atom is usually coordinated by thiolate groups (deprotonated form of cysteine), or the Nδ atoms of histidines or the carboxylate anions of acidic residues present in the polypeptide. In these proteins the iron provides redox activity and the surrounding aminoacidic and structural environment confer the specificity for different substrates. The characteristics and functions of a number of iron-centered proteins from trypanosomatids are addressed below.

3.2.1 Energy metabolism: Alternative oxidase

The bloodstream form of the parasite lacks cytochrome activity yet they "respirate" at high rates (Priest & Hajduk, 1994). The molecular entity responsible for this is a plant-like mitochondrial ubiquinol oxidase (EC 1.10.3.10), known as trypanosomal alternative oxidase (TAO; Clarkson *et al.*, 1989). The enzyme is imported into the mitochondrion of bloodstream and procyclic parasites by distinct mechanisms involving external ATP supply and inner membrane potential, respectively (Williams *et al.*, 2008). It localizes at the outer membrane of the organelle where it transfers electrons from ubiquinol to oxygen without proton translocation or ATP generation (Chaudhuri *et al.*, 2006), resulting in the reoxidation of NADPH produced during glycolysis. TAO genes have been identified in the genome of all the subspecies forming the "*brucei*" clade but are absent in related trypanosomatids such as *Leishmania* spp. or *T. cruzi* (Chaudhuri *et al.*, 2006; Nakamura *et al.*, 2010). In agreement with its metabolic function (NADP/NAPDH-shunt during carbohydrate catabolism), TAO is developmentally regulated (Chaudhuri *et al.*, 2002) achieving ~100 times higher levels in bloodstream parasites than in procyclic cells (Tsuda *et al.*, 2005; Tyler *et al.*, 1997). The essential role of TAO in the physiology of infective *T. brucei* was recognized early using the iron chelator salicyl hydroxamic acid (2-hydroxybenzhydroxamic acid, SHAM) and glycerol to alter the metabolic output (Clarkson & Brohn, 1976; Grant & Sargent, 1960). On the other hand, recent studies show that TAO plays an important role in preventing oxidant-induced programmed cell death of long-slender bloodstream parasites (Tsuda *et al.*, 2005, 2006). This antioxidant function of TAO resembles that proposed for the orthologue enzyme from plants (Maxwell *et al.*, 1999). In trypanosomes, apoptosis is a highly regulated process deeply associated with the accumulation of quiescent parasite forms (short stumpy) in the preparation for transmission to the insect vector (Welburn *et al.*, 2006). It is therefore tempting to speculate that, at least in bloodstream trypanosomes, TAO might be an important checkpoint connecting metabolic status ($NADP^+$/NAPDH ratio) with programmed cell death and differentiation. In procyclic forms, TAO has been shown to compensate for a depletion of complex III or IV activities in the mitochondrial electron transfer chain (Horváth *et al.*, 2005). Despite this backup role in respiration, the enzyme appears to fulfill a yet unknown but essential function in this parasite stage (Tsuda *et al.*, 2005; Tyler *et al.*, 1997).

Although no structures are available for TAO or any other related alternative oxidase, current structural models (Moore & Albury, 2008) and proteomic data (Acestor *et al.*, 2009) indicate that it is an interfacial membrane protein that interacts with a single leaflet of the lipid bilayer, and contains a non-heme di-iron carboxylate center bounded by two highly conserved EXXH motifs (Kido *et al.*, 2010a, 2010b). The iron-dependence of TAO was established working *in vitro* with chelating agents and mutant forms of the protein (Ajayi *et al.*, 2002; Chaudhuri *et al.*, 1998).

3.2.2 Oxidant defense: Iron-dependent superoxide dismutases

Aerobic respiration produce partly reduced oxygen intermediates that leak from several protein complexes from the electron transport chain. The most important radical species formed is the anion superoxide ($O_2^{\bullet-}$), the one-electron reduction product of molecular oxygen. Superoxide can reduce or oxidize biological targets *in vivo*, or dismutate to the less reactive but highly diffusible oxidant hydrogen peroxide (Halliwel & Gutteridge, 1999). Despite hydrogen peroxide is biologically more toxic than $O_2^{\bullet-}$, active removal of this anion radical is necessary to prevent formation of the most reactive and harmful radical product, hydroxyl radical ($OH^{\bullet}$), which originates from a physiological reaction involving iron and known as Fenton reaction[5]. To accomplish this, all living organisms contain enzymes devoted to the $O_2^{\bullet-}$ dismutation, called superoxide dismutases (EC 1.15.1.1). There are three major families of SODs, depending on the metal cofactor. Most of the cytosolic eukaryotic SODs use a bimetallic active site with copper and zinc (CuZn-SODs) while the mitochondria harbor a bacterial-related Mg-dependent SOD. In prokaryotes and plastids most of the SODs are Fe-dependent (Abreu & Cabelli, 2010).

Trypanosomes express four different isoforms of SODs (Dufernez *et al.*, 2006; Kabiri & Steverding, 2001; Le Trant *et al.*, 1983; Wilkinson *et al.*, 2006) that, in contrast to homologues from prokaryotes and eukaryotes, show a restricted metal dependency all of them being Fe-dependent enzymes (Wilkinson *et al.*, 2006; Bachega *et al.*, 2009). In *T. brucei*, SOD-A and SOD-C localize at the mitochondrion whereas SOD-B1 and SOD-B2 are mostly compartmentalized within the glycosome and less abundantly at the cytosol (Dufernez at al., 2006). A similar localization was reported for SOD-B enzymes from *L. chagasi* (Plewes *et al.*, 2003). RNAi-mediated knockdown of SOD-A and SOD-C revealed that under normal growth conditions the mitochondrial isoforms are dispensable for bloodstream *T. brucei* (Prathalingham *et al.*, 2007; Wilkinson *et al.*, 2006). However, the biological importance of SOD-A was put in evidence when parasites depleted in this isoform showed a higher sensitivity towards paraquat, an $O_2^{\bullet-}$-generating compound (Wilkinson *et al.*, 2006). Consistent with a role in oxidant defense for mitochondrial Fe-SOD, transgenic *T. cruzi* overexpressing a mitochondrial isoform was found to be more resistant to fresh human serum, a death stimuli mediated by oxidative stress (Piacenza *et al.*, 2007). In contrast, the SOD B-type enzymes are indispensable for infective *T. brucei* grown under normal culture conditions (Wilkinson *et al.*, 2006), which poses the question to the glycosomal source of $O_2^{\bullet-}$, a charged molecule that does not diffuse through lipid membranes. In this respect, unwanted $O_2^{\bullet-}$ might leak as byproduct from a variety of metabolic activities occurring in this organelle, such as glycolysis, oxidation of fatty acids, lipid biosynthesis, and purine salvage (Michels *et al.*, 2006). Further dissection of the functional relevance of SOD-B isoforms was achieved by means of targeted gene replacement, which demonstrates that SOD-B1 and not SOD-B2 is critical to withstand exposure to nifurtimox and benznidazole (Prathalingham *et al.*, 2007), two anti-trypanosomal drugs whose mechanism of action involves the generation of reactive oxygen intermediates (Maya *et al.*, 2003 and 2007). Also the homologue isoforms present in *L. chagasi* and *L. tropica* were earlier reported to be important for parasite survival in mouse or human macrophages as well as under paraquat insult (Plewes *et al.*, 2003; Ghosh *et al.*, 2003). Interestingly, *T. brucei* SOD-B1 has been shown to be developmentally regulated with higher intracellular concentration in proliferating stages (Kabiri & Steverding, 2001). This particular expression pattern led the authors to propose that the role of SOD-B1 in dividing cells is to counteract the formation of superoxide radicals released during the generation of the iron-tyrosyl free-radical centre in the small subunit (R2) of ribonucleotide reductase, other iron-containing enzyme (see next section). Unexpectedly, a 5- to 8-fold increase in SOD-B1 activity in transgenic *T. cruzi* was accompanied by a significant sensitization of parasites against two pro-oxidant compounds namely gentian violet and benznidazole (Temperton *et al.*, 1998). This striking behavior was

[5] $H_2O_2 + O_2^{\bullet-} \xrightarrow{Fe^3} OH^- + OH^{\bullet} + O_2$

interpreted as a consequence of an imbalance in the redox homeostasis of the parasite resulting from the overexpression of Fe-SOD, a hypothesis that deserves further investigation.

In summary, trypanosomal SODs diverged from their human homologues by using iron as cofactor. They apparently evolved to protect parasites against toxic $O_2^{\bullet -}$ produced in the glycosomes and/or mitochondrion as a result of sudden changes in metabolism or originated from the different environment they live in (*e.g.*, insect midgut, macrophages, epithelium, mammal bloodstream).

3.2.3 Cell proliferation: Ribonucleotide reductase

Ribonucleotide reductase (RNR, EC 1.17.4.1-2) catalyses the reduction of ribonucleotides to deoxyribonucleotides needed for DNA synthesis. There are three different classes of RNR being class I the most abundant in eukaryote organisms. Class I RNR are heterotetrameric enzymes formed by the association of two related but not identical polypeptides known as subunit R1 and R2. The large R1 subunit binds substrates and allosteric effectors, conferring specificity and regulatory potential, while the small R2 subunit contains the catalytic center composed of two high spin Fe^{3+} atoms antiferromagnetically coupled to each other through a μ-oxo bridge, a highly conserved tyrosine residue and two cysteines (Cotruvo & Stubbe, 2011). The di-iron center generates a free radical on this catalytic tyrosine through electron donation. In a reaction involving several intermediate states, the tyrosine radical attacks the nucleotide resulting in reduction of the 2′-OH group of ribonucleoside and the formation of a disulfide. Regeneration of active RNR is finally achieved *via* reduction of this disulfide mainly by thioredoxin (Trx), which is subsequently reduced at expenses of NADPH (Cotruvo & Stubbe, 2011).

The biochemical information about parasite RNR is rather limited. Both subunits of RNR from *T. brucei* were cloned, expressed (Dormeyer *et al.*, 1997; Hofer *et al.*, 1997) and kinetically characterized (Hofer el al., 1998). The parasite-specific thioredoxin-like oxidoreductase tryparedoxin (TXN, Lüdemann *et al.*, 1998) and, in contrast to all other RNR from eukaryotes, also the low-molecular weight dithiol $T(SH)_2$ (Dormeyer *et al.*, 2001) but less likely glutaredoxins (Ceylan *et al.*, 2010) proved to be physiological reductants of recombinant RNR. The activity of the enzyme appears to be post-transcriptionally regulated by a redox mechanism (Dormeyer *et al.*, 2001) and by the selective expression of its catalytic subunit R2. For example, whereas the R1 protein is actively expressed throughout the whole life cycle of the parasite, the R2 protein is not detected in cell cycle-arrested short stumpy trypanosomes (Breidbach *et al.*, 2000). How iron is incorporated into the R2 subunit is yet elusive (Cotruvo & Stubbe, 2011). Recent findings suggest that, at least in yeast, the di-iron non-heme incorporation into apo-proteins is tightly related to the Fe/S cluster biogenesis machinery both from the cytosol and mitochondria (see section 3.3) (Cotruvo & Stubbe, 2011; Mühlenhoff *et al.*, 2010) and in particular to the cytosolic monothiol glutaredoxins (Grx3/4), discussed later in this review (see section 3.3.2). In trypanosomes, the only link between iron and RNR came from experiments in which parasites treated with the iron chelator deferoxamine (DFX) show an extremely reduced [^{3}H]-timidine incorporation, pointing to an essential role of iron in DNA synthesis (Breidbach *et al.*, 2002).

3.2.4 Lipid biosynthesis: Stearoyl-CoA desaturase

Stearoyl-CoA desaturases (SCD) from eukaryotes are di-iron containing proteins responsible for the *de novo* synthesis of monounsaturated fatty acids from saturated fatty acids. The iron is usually coordinated by 8 histidine residues that form the active site (Man *et al.*, 2006). They are integral membrane proteins anchored in the endoplasmic reticulum. Recent genetic and chemical validation of the orthologue enzyme from *T. brucei* demonstrated its indispensability for *in vivo* survival of bloodstream forms, as well as for the procyclic stage (Alloati *et al.*, 2010, 2011).

3.3 Iron-sulfur cluster proteins[6]

The name iron-sulfur proteins refer to a broad group of proteins. A class of them contains mononuclear Fe centers coordinated directly by cysteine residues (e. g., rubredoxins and related proteins). A second class ligates a complex between iron and inorganic sulfur through side-chain atoms provided mainly by the aminoacid cysteine, or eventually histidine or aspartate. These centers are known as Fe/S clusters (Lill & Mühlenhoff, 2008). Fe/S centers are ubiquitous inorganic cofactors present in all forms of life and are probably the most ancient cofactors and catalysts in the prebiotic world. Among them, the [2Fe-2S] is the simplest and most common cluster found *in vivo*, whereas Fe/S clusters of higher complexity require further "maturation" (Lill & Mühlenhoff, 2008; Lill, 2009; Py & Barras, 2010). In eukaryotes, the list of Fe/S dependent proteins has nearly one hundred members (Rouault & Tong, 2005; Ye & Rouault, 2010). In general, this cofactor enables electron transfer reactions due to the propensity of the iron atoms to switch between reduced (Fe^{2+}) and oxidized (Fe^{3+}) states. In addition, the redox potential of the cluster can be finely tuned by the protein environment covering a wide range of potentials, from very reducing (~-500 mV) to highly oxidizing (~+300 mV) (Lill, 2009; Xu & Møller, 2011). In consequence, Fe/S clusters are essential components of the most important biological electron transport chains, *i.e.* photosynthesis and mitochondrial respiration. But the role Fe/S clusters can play in proteins goes far beyond their redox properties. For instance, they act as important structural or regulatory moieties of some proteins from the DNA metabolism and as cofactors in enzymes of the amino acid biosynthesis or Krebs cycle (Lill & Mühlenhoff, 2006; Lill, 2009; Netz *et al.*, 2010; Py & Barras, 2010; Ye & Rouault, 2010a, 2010b).

3.3.1 Biogenesis of iron-sulfur clusters and proteins

Despite the chemical simplicity of these cofactors, their biosynthesis and insertion into apoproteins within the cell requires devoted machineries that are are highly conserved from bacteria to humans (Lill & Mühlenhoff, 2006, 2008; Xu & Møller, 2011). In bacteria, there are three different systems for the biogenesis of Fe/S proteins, all encoded in specific operons and tightly regulated. The "nitrogen fixation" (NIF) system was the first Fe/S cluster biogenesis mechanism described and is exclusively dedicated to the maturation of nitrogenase enzymes from certain bacterias. On the contrary, the "iron-sulfur cluster" (ISC)

[6] Due to the high amount of literature on this topic, this section contains mainly quotations to the most recent reviews, facilitating further reading for interested lectors. We therefore apologize to the authors of the original contributions.

and "sulfur utilization factor" (SUF) systems are widely distributed among bacteria and are responsible for the biosynthesis of Fe/S proteins in basal and stressed conditions, respectively (Xu & Møller, 2011). The mitochondria and plastids of eukaryotes have inherited the ISC and SUF systems, respectively, from ancient symbionts (Balk & Lobréaux, 2005; Balk & Pilon, 2011; Xu & Møller, 2011). Additionally, maturation of Fe/S cluster proteins in eukaryotes can be accomplished in the cytosol by a specific set of proteins that constitute the *c*ytosolic *i*ron sulfur cluster *a*ssembly (CIA) machinery. In this section we will summarize the most relevant aspects of the mitochondrial machinery related to the bacterial ISC system, and will introduce the limited information available for the CIA system. Most of the reports published stem from studies with the budding yeast *Saccharomyces cerevisiae*, and we will refer to them before describing what is known for Fe/S protein biogenesis in trypanosomes (Section 3.3.2).

The building blocks for the biosynthesis of Fe/S clusters are: iron atoms (in the reduced form, Fe^{2+}), sulfide (S^{2-}), reducing power and proteins, which act as scaffolds to assemble the Fe/S cluster that is being formed (Py & Barras, 2010; Lill & Mühlenhoff, 2006). Sulfide is generated from cysteine by the pyridoxal-5-phosphate-dependent cysteine desulfurase (eukaryotic Nfs1 or the bacterial NifS, IscS and SufS). This reaction produces alanine and leaves a protein-bound cysteine persulfide intermediate, which is presumably reduced by the ferredoxin system (NADPH-dependent ferredoxin reductase and ferredoxin) leading to release of S^{2-}. Ferredoxin is a Fe/S protein that in mammals is also known as adrenodoxin, an essential component of the thyroid hormone production. Recent studies identified an accessory protein, Isd11, that is essential for *in vivo* Fe/S biogenesis in eukaryotes (Adam *et al.*, 2006; Shi *et al.*, 2009; Wiedemann *et al.*, 2006). Isd11 forms a tight complex with Nfs1 that renders the cysteine desulfurase active (Xu & Møller, 2011). The iron-carrying protein Yfh1, known in humans as frataxin or CyaY in bacteria, participates in the delivery of iron for Fe/S cluster biosynthesis but whether this protein is or not the direct iron-carrier is still a matter of debate. Frataxin dysfunction is responsible for the most common form of inherited ataxia in humans, namely "Friederich ataxia" (Py & Barras, 2010; Lill & Mühlenhoff., 2006, 2008; Stemmler *et al.* 2010). The next step involves the transient assembly of the newly synthesized Fe/S cluster into "scaffold" proteins. These macromolecules are ubiquitous to most living organisms and contain conserved cysteine residues that bind Fe/S clusters in a labile manner, allowing the complex to be readily transferred to target proteins. The most conserved ones are the U-type scaffold proteins (*e.g.*, bacterial IscU and SufU and eukaryotic Isu1), and other include the bacterial NifU, plastid NFU and the A-type scaffolds (*e.g.*, IscA and SufA; Lill, 2009; Xu & Møller, 2011), which are supposed to work downstream the U-type ones or to subrogate their function in specific situations (*e.g.*, heme biosynthesis in mammals; Ye & Rouault, 2010b). Whereas the mitochondrial ISC system has more than 15 proteins identified (Lill & Mühlenhoff, 2008), Nfs1-Ids11, Isu1/Isu2 and Yfh1 are the core elements for Fe/S cluster biogenesis in eukaryotic mitochondria (Fig 2; Lill & Mühlenhoff, 2006).

The transference of the Fe/S cluster to the target apoprotein is assisted by a set of proteins and consumes energy (Amutha *et al.*, 2008; Subramanian *et al.*, 2011). The minimal components are: a dedicated chaperone from the HSP70 family termed Ssq1, the DnaJ-like chaperon Jac1, the nucleotide exchange factor Mge1 and a mitochondrial monothiol glutaredoxin (Grx5 in humans and yeast; Fig. 2). The requirement for a glutaredoxin-like protein, formerly considered an oxidoreductase (Lillig *et al.*, 2008; Rouhier *et al.*, 2010), in Fe/S cluster biogenesis was initially suggested by studies in a yeast Grx5 deletion mutant. These cells displayed deficient cluster assembly for at least two Fe/S proteins (aconitase and succinate dehydrogenase), leading to impaired respiratory growth and increased sensitivity to oxidative stress with accumulation of free iron in the cell (Rodríguez-Manzaneque *et al.*, 1999 and 2002). Although the precise function of monothiol glutarredoxins within the iron metabolism remain to be established, they are critical components of the ISC biosynthetic pathway in distantly related organisms such as bacteria (Fernandes *et al.*, 2005), protists (Comini *et al.*, 2008) and vertebrates (Xu & Møller, 2011; Ye *et al.*, 2010; Ye & Rouault, 2010b).

The CIA machinery was first discovered in yeast when seeking for cytosolic proteins essential for Fe/S cluster assembly on aconitase (Fig. 2). Nowadays, several components are recognized: i) two P-loop NTPases (Cfd1 and Nbp35) that form a stable heterotetrameric complex with a [4Fe-4S] cluster bound to the C-terminal region, suggesting a scaffold role for cluster assembly; ii) Nar1, a Fe/S-dependent protein related to bacterial iron-containing hydrogenases, iii) WD40 β-propeller protein Cia1, which preferentially localizes in the nucleus and assists cluster delivery to Nbp35 (Lill & Mühlenhoff, 2008; Sharma *et al.*, 2010; Xu & Møller, 2011), and iv) redox components of the CIA machinery (Tah18, Dre2 and monothiol glutaredoxins 3 and 4). In yeast, intracellular iron level is sensed by the transcription factor Aft1 and requires the regulatory proteins Fra1-Fra2 that interact with the cytosolic-nuclear monothiol glutaredoxins Grx3 or Grx4 through the formation of heterodimers linked by a Fe/S cluster (Kumánovics *et al.*, 2008; Mühlenhoff *et al.*, 2010; Pujol-Carrion *et al.*, 2006). Interestingly, besides the existence of specific and compartmentalized machineries, Fe/S cluster biogenesis in the cytosol has been confirmed to depend on the mitochondrial system. A still unknown essential compound (noted as "X" in Fig. 2) is exported from mitochondria *via* the inner mitochondrial membrane ATP-binding cassette (ABC) transporter Atm1 and the intermembrane space protein Erv1, in a process that requires GSH (Netz *et al.*, 2010; Sharma *et al.*, 2010; Xu & Møller, 2011). As pointed by Ye and Rouault (2010a, 2010b) the next frontier in Fe/S cluster biogenesis will consist in unraveling how the monothiol glutaredoxin 5 and ABCB7 transporter are involved in the mitochondrial synthesis and export to the cytosol/nucleus of a still unknown factor that connects these processes in both compartments. Moreover, it remains to be studied how the system operates as a whole (Mühlenhoff *et al.*, 2010; Netz *et al.*, 2010; Zhang *et al.*, 2008).

3.3.2 Biogenesis of iron-sulfur clusters in trypanosomes

The characterization of the Fe/S biogenesis in trypanosomes was driven by the completion of the genome sequencing of three trypanosomatid species (Berriman *et al.*, 2005; El Sayed *et al.*, 2005; Ivens *et al.*, 2005). As noted previously, the mitochondrion is a key organelle in Fe/S cluster biosynthesis that undergoes important metabolic and morphological changes in trypanosomatids, especially in African trypanosomes, during life cycle. For instance, several mitochondrial respiratory-chain proteins that depend on these cofactors are developmentally synthesized in insect stage parasites (Alfonzo & Lukeš, 2011; Tyler et al, 1997). Based on sequence comparison with identified Fe/S cluster biogenesis proteins from yeast, plants and humans, a number of members of the ISC system are conserved in trypanosomatids (see Fig. 2). Smíd *et al.* (2006) characterized two major components of this machinery present in *T. brucei*: a cysteine desulfurase (*Tb*IscS2, related to Nfs1) and one U-type scaffold protein (*Tb*IscU, related to Isu1). Both proteins proved to be essential for the mitochondrial biogenesis of Fe/S proteins (Smíd *et al.*, 2006). In agreement with phenotypes observed in yeast mutants, down-regulation of *Tb*IscS2 in procyclic parasites by RNAi results in inhibition of Fe/S cluster dependent processes both in the mitochondrion and cytosol, with a concomitant impairment in ATP production, cellular respiration and growth (Smíd *et al.*, 2006; Paris *et al.*, 2009). The occurrence of this protein in the rudimentary mitochondrion of bloodstream parasites was still not addressed but appears reasonable considering that this stage relies on important Fe/S protein activities (Comini *et al.*, 2008). As mentioned above, a stable tricomponent system between Nfs1, Isd11 and IscU have to be formed to enable the formation of Fe/S cluster on IscU. An Isd11 homologue is actively expressed by both life stages of *T. brucei* and, as expected, is critical for cytosolic and mitochondrial Fe/S cluster biosynthesis in trypanosomes (Paris *et al.*, 2010). A second Nfs-like gene was identified in *T. brucei* (Smíd *et al.*, 2006) and characterized as a selenocysteine lyase (SLC; Poliak *et al.*, 2010), an enzyme that cleaves selenocysteine into alanine and selenium during selenoprotein metabolization. Supporting the experimental evidences on the dispensability of the selenoproteome for this parasite (Aeby et al, 2009), down-regulation of SLC is not detrimental for *T. brucei*, at least under cultivation (Poliak *et al.*, 2010). A single-copy gene with a significant sequence similarity to eukaryotic frataxin was identified in *T. brucei* genome (*Tb*FXN; Long *et al.*, 2008b). Abrogation of frataxin function in the mitochondrion of procyclic cells induces a growth-retardation phenotype with a marked inhibition of Fe/S-dependent processes, *e.g.*, aconitase activity (Long *et al.*, 2008a, 2008b). Interestingly, *Tb*FXN was also identified in the bloodstream form of the parasite but its biological relevance was not addressed (Long *et al.*, 2008b). Works with the fission yeast indicate that thiolation of tRNA depends on components from the mitochondrial and cytosolic ISC systems (Lill & Mühlenhoff, 2006, 2008). A similar link between both pathways has recently been disclosed for trypanosomes (Alfonzo & Lukeš, 2011; Bruske *et al.*, 2009). More recently, two A-type scaffold proteins from *T. brucei* were characterized and their function rated as essential for the growth and Fe/S cluster metabolism of procyclic but not of bloodstream parasites (Long *et al.*, 2011), suggesting specificity for Fe/S protein acceptors that are developmentally regulated. The final step in mitochondrial Fe/S cluster biogenesis consists in the delivery of the cluster to acceptor proteins, in an ATP-depedent process assisted by mitochondrial HSP70 and monothiol glutaredoxins, interestingly, the last being Fe/S proteins (Comini *et al.*, 2008; Manta *et al.*, unpublished). Three sequences for putative monothiol glutaredoxins, named 1-C-Grx1 to 3, are present in the genome of different trypanosomatids (Berriman *et al.*, 2005; El Sayed *et al.*, 2005; Ivens *et al.*, 2005). The proteins from *T. b. brucei* are the best studied so far. 1-C-Grx1 and 1-C-Grx2 localizes at the parasite mitochondrion (Filser *et al.*, 2007; Comini *et al.*, 2008; Manta *et al.* unpublished), whereas 1-C-Grx3, a hybrid protein containing an N-terminal Trx domain, is probably cytosolic. 1-C-Grx1 and 1-C-Grx3, but not 1-C-Grx2, are abundant proteins in bloodstream parasites and reach maximum levels in stationary phase cultures (Comini *et al.*, 2008). Strikingly, targeting these proteins to the mitochondria of *S. cerevisiae* defective in Grx5 did not rescue the mutant phenotype, suggesting the existence of structural or biochemical differences between the trypanosomal and eukaryote/prokaryotes orthologues (Filser *et al.*, 2007). Indeed, *in vitro* all three proteins are capable to coordinate an Fe/S cluster at expenses of a protein thiol and low molecular mass thiols that are parasite-specific, namely $T(SH)_2$ and monoglutathionilspermidine (Comini *et al.*, 2008; Manta *et al.* unpublished). We observed a similar behavior for *T. cruzi* 1-C-Grx1 (Fleitas *et al.*, unpublished). 1-C-Grx1 is indispensable for infective *T. brucei* with an important function in parasite iron homeostasis and no role in protection against oxidants (Comini *et al.*, 2008; Manta *et al.*, unpublished), as previously proposed for yeast Grx5 (Rodriguez-Manzaneque *et al.*, 1999). Overexpression of a functional apo-mutant of 1-C-Grx1 impairs parasite survival inside an animal host (Manta *et al.*, unpublished). Also overexpression of a wildtype form of 1-C-Grx1 was detrimental for parasite survival either *in vitro* (under iron deprivation or oxidative stress conditions) and *in vivo* (mice), indicating that iron homeostasis in African trypanosomes is tightly controlled with this protein playing an important role. Altogether, this provides the first evidence for a critical physiological role of iron and Fe/S cluster metabolism for *T. brucei* survival during infection. The information concerning Fe/S cluster biogenesis in the cytosol of trypanosomes is very scarce. So far, only a putative orthologue of ABCB7 was identified in *T. brucei* genome (Sauvage *et al.*, 2009) and, as outlined above, the occurrence of a putative cytosolic monothiol glutaredoxin orthologue of yeast Grx3/Grx4 was described (Smíd *et al.*, 2006; Filser *et al.*, 2007; Comini *et al.*, 2008). Further investigations are required to establish whether trypanosomal 1-C-Grx3 shares a regulatory function on iron- and iron-sulfur-homeostasis as their yeast counterparts.

As noted by Long *et al.* (2011), following the identification of several components of the ISC system in *T. brucei* and owing to the high degree of evolutionary conservation for this important pathway it is reasonable to assume a similar complexity for the Fe/S cluster assembly machinery in this unicellular eukaryote with respect to that of yeast or even human. Nevertheless, certain structural or biochemical specialization in some of it molecular components may be envisaged (Filser *et al.*, 2007; Comini *et al.*, 2008; Manta *et al.*, unpublished). The regulation of Fe/S biogenesis in trypanosomes is equally unexplored yet. Considering the Fe/S metabolic repertoire of each developmental stage of the parasite, it makes sense to consider multiple and inter-dependent mechanisms controlling substrate supply, Fe/S-biosynthesis and turnover, all important issues that await elucidation. Another challenging question raised by Smíd *et al.* (2006) deals with the identification of the factor(s) triggering Fe/S-cluster and -protein synthesis during differentiation.

3.3.3 Examples of iron-sulfur proteins in trypanosomes

3.3.3.1 Aconitase

The enzyme aconitase (EC 4.2.1.3) is an essential component of the mitochondrial tricarboxylic acid cycle that catalyzes the reversible conversion of citrate to isocitrate through the intermediary formation of the tricarboxylic acid *cis*-aconitate. Aconitase contains an [2Fe-2S] center that acts both in substrate binding and catalytic addition or removal of H_2O, but not in electron transfer reactions. In addition to this enzymatic activity, cytosolic isoforms of apo-aconitase participate in regulation of cellular iron homeostasis, therefore, receiving also the name of iron-regulatory proteins (IRP). In its apo-form (non-cluster bound) aconitase undergoes a conformational change that confers the protein with affinity to bind the 3′- or 5′- untranslated regions, known as IRE (iron-response elements), present in the mRNA encoding for several proteins related to iron uptake and metabolization. Under iron starvation the ratio apo:holo aconitase increases and, hence, IRP activation takes over the post-translational response that triggers iron mobilization, uptake and utilization (Hentze *et al.*, 2010).

As mentioned previously, the bloodstream form of *T. brucei* possess a rudimentary mitochondrion with most enzymes from the Krebs cycle repressed (Saas *et al.*, 2000). In this parasite, aconitase is encoded by a single gene whose sequence resembles that of the cytosolic isoform of mammalian aconitase (Fast *et al.*, 1999; Saas *et al.*, 2000). The protein localizes within both the cytosol and mitochondrion (Saas *et al.*, 2000). While the mRNA abundance is almost unaffected during development, the protein content increases several times during transformation from dividing to arrested bloodstream form (Overath *et al.*, 1986), in concordance with the morphological and biochemical events that occur in the preparation of the parasite to differentiate to the insect stage (Saas *et al.*, 2000). The protein is not essential for infective or procyclic parasites (van Weelden *et al.*, 2003) neither involved in the regulation of the transferrin receptor (Fast *et al.*, 1999), as occurs in mammals. Moreover, genome survey indicated the absence of sequences with homology to IREs in trypanosomes (Berriman *et al.*, 2005; Ivens *et al.*, 2005; El-Sayed *et al.*, 2005), which in principle agrees with the low aconitase activity detected in bloodstream parasites and its dispensability for procyclic forms. The discovery that insect stage *T. brucei* does not rely on Krebs cycle for pyruvate metabolisation has set a new metabolic paradigm for this parasite species. Despite *T. brucei* aconitase has never been shown *in vitro* to be a Fe/S-dependent protein, its high sequence conservation (Saas *et al.*, 2000) and several biological data supports its Fe/S nature. For instance, knockdown of IscS, IscU (Smíd *et al.*, 2006) and Isd11 (Paris *et al.*, 2010) was followed by down-regulation of aconitase activity both in the mitochondria and cystosol. The final answer for the physiological (in)dispensability of aconitase in infective parasites will have to await experiments in animal infection models.

3.3.3.2 Fumarate hydratases

Fumarases, also called fumarate hydratases (FHs, E.C. 4.2.1.2), are ubiquitous enzymes that catalyze the stereospecific reversible hydration of fumarate to malate. Most prokaryotes and eukaryotes express two isoforms of fumarases. In eukaryotes, the mitochondrial isoform is a component of the tricarboxylic acid cycle and, hence, central to aerobic respiration. The cytosolic isoform is probably involved in the metabolism of fumarate that stem from a number of reactions occurring in the cytosol. Two distinct classes of fumarases, class I and class II, have been identified so far. The proteins lack sequence homology but are functionally related. Class II fumarases (or *fumC* enzymes) are iron-independent enzymes. They occur in several bacteria and in eukaryotes, such as fungi, mammals, and higher plants. In contrast, class I fumarases are Fe/S-containing enzymes. Bacteria but also unicellular eukaryotes contain class I fumarases. The characterization of two class I fumarases in *T. brucei* revealed that two single copy genes code for mitochondrial and cytosolic isoforms that are expressed in procyclic but not in bloodstream parasites (Coustou *et al.*, 2006). Simultaneous downregulation of both transcripts was deleterious for the viability of procyclic trypanosomes, a phenotype that was counteracted by the addition of extracellular fumarate, highlighting the essential and stage-specific role of this metabolite (Coustou *et al.*, 2006). Taking into account that secretion of succinate has been described for the infective stage of *Leishmania* spp. and *T. cruzi* grown in glucose-supplemented medium

(Cazzulo, 1992), the authors proposed the occurrence of FHs in these trypanosomatids. Nevertheless, if any, their biochemical importance awaits elucidation.

4. Heme uptake and utilization

Heme is an essential cofactor for various proteins. It can perform diverse functions such as oxygen transport and storage (hemoglobin and myoglobin), mitochondrial electron transport (Complex II–IV), xenobiotic detoxification and steroid metabolism (cytochromes), signal transduction (nitric oxide synthases, soluble guanylate cyclases), and regulation of antioxidant defense enzymes, since many enzymes like peroxidases, catalases, and the large group of cytochrome P450 (CYP450) rely on heme as a prosthetic group. Heme-proteins have also been implicated in microRNA processing and microbicide defense (Mochizuki *et al.*, 2010; Roberts & Montfort, 2007).

Heme consists of a cyclic tetrapyrrole ring structure (protoporphyrin IX) that coordinates an iron atom which can adopt Fe^{+3} or Fe^{+2} oxidation states. Different substitutions over the pyrrolic moieties originate the different types of heme (a, b and c; Severance & Hamza, 2009; Tripodi *et al.*, 2011). As stated earlier, African trypanosomes are extracellular parasites that depend on heme uptake to face their metabolic needs (Fig. 3), thus, the biosynthetic pathway operating in the host will be briefly outlined. The complete heme biosynthetic pathway involves eight-steps. Although the synthesis of δ-aminolevulinic acid (ALA), the first heme precursor, may differ between organisms the remaining seven steps of the pathway (from ALA to heme b) are strictly conserved. In most heterotrophic eukaryotes the biosynthesis alternates between the mitochondria and the cytosol while in photosynthetic organisms heme is exclusively produced in the chloroplasts (Korený *et al.*, 2010). Despite its essentiality and versatility, iron and porphyrins are highly toxic to cells due to iron-induced pro-oxidant effect on DNA, proteins and membrane lipids. Therefore, its biosynthesis and storage is tightly regulated in order to reduce the level of free heme inside the cell.

Certain organisms lack some components of the biosynthetic pathway from ALA to protoporphyrin IX and have developed strategies to obtain heme from other sources. The tick *Boophilus microplus* (Braz *et al.*, 1999), the filarial nematode *Brugia malayi* (Wo *et al.*, 2009), the free-living nematode *Caenorhabditis elegans* (Rao *et al.*, 2005) and most kinetoplastid parasites are examples of eukaryotes that are partially or completely unable to synthesize heme despite some of their developmental stages depend on oxidative fosforilation (*i.e.*, cytochromes) to obtain energy. The order Kinetoplastida contains species where the complete biosynthetic pathway is absent (*e.g.* most members of the genus *Trypanosoma*), and others, such as *Leishmania* spp. or *Crithidia* spp., able to perform only the last three biosynthetic steps (Chang *et al.*, 1975; Salzman *et al.*, 1982). Although it is very likely that a kinetoplastid's ancestor harbored a complete set of eukaryotic genes for heme synthesis, during evolution these genes have been either lost (*e.g. Trypanosoma* genus) or subsequently rescued from a γ-proteobacterium endosymbiont by horizontal gene transfer, as proposed for the non-Trypanosoma trypanosomatids (Korený *et al.*, 2010). As a general consequence, trypanosomatids must scavenge heme or precursors from their hosts. At this point, it is important to note that there are several species of trypanosomatids that parasitize insects, including *Herpetomonas roitmani, Crithidia deanei, C. desouzai, C. oncopelti* and *Blastocrithidia*

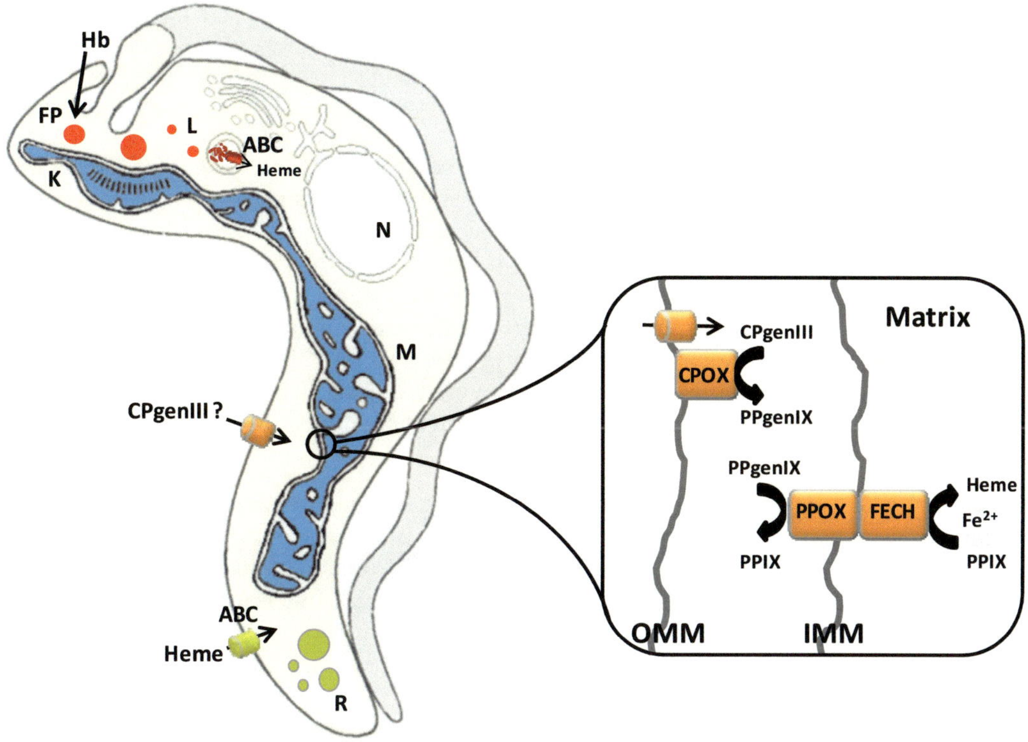

Fig. 3. Pathways for heme incorporation and biosynthesis in trypanosomes.
Although two possible routes for heme internalization have been described in *T. cruzi*, so far none of the putative transporters has been characterized. In *T. brucei*, hemoglobin (Hb, upper left) endocytosis was shown to depend on a haptoglobin-hemoglobin receptor (HpHbR) localized at the flagellar pocket (FP) and expressed exclusively in the bloodstream form of the parasite. An ABC transporter (ABCG5 in *L. major*) has been shown to rescue heme after lysosomal (L) degradation of Hb. On the other hand, in *T. cruzi* a non-endocytic route was described for free forms of heme (lower part, in green). This is an active process mediated by ABC transporters that leads to accumulation of heme inside storage organelles, the reservosomes (R). Specific inhibitors for ABC transporters (cyclosporin A, verapamil and indomethacin) reduce significantly heme uptake (Peixoto Cupelloa *et al.*, 2011). Intracellular parasites endowed with the last three enzymes of heme biosynthesis, such as *Leishmania* spp., are capable to incorporate heme precursors, such as coproporphobilinogen III (CPgenIII), which upon transport to the mitochondrial intermembrane space can undergo a serie of oxidative reactions leading to the formation of protoporphyrin IX (PPIX) that is finally converted into heme by addition of iron through a ferrochelatase (FECH) facing the mitochondrial matrix (middle part and insert, orange). Additional subcellular structures and biosynthetic components are abbreviated as follows: nucleus (N), kinetoplast (K), mitochondrion (M), outer mitochondrial membrane (OMM), inner mitochondrial membrane (IMM), coproporphyrinogen oxidase (CPOX), protoporphyrinogen IX (PPgenIX), protoporphyrinogen oxidase (PPOX).

culicis, which have been found to contain symbiotic bacteria that may supply the protists with heme and other essential nutrients (Chang & Trager, 1974). The bacterial symbiotes would be subject of regulation by their hosts, hence, functioning as cell organelles rather than as independent living entities (Chang *et al.*, 1975).

Heme's transport and distribution in trypanosomatids remain elusive. Diffusion across the lipid bilayer is hampered for heme due to its anionic carboxylate side-chains. Instead, high affinity heme-binding proteins in the cell surface of *T. cruzi* (Lara *et al.*, 2007), procyclic forms of *T. brucei* (Vanhollebeke *et al.*, 2008) and *L. donovani* (Campos-Salinas *et al.*, 2011) allows for active heme uptake. In *T. cruzi* epimastigotes, both endocytotic and non-endocytotic mechanisms of heme internalization have been confirmed. *L. donovani* can also incorporate heme by receptor-mediated endocytosis followed by lysosomal degradation of hemoglobin. An ABC transporter localized in membranes of multivesicular structures is probably related to intracellular heme trafficking after hemoglobin degradation. Porphyrin trafficking in trypanosomatids is yet an uncovered subject but intracellular transport appears to involve membrane-bound vesicles as carriers (Severance & Hamza, 1982; Tripodi *et al.*, 2011).

In summary, pathogenic trypanosomatids are auxotrophic for heme and have to adapt their heme-dependent metabolic pathways (*i.e.* biosynthesis of sterols and polyunsaturated fatty acids, respiration, oxidative stress response and detoxification) to fluctuations in nutrient availability across their life cycle. The most relevant cellular functions requiring heme in trypanosomatids are discussed in the next sections.

4.1 Heme in oxidative defense

Trypanosomes lack catalase and selenium-dependent glutathione peroxidases but instead express two types of trypanothione/tryparedoxin dependent peroxidases to decompose endogenous and exogenously produced oxidants (rewieved in Schlecker *et al.*, 2007 and Krauth-Siegel & Comini, 2008) and some species have an additional plant-like ascorbate-dependent hemoperoxidase (APX; Adak & Datta, 2005; Wilkinson *et al.*, 2002a). Interestingly, APX is present in intracellular trypanosomatids (*T. cruzi* and *Leishmania* spp.) but absent in parasites with an extracellular life style in the mammal host, namely *T. brucei*. This feature has been attributed to the major demand for anti-oxidant capacity that intracellular parasites need during infection (Wilkinson *et al.*, 2005; Dolai *et al.*, 2009). APX localizes to the endoplasmic reticulum (ER; Wilkinson *et al.*, 2002a) and cell membrane (M. Hugo *et al.*, personal communication) of *T. cruzi* and in the intermembrane space of the mitochondrial inner membrane in the case of *L. major* (Dolai *et al.*, 2008). Both enzymes are reduced by ascorbate or, alternatively, cytochrome c (Wilkinson *et al.*, 2002a; Dolai *et al.*, 2008; M. Hugo *et al.*, personal communication). The regeneration of reduced ascorbate occurs upon spontaneous reaction of dehydroascorbate with $T(SH)_2$ (Krauth-Siegel & Lüdemann, 1996). With respect to the source of ascorbate, in contrast to humans, African and American trypanosomes can synthesize this metabolite *de novo*, a process that takes place in the glycosome (Wilkinson *et al.*, 2005). *T. cruzi* cannot take up ascorbate from the environment, as *T. brucei* does, and therefore relies entirely on its biosynthesis to fuel other unknown cellular functions, in addition to oxidant detoxication (Logan *et al.*, 2007).

The biological role of APX is consistently related to oxidant defense. Overexpression of APX in *T. cruzi* and *L. major* enhances tolerance against oxidative stress induced by exogenous hydrogen peroxide (Wilkinson *et al.*, 2002a and 2005) and mitochondrial cardiolipin oxidation, providing thus protection towards programmed cell death and protein damage (Dolai *et al.*, 2008, 2009). This function appears to be redundant with that performed by the ER glutathione-like trypanothione-dependent peroxidase of *T. cruzi* (GPxII; Wilkinson *et al.*, 2002a) and the mitochondrial trypanothione-dependent peroxiredoxin (mTXNPx) from *Leishmania* spp. However, an explanation for this may lie on different substrate specificities (*e.g.*, GpxII reduces fatty acid and phospholipid hydroperoxides; Wilkinson *et al.*, 2002b) or the macromolecular targets these enzymes have.

4.2 Heme in polyunsaturated fatty acids biogenesis

Fatty acid biosynthesis in trypanosomatids seems to be an essential pathway for the parasite life cycle. As stated earlier, differentiation involves dramatic morphological changes in the cell and its organelles that certainly require membrane fluidity. The biosynthesis of unsaturated fatty acids is another plant-like pathway inherited by trypanosomatids. In this respect, lipid desaturation occurs at the methyl end of the molecule, in contrast to mammals, in which a double bond is generated at the carboxy end of the molecule.

T. cruzi and both life stages of *T. brucei* are able to synthesize fatty acids, although *T. brucei* bloodstream form was formerly thought to depend on lipid uptake from their host. Short and medium chain fatty acids are usually synthesized by means of the soluble fatty-acid synthetase system and subsequently elongated by the elongase system that resides in the ER. *T. brucei* can elongate fatty acids up to stearate (C18:0). *T. cruzi* can further elongate C18 to C24 and C26 fatty acids required in the synthesis of anchors for surface macromolecules. The stearate is mainly converted into linoleate (C18:2), which represents near 30% and 40% of total fatty acids in *T. brucei* and *T. cruzi*, respectively. Moreover, unsaturated fatty acids can represent up to 70% of total fatty acid content depending on the parasite species and life cycle stage (Alloatti *et al.*, 2010).

T. brucei oleate desaturase shares high similarity with $\Delta 12$ desaturases and, to a lesser extent, with $\omega 3$ desaturases although the parasite enzyme lacks $\omega 3$ desaturase activity. Fatty acid desaturases require an electron donor, that can be either ferredoxin in plastids and bacteria or cytochrome *b*5 (cyt*b*5) in the ER, as it is the case for the orthologue from *T. brucei* (Uttaro, 2006). Since *T. brucei* oleate desaturase lacks a consensus sequence for the covalent binding of cyt*b*, it has been suggested that electron donation occurs *via* complex formation with another desaturase capable to bind cyt*b*5 (Petrini *et al.*, 2004). The drastic growth defect observed upon partial ablation of enzyme activity (even an 8% reduction) by RNAi is a strong indication of the essentiality of this pathway for infective parasites (see also section 3.2.4; Alloatti *et al.*, 2010)

4.3 Trypanosomes contain unusual single-cys cytochromes

Cytochromes are heme-containing complexes that participate in many electron transfer reactions including oxidative phosphorylation in the respiratory chain (cytochromes type c, cyt*c* and cytochromes type c1, cyt*c*1), desaturation of fatty acids or xenobiotic detoxification (Comini *et al.*, 2011). In cyt*c* heme is covalently attached through thioether bonds between the vinyl groups of the heme and the thiols of two cysteine residues in a conserved CXXCH motif, in which the histidine functions as an axial ligand for heme iron. Mitochondrial cyt *c* is the best known example of this type of protein. It is located in the intermembrane space and transfers electrons from the cytochrome *bc*1 complex to the cytochrome *aa*3 oxidase. Cytochrome *c*1 of the *bc*1 complex (cytochrome reductase) is also a *c*-type cytochrome. Heme coordination by cyt*c* and cyt*c*1 from euglenoids (*e.g.* the green flagellated algae *Euglena gracilis*) and trypanosomatids occurs through a single thioether bond involving the single thiol group from their binding motifs AAQCH and FAPCH, respectively (Priest & Hajduk, 1994). As another example of a metabolic trait that trypanosomatids share with higher plants, plastids contain *b*6f-type cytochromes with heme covalently attached through a single thioether bond (Allen *et al.*, 2004; Tripodi *et al.*, 2011). The biogenesis of holo cytochrome *c* is a catalyzed process that involves different mechanisms and enzymatic components that can be grouped into five major systems (Tripodi *et al.*, 2011). The cytochrome *c* maturation machinery employed by kinetoplatids remains unidentified and is possibly unique to this and the entire euglenid taxon (Allen *et al.*, 2004; Tripodi *et al.*, 2011). Based on the metabolic repertoire of each developmental stage, the relevance of cytochrome activity for energy production appears to be restricted to the procyclic form of the parasite.

4.4 Heme in sterol biogenesis

Cholesterol, ergosterol and sitosterol are essential structural components of plasma membranes from mammals, fungi and plants, respectively. They stabilize membranes, determine their fluidity and permeability, and modulate the activity of membrane-bound enzymes and ion channels. *T. cruzi* and *T. brucei* encode all sterol biosynthetic enzymes, including sterol 14-α-demethylase (CYP51), a member of the CYP450 superfamily that operates at the initial phase (post-squalene stage) of the pathway that drives the oxidative removal of the 14-α-methyl group from the newly cyclized sterol precursors. Azole-based compounds, common in antifungal therapies (*e.g.*, posaconazole) proved to be potent inhibitors of CYP51 by interacting with the enzyme active site and its prosthetic group (Chen *et al.*, 2010). Inhibition of CYP51 leads to accumulation of 14α-methylated sterols, which are unable to replace ergosterol in the membrane because of steric hindrance, followed by growth arrest and cell death (Lepsheva *et al.*, 2007; Vanden Bosschef *et al.*, 1995). In contrast to *T. cruzi* and *Leishmania* spp., ergosterol has been thought to be dispensable for *T. brucei*. However, the observation that antifungals are also detrimental for this parasite lead to the proposal that sterol derivatives may additionally serve as precursors for bioactive molecules that act as regulators of cell cycle and development (Lepsheva *et al.*, 2007).

Other CYP450s possess a monooxygenase activity that, upon oxygen activation, catalyzes the addition of an oxygen atom into an organic substrate and the reduction of the second one to water. After each catalytic cycle, CYPs must be restored to their reduced state by a CYP450 reductase (CPR), a NADPH-dependant diflavin (FAD/FMN) enzyme that couple a two-electron donor (NADPH) with one-electron acceptors, supplying the electrons one at a time. CYPs and CPR are involved in the metabolism of a wide range of endogenous compounds and xenobiotics including fatty acids, steroids, drugs, alkanes, polycyclic hydrocarbons, insecticides and other environmental contaminants (Murataliev *et al.*, 2004). In mammals, there is only one CPR gene. However, *T. cruzi* and *L. major* encode three different CPR genes (CPR-A, CPR-B and CPR-C), while *T. brucei* possesses four sequences, all of them sharing a high sequence identity. Similar to some higher plant species

(Koopmann & Hahlbrock, 1997; Ro *et al.*, 2002; Urban *et al.*, 1997), *T. cruzi* CPRs are encoded by a small gene family, with differential regulation and subcellular localization (Portal *et al.*, 2008). *Tc*CPR-B is localized mainly in reservosomes, *Tc*CPR-C is mostly found in the ER while *Tc*CPR-A displays a more ubiquitous distribution pattern (De Vas *et al.*, 2011). The presence of multiple isoforms argues for a well-supported P450-mediated molecular system. Portal *et al.* (2008) showed that CPR-B overexpression in *T. cruzi* confers increased resistance to nifurtimox and, more significantly, to benznidazole. In addition, increased levels of CPRs are observed in trypomastigotes, a stage that is particularly exposed to stress during cell invasion supporting a role for CPRs in oxidative stress defense (Portal *et al.*, 2008). Moreover, CPR-B and CPR-C overexpression increases the synthesis of ergosterol, with the concomitant augmentation in membrane rigidity and decrease in endocytic activity. Modification in cell membrane fluidity could result in alteration of drug uptake and, as a consequence, in the observed drug resistance (De Vas *et al.*, 2011).

5. Iron and infection

As noted in the introductory section, African trypanosomiasis is a parasitic disease of medical and veterinary importance that has adverse impact in the health and economical development of the sub-Saharian region of Africa (Maudlin, 2006; Stijlemans *et al.*, 2008, 2010a). Since African trypanosomes multiply predominantly in the bloodstream as extra-cellular parasites, they are continuously dependent on host nutrient supply and exposed to host immune attack. As will be addressed next, the response mounted by the mammalian host towards infection includes the activation of both arms of the immune system.

Beyond the aforementioned clinical outcomes for HAT (Section 1), the most prominent immunopathological disease-related feature of trypanosomiasis is anemia. In fact, anemia is the major cause of death in bovine trypanosomiasis and an important debilitating symptom in HAT (Stijlemans *et al.*, 2008). Anemia of inflammation, also termed anemia of chronic disease (ACD), is frequent among patients suffering chronic inflammatory disorders (*e. g.*, autoimmune diseases) or chronic infections (Camaschella & Strati, 2010). ACD is the consequence of a persistent activated inflammatory immune response and is considered to be a defense mechanism where the host establishes an iron "withholding" strategy to limit the availability of essential iron for the pathogens (Lalonde & Holbein, 1984; Stijlemans *et al.*, 2008; Sutak *et al.*, 2008). Stijlemans and coworkers (Stijlemans *et al.*, 2008, 2010a, 2010b; Vankrunkelsven *et al.*, 2010) studied the immunological and hematological development of *T. brucei* infection using animal models (cattle and mice). Despite mouse models show limitations and artifacts, like the extremely high parasitemia levels reached compared to infection in the natural host, they have contributed significantly to our current understanding of trypanosomiasis patho-physiology (Magez & Caljon, 2011). The molecular mechanism underlying the development of ACD during trypanosomiasis resembles that observed in other infectious diseases. Briefly, during the early stage of the infection trypanosomes stimulate T-cells to secrete interferon-γ resulting in the activation of macrophages (type I cellular immune response) that liberate pro-inflammatory mediators like tumor necrosis factor, interleukin (IL) -1, IL-6 and •NO (Stijlemans *et al.*, 2010b). This response leads to parasite clearance but also enhances erythrophagocytosis by activated macrophages within the spleen and liver (Kupffer cells). At this point it is important to recall that under physiological conditions Kupffer cells recycle iron from engulfed senescent erythrocytes (see Section 2; Hentze *et al.*, 2010). Thus, enhanced removal of red blood cells from systemic fluids by the reticuloendothelial system will contribute to deprive host of iron. In addition, hepcidin (Section 2) is secreted in response to pro-inflammatory mediators, blocking iron release from macrophages and iron intake by enterocytes (Nishimura *et al.*, 2011), which decreases plasma iron levels and limits host and pathogen accessibility to the metal (Taylor & Kelly, 2010). The upregulation of several iron-related molecules (*e.g.* hemooxygenase 1, ferritin and ferroportin) provides additional evidence for the strong type I immune response, augmented liver iron-metabolism and accelerated senescence of erythrocytes that takes place during trypanosomal infection (Nishimura *et al.*, 2011; Omotainse & Anosa, 1992; Stijlemans *et al.*, 2010a; see Section 2). The class of anemia originated during the acute phase of trypanosomiasis is a typical non-haematopoietic anemia. However, if at the long term the type I response persists, then iron will be sequestered intracellularly, resulting in a marked iron deprivation with compromise of erythropoiesis and development of ACD (Mwangi *et al.*, 1995; Omotainse & Anosa, 1992; Stijlemans *et al.*, 2010b). Despite its adverse effects, if sustained on time, limited iron bioavailability can be considered a reasonable host response to control parasitemia (Ganz, 2009). In the last years, several evidences point to the possibility that the parasite deliberately manipulates the mammalian host immune response. Activation of a strong type I immune response in early stages of the infection promotes erythrophagocytosis (Igbokwe *et al.*, 1994), a strategy that yields abundant iron and lipids (*e.g.* myristic acid), the last needed for GPI biosynthesis and VSG coating (Stijlemans *et al.*, 2010a, 2010b). It is important to stress that the trypanosome body is totally covered by a dense GPI-anchored coat of VSGs that plays an important protective (physical and immunological barrier) function in bloodstream parasites (Comini *et al.*, 2011).

A large number of microbial pathogens have been reported to affect the morbidity and mortality of patients with high iron content, a physiopathological state characterized by the presence of non-transferrin bound iron in plasma. Moreover, iron overload due to genetic predisposition, therapeutic intervention or nutritional status is known to increase the risk of several infections (Kontoghiorghes *et al.*, 2010). It is worth to note that human iron overload is common in rural populations inhabiting sub-Saharan regions of Africa, the "tsetse belt", with a high incidence of HAT (Gordeuk, 2002; McNamara *et al.*, 1999). Originally, this chronic condition was supposed to be an exclusive consequence of an iron-rich diet based on the large consumption of homebrewed beers, but recent studies of pedigrees suggest the presence of genetic components (Gordeuk, 2002; Moyo *et al.*, 1998). It remains to be investigated whether there is a co-evolutionary development of iron overload and HAT, as it is the case for glucose-6-phosphate dehydrogenase deficiency and malaria.

Considering the well-known role of iron in *T. brucei* infection and the fact that *in vitro* iron deprivation with chelating agents cause growth retardation of bloodstream *T. brucei* (Fast *et al.*, 1999; Breidbach *et al.*, 2002; Comini *et al.*, 2008), it is surprising the absence of works studying the therapeutic potential of iron chelation against *T. brucei* (Tayor & Kelly, 2010). This is not the case for *T. cruzi*, for which the chelating agent deferoxamine (DFX) proved its efficacy to halt replication of intra-macrophage amastigotes (Arantes *et al.*, 2011; Lalonde & Holbein, 1984; Jones *et al.*, 1996), and to decrease parasitemia and mortality of infected mice (Loo & Lalonde, 1984). However, in contrast to extracellular *T. brucei*, the possible success of chelating therapies against *T. cruzi* infection are hampered by the intracellular nature of the infective stage of this parasite, which, if not specifically targeted to the pathogen, will imply a high dosage or a long-term treatment, both deleterious for the host. Based on the demonstration that iron metabolism is crucial for parasite survival in the host (Manta *et al.*, unpublished; see section 3.3.2), our group has recently evaluated the therapeutic effect of intraperitoneal (i.p.) and oral administration of DFX to *T. brucei* infected mice. Preliminary results show a marked increase in life span of the animal group receiving i.p. treatment (200 mg/Kg for ~10 days) and almost no side effects (red blood cell and reticulocyte counts) on animals treated but non-infected (Manta *et al.*, unpublished). However, DFX displayed a cytostatic effect against acute infection by *T. brucei,* which implies that a successful therapeutic regimen will require drug association.

6. Summary and outlook

As any other living organism on earth, trypanosomes depend on iron to fulfill critical cellular functions (DNA and lipid biosynthesis, oxidant protection and energy generation). Their complex life cycle has added an additional problem in the struggle for the supply of (micro)nutrients. However, these organisms have developed different strategies and mechanisms in order to ensure a physiological iron status within the distinct hosts. Moreover, host-parasite co-evolution has resulted in the development of well-balanced growth regulation systems, allowing the parasite to survive sufficiently long without killing its mammalian host and ensuring an efficient transmission cycle. Interruption of this cycle is necessary to abolish the devastating disease these parasites produce to humans and livestock. In this respect, the iron metabolism of trypanosomatids should be considered as a promising target for effective antiparasitic treatments. Although metal-chelating compounds are, obviously, not innocuous to the host, in general they are less toxic than the drugs actually used for the treatment of HAT and their side effect is fully reversible upon dietary supplementation. In addition, several chelating agents are approved for the treatment of human pathologies, some of them are relatively cheap and available for oral administration (Sharma & Pancholi, 2010). The risk/benefit assessment for the use of iron chelating drugs as antiparasitic therapeutic depends on many factors not addressed yet.

Moreover, beyond the relevance of iron homeostasis for parasite survival, some components of this metabolism and/or iron-, Fe/S cluster- or heme-proteins offer excellent opportunities for the design of more specific and efficacious drugs. For instance, the enzymes involved in fatty acids biogenesis (oleate desaturase and stearoyl-CoA-desaturase) and sterol biosynthesis (CYP51); in defense against oxidants (the plant-like ascorbate peroxidase) and xenobiotics (CYP450 reductases); in cell proliferation (ribonucleotide reductase); and in Fe/S cluster biogenesis. Alternatively, chemical downregulation of the functions these proteins fulfill in the cell can be complemented by the action of first line drugs currently used in chemotherapy. A combined therapy would have the advantage of reducing dosage, shortening treatment and loweing the possibility for development of drug resistance. The specificity of the transferrin receptor is another target to be exploited as an efficient mechanism to deliver toxic molecules inside the parasite

The future prospects look promising in terms of finding novel therapeutic options to fight trypanosomiasis. However as depicted in Fig. 2 and Fig. 3, there are still several open questions that deserve to be investigated in detail to disclose atomic and functional divergences within the components of the parasite and host iron metabolism that can lead to the development of safer and efficacious drugs.

7. References

Abreu IA & Cabelli DE. (2010) Superoxide dismutases-a review of the metal-associated mechanistic variations. *Biochim. Biophys. Acta.* Vol. 1804, No. 2, pp. 263–274.

Acestor N, Panigrahi AK, Ogata Y, Anupama A & Stuart KD. (2009) Protein composition of *Trypanosoma brucei* mitochondrial membranes. *Proteomics.* Vol. 9, No. 24, pp. 5497–5508.

Adak S & Datta AK. (2005) *Leishmania major* encodes an unusual peroxidase that is a close homologue of plant ascorbate peroxidase: a novel role of the transmembrane domain. *Biochem. J.* Vol. 390, pp. 465-474.

Adam AC, Bornhövd C, Prokisch H, Neupert W & Hell K. (2006) The Nfs1 interacting protein Isd11 has an essential role in Fe/S cluster biogenesis in mitochondria. *EMBO J.* Vol. 25, No. 1, pp. 174–183.

Adl SM, Simpson AGB, Farmer MA, Andersen RA, Anderson OR, Barta JR, Bowser SS, Brugerolle G, Fensome RA, Fredericq S, James TY, Karpov S, Kugrens P, Krug J, Lane CE, Lewis LA, Lodge J, Lynn DH, Mann DG, McCourt RM, Mendoza L, Moestrup O, Mozley-Standridge SE, Nerad TA, Shearer CA, Smirnov AV, Spiegel FW & Taylor MF. (2005) The new higher level classification of eukaryotes with emphasis on the taxonomy of protists. *J. Eukaryot. Microbiol.* Vol. 52, No. 5, pp. 399–451.

Adl SM, Leander BS, Simpson AGB, Archibald JM, Anderson OR, Bass D, Bowser SS, Brugerolle G, Farmer MA, Karpov S, Kolisko M, Lane CE, Lodge DJ, Mann DG, Meisterfeld R, Mendoza L, Moestrup Ø, Mozley-Standridge SE, Smirnov AV & Spiegel F. (2007) Diversity, nomenclature, and taxonomy of protists. *Syst. Biol.* Vol. 56, No 4, pp. 684–689.

Aeby E, Seidel V & Schneider A. (2009) The selenoproteome is dispensable in bloodstream forms of *Trypanosoma brucei. Mol. Biochem. Parasitol.* Vol. 168, No. 2, pp. 191–193.

Ajayi WU, Chaudhuri M & Hill GC. (2002) Site-directed mutagenesis reveals the essentiality of the conserved residues in the putative diiron active site of the trypanosome alternative oxidase. *J. Biol. Chem.* Vol. 277, No. 10, pp. 8187–8193.

Alfonzo JD & Lukeš J. (2011) Assembling Fe/S-clusters and modifying tRNAs: ancient co-factors meet ancient adaptors. *Trends Parasitol.* Vol. 27, No. 6, pp. 235–238.

Allen JWA, Gringer ML & Ferguson SJ. (2004) Maturation of the unusual single-cysteine (XXXCH) mitochondrial c-type cytochromes found in trypanosomatids must occur through a novel biogenesis pathway. *Biochem. J.* Vol. 383, pp. 537-542.

Alloatti A, Gupta S, Gualdrón-López M, Igoillo-Esteve M, Nguewa PA, Deumer G, Wallemacq P, Altabe SG, Michels PAM & Uttaro AD. (2010) Genetic and chemical evaluation of *Trypanosoma brucei* oleate desaturase as a candidate drug target. *PLoS ONE* Vol. 5, No. 12, pp. 1-10, e14239

Alloatti A, Gupta S, Gualdrón-López M, Nguewa PA, Altabe SG, Deumer G, Wallemacq P, Michels PA & Uttaro AD. (2011) Stearoyl-CoA desaturase is an essential enzyme for the parasitic protist *Trypanosoma brucei. Biochem. Biophys. Res. Commun.* Vol. 412, No. 2, pp. 286-290.

Alvarez MN, Peluffo G, Piacenza L & Radi R. (2011) Intraphagosomal peroxynitrite as a macrophage-derived cytotoxin against internalized *Trypanosoma cruzi*: consequences for oxidative killing and role of microbial peroxiredoxins in infectivity. *J. Biol. Chem.* Vol. 286, No. 8, pp. 6627–6640.

Amutha B, Gordon DM, Gu Y, Lyver ER, Dancis A & Pain D. (2008) GTP is required for iron-sulfur cluster biogenesis in mitochondria. *J. Biol. Chem.* Vol. 283, No. 3, pp. 1362–1371.

Anderson GJ & Vulpe CD. (2009) Mammalian iron transport. *Cell. Mol. Life Sci.* Vol. 66, No. 20, pp. 3241-3261.

Andrews SC. (2010) The Ferritin-like superfamily: Evolution of the biological iron storeman from a rubrerythrin-like ancestor. *Biochim. Biophys. Acta.* Vol. 1800, No. 8, pp. 691–705.

Arantes JM, Francisco AF, de Abreu Vieira PM, Silva M, Araújo MSS, de Carvalho AT, Pedrosa ML, Carneiro CM, Tafuri WL, Martins-Filho AO & Elói-Santos SM. (2011) *Trypanosoma cruzi*: desferrioxamine decreases mortality and parasitemia in infected mice through a trypanostatic effect. *Exp. Parasitol.* Vol. 128, No. 4, pp. 401–408.

Atanasiu V, Manolescu B & Stoian I. (2007) Hepcidin: central regulator of iron metabolism. *Eur. J. Haematol.* Vol. 78, No. 1, pp. 1–10.

Bachega JFR, Navarro MVAS, Bleicher L, Bortoleto-Bugs RK, Dive D, Hoffmann P, Viscogliosi E & Garratt RC. (2009) Systematic structural studies of iron superoxide dismutases from human parasites and a statistical coupling analysis of metal binding specificity. *Proteins.* Vol. 77, No. 1, pp. 26–37.

Balk J & Lobréaux S. (2005) Biogenesis of iron-sulfur proteins in plants. *Trends Plant Sci.* Vol. 10, No. 7, pp. 324–331.

Balk J & Pilon M. (2011) Ancient and essential: the assembly of iron-sulfur clusters in plants. *Trends Plant Sci.* Vol. 16, No. 4, pp. 218–226.

Balmer O, Beadell JS, Gibson W, & Caccone, A. (2011). Phylogeography and taxonomy of *Trypanosoma brucei*. *PLoS Negl. Trop. Dis.* Vol. 5, e961.

Barrett MP, Burchmore RJS, Stich A, Lazzari JO, Frasch AC, Cazzulo JJ, & Krishna S. (2003) The trypanosomiases. *Lancet.* Vol. 362, No. 9394, pp. 1469–1480.

Batista JS, Riet-Correa F, Teixeira MMG, Madruga CR, Simões SDV & Maia TF. (2007) Trypanosomiasis by *Trypanosoma vivax* in cattle in the Brazilian semiarid: Description of an outbreak and lesions in the nervous system. *Vet. Parasitol.* Vol. 143, No. 2, pp.174–181.

Batista JS, Oliveira AF, Rodrigues CMF, Damasceno CAR, Oliveira IRS, Alves HM, Paiva ES, Brito PD, Medeiros JM, Rodrigues AC & Teixeira MM. (2009) Infection by *Trypanosoma vivax* in goats and sheep in the Brazilian semiarid region: from acute disease outbreak to chronic cryptic infection. *Vet. Parasitol.* Vol. 165, No. 1-2, pp.131–135.

Berriman, M., Ghedin, E., Hertz-Fowler, C., Blandin, G., Lennard, N.J., Bartholomeu, D., Renauld, H.J., Caler, E., Hamlin, N., Haas, B., Harris, B.R., Hannick, L., Barrell, B., Donelson, J., Hall, N., Fraser, C.M., Melville, S.E., El-Sayed, N., Böhme, U.C., Shallom, J., Aslett, M., Hou, L., Atkin, B., Barron, A.J., Bringaud, F., Brooks, K., Cherevach, I., Chillingworth, T., Churcher, C., Clark, L.N., Corton, C.H., Cronin, A., Davies, R., Doggett, J., Djikeng, A., Feldblyum, T., Fraser, A., Goodhead, I., Hance, Z., Harper, A.D., Hauser, H., Hostetler, J., Jagels, K., Johnson, D., Johnson, J., Jones, C., Kerhornou, A., Koo, H., Larke, N., Larkin, C., Leech, V., Line, A., MacLeod, A., Mooney, P., Moule, S., Mungall, K., Norbertczak, H., Ormond, D., Pai, G., Peterson, J., Quail, M.A., Rajandream, M.A., Reitter, C., Sanders, M., Schobel, S., Sharp, S., Simmonds, M., Simpson, A.J., Tallon, L., Turner, C.M., Tait, A., Tivey, A., Van Aken, S., Walker, D., Wanless, D., White, B., White, O., Whitehead, S., Wortman, J., Barry, J.D., Fairlamb, A.H., Field, M.C., Gull, K., Landfear, S., Marcello, L., Martin, D.M., Opperdoes, F., Ullu, E., Whickstead, B.,

Alsmark, C., Arrowsmith, C., Carrington, M., Embley, T.M., Ivens, A., Lord, A., Morgan, G.M., Peacock, C.S., Rabbinowitsch, E., Salzberg, S., Wang, S., Woodward, J., Adams, M.D., Embley, T.M., Gull, K., Ullu, E., Barry, J.D., Fairlamb, A.H., Opperdoes, F., Barrell, B.G., Donelson, J.E., Hall, N., Fraser, C.M., Melville, S.E. & El-Sayed, N.M. (2005). The genome of the African trypanosome, *Trypanosoma brucei*. *Science*. Vol. 309, *No. 5733*, pp. 416-422.

Birkholtz L-M, Williams M, Niemand J, Louw AI, Persson L & Heby O. (2011) Polyamine homoeostasis as a drug target in pathogenic protozoa: peculiarities and possibilities. *Biochem. J.* Vol. 438, No. 2, pp. 229–244.

Bitter W, Gerrits H, Kieft R & Borst P. (1998) The role of transferrinreceptor variation in the host range of *Trypanosoma brucei*. *Nature*. Vol. 391, No. 6666 pp. 499-502.

Bocedi A, Dawood KF, Fabrini R, Federici G, Gradoni L, Pedersen JZ & Ricci G. (2010) Trypanothione efficiently intercepts nitric oxide as a harmless iron complex in trypanosomatid parasites. *FASEB J.* Vol. 24, No. 4, pp. 1035–1042.

Bosworth CA, Toledo JC Jr, Zmijewski JW, Li Q & Lancaster JR Jr. (2009) Dinitrosyliron complexes and the mechanism(s) of cellular protein nitrosothiol formation from nitric oxide. *Proc. Natl. Acad. Sci. USA*. Vol. 106, No. 12, pp. 4671-4676.

Braz, GRC, Coelho HSL, Masuda H & Oliveira PL. (1999) A missing metabolic pathway in the cattle tick *Boophilus microplus*. *Curr. Biol.* Vol. 9, No. 13, pp. 703-706.

Breidbach T, Krauth-Siegel RL & Steverding D. (2000) Ribonucleotide reductase is regulated via the R2 subunit during the life cycle of *Trypanosoma brucei*. *FEBS Lett.* Vol. 473, No. 2, pp. 212–216.

Breidbach T, Scory S, Krauth-Siegel RL & Steverding D. (2002) Growth inhibition of bloodstream forms of *Trypanosoma brucei* by the iron chelator deferoxamine. *Int. J. Parasitol.* Vol 32, No. 4, pp. 473–479.

Bruske EI, Sendfeld F & Schneider A. (2009) Thiolated tRNAs of *Trypanosoma brucei* are imported into mitochondria and dethiolated after import. *J. Biol. Chem.* Vol. 284, No. 52, pp. 36491–36499.

Camaschella C & Strati P. (2010) Recent advances in iron metabolism and related disorders *Intern. Emerg. Med.* Vol. 5, No. 5, pp. 393–400.

Campos-Salinas J, Cabello-Donayre M, García-Hernández R, Pérez-Victoria I, Castanys S, Gamarro F & Pérez-Victoria JM. (2011) A new ATP-binding cassette protein is involved in intracellular haem trafficking in *Leishmania*. *Molec. Microbiol.* Vol. 79, No. 6, pp. 1430-1444.

Cavalli A & Bolognesi ML. (2009) Neglected tropical diseases: multi-target-directed ligands in the search for novel lead candidates against *Trypanosoma* and *Leishmania*. *J. Med. Chem.* Vol. 52, No. 23, pp. 7339–7359.

Cazzulo JJ. (1992) Aerobic fermentation of glucose by trypanosomatids. *FASEB J.* Vol. 6, pp-3153-3161.

Ceylan S, Seidel V, Ziebart N, Berndt C, Dirdjaja N & Krauth-Siegel RL. (2010) The dithiol glutaredoxins of african trypanosomes have distinct roles and are closely linked to the unique trypanothione metabolism. *J. Biol. Chem.* Vol. 285, No. 45, pp. 35224–35237.

Chang KP & Trager W. (1974) Nutritional Significance of Symbiotic Bacteria in Two Species of Hemoflagellates. *Science* Vol. 183, pp. 531-532.

Chang KP, Chang CS & Sassa S. (1975) Heme biosynthesis in bacterium-protozoon symbioses: enzymic defects in host hemoflagellates and complemental role of their intracellular symbiotes. *Proc. Nat. Acad. Sci.* Vol. 72, No. 8, pp. 2979-2983.

Chaudhuri M, Ajayi W & Hill GC. (1998) Biochemical and molecular properties of the *Trypanosoma brucei* alternative oxidase. *Mol. Biochem. Parasitol.* Vol. 95, No. 1, pp. 53–68.

Chaudhuri M, Sharan R & Hill GC. (2002) Trypanosome alternative oxidase is regulated post-transcriptionally at the level of RNA stability. *J. Eukaryot. Microbiol.* Vol. 49, No. 4, pp. 263–269.

Chaudhuri M, Ott RD & Hill GC. (2006) Trypanosome alternative oxidase: from molecule to function. *Trends Parasitol.* Vol. 22, No. 10, pp. 484–491.

Chisi JE, Misiri H, Zverev Y, Nkhoma A & Sternberg JM (2004). Anaemia in human African trypanosomiasis caused by *Trypanosoma brucei rhodesiense. East Afr. Med. J.* Vol. 81, No. 10, pp. 505-508.

Chen CK, Leung SSF, Guilbert C, Jacobson MP, Mckerrow JH & Podust LM. (2010) Structural characterization of CYP51 from *Trypanosoma cruzi* and *Trypanosoma brucei* bound to the antifungal drugs posaconazole and fluconazole. *PLoS Neglected Tropical Diseases*, 4(4): e651.

Clarkson AB Jr & Brohn FH. (1976) Trypanosomiasis: an approach to chemotherapy by the inhibition of carbohydrate catabolism. *Science.* Vol. 194, No. 4261, pp. 204–206.

Clarkson AB Jr, Bienen EJ, Pollakis G & Grady RW. (1989) Respiration of bloodstream forms of the parasite *Trypanosoma brucei* brucei is dependent on a plant-like alternative oxidase. *J. Biol. Chem.* Vol. 264, No. 30, pp. 17770–17776.

Colombo FA, Odorizzi RM, Laurenti MD, Galati EA, Canavez F & Pereira-Chioccola VL. (2011) Detection of *Leishmania* (Leishmania) *infantum* RNA in fleas and tickscollected from naturally infected dogs. *Parasitol. Res.* Vol. 109, No. 2, pp. 267-274.

Comini MA, Rettig J, Dirdjaja N, Hanschmann E-M, Berndt C & Krauth-Siegel RL. (2008) Monothiol glutaredoxin-1 is an essential iron-sulfur protein in the mitochondrion of African trypanosomes. *J. Biol. Chem.* Vol. 283, No. 41, pp. 27785–27798.

Comini MA, Medeiros AM & Manta B. (2011) Stress response in the infective stage of *Trypanosoma brucei.* In: Stress response in microbiology. Ed. José M. Requena. Horizon Scientific Press, Norwich, UK. *In press*

Coustou V, Biran M, Besteiro S, Rivière L, Baltz T, Franconi JM & Bringaud F. (2006) Fumarate is an essential intermediary metabolite produced by the procyclic *Trypanosoma brucei. J. Biol. Chem.* Vol. 281, No. 37, pp. 26832-26846.

Cotruvo JA & Stubbe J. (2011) Class I ribonucleotide reductases: metallocofactor assembly and repair in vitro and in vivo. *Annu. Rev. Biochem.* Vol. 80, pp. 733–767.

Dantas-Torres F. (2011) Ticks as vectors of *Leishmania* parasites. *Trends Parasitol. Vol. 27, No. 4, pp.155-159.*

Da Silva AS, Garcia Perez HA, Costa MM, França RT, De Gasperi D, Zanette RA, Amado JA, Lopes ST, Teixeira MM & Monteiro SG. (2011) Horses naturally infected by *Trypanosoma vivax* in southern Brazil. *Parasitol. Res.* Vol. 108, No. 1, pp. 23–30.

Dávila AM & Silva RA. (2000) Animal trypanosomiasis in South America. Current status, partnership, and information technology. *Ann. N. Y. Acad. Sci.* Vol. 2000, No. 916, pp. 199–212.

De Vas MG, Portal P, Alonso GD, Schleinger M, Flawiá MM, Torres HN, Fenrández Villamil S & Paveto C. (2011) The NADPH–cytochrome P450 reductase family in *Trypanosoma cruzi* is involved in the sterol biosynthesis pathway. *Int. J. Parasitol.* Vol. 41, pp. 99-108.

Delespaux V & de Koning HP. (2007) Drugs and drug resistance in African trypanosomiasis. Drug *Resist. Updat.* Vol 10, No. 1-2, pp. 30–50.

Dolai S, Yadav RK, Pal S & Adak S. (2008) *Leishmania major* ascorbate peroxidase overexpression protects cells against reactive oxigen species-mediated cardiolipin oxidation. *Free Rad. Biol. Med.* Vol. 45, pp. 1520-1529.

Dolai S., Yadav R. K., Pal S. & Adak S. (2009) Overexpression of mitochondrial Leishmania major ascorbate peroxidase enhances tolerance to oxidative stress-induced programmed cell death and protein damage. *Eukaryot. Cell.* Vol. 8. No. 11, pp. 1721-1731.

Dormeyer M, Schöneck R, Dittmar GA & Krauth-Siegel RL. (1997) Cloning, sequencing and expression of ribonucleotide reductase R2 from *Trypanosoma brucei*. *FEBS Lett.* Vol. 414, No. 2, pp. 449–453.

Dormeyer M, Reckenfelderbäumer N, Ludemann H & Krauth-Siegel RL. (2001) Trypanothione-dependent synthesis of deoxyribonucleotides by *Trypanosoma brucei* ribonucleotide reductase. *J. Biol. Chem.* Vol. 276, No. 14, pp. 10602–10606.

Dufernez F, Yernaux C, Gerbod D, Noël C, Chauvenet M, Wintjens R, Edgcomb VP, Capron M, Opperdoes FR & Viscogliosi E. (2006) The presence of four iron-containing superoxide dismutase isozymes in trypanosomatidae: characterization, subcellular localization, and phylogenetic origin in *Trypanosoma brucei*. *Free Radic. Biol. Med.* Vol. 40, No. 2, pp. 210–225.

El-Sayed NM, Myler PJ, Bartholomeu DC, Nilsson D, Aggarwal G, Tran AN, Ghedin E, Worthey EA, Delcher AL, Blandin G, Westenberger SJ, Caler E, Cerqueira GC, Branche C, Haas B, Anupama A, Arner E, Aslund L, Attipoe P, Bontempi E, Bringaud F, Burton P, Cadag E, Campbell DA, Carrington M, Crabtree J, Darban H, da Silveira JF, de Jong P, Edwards K, Englund PT, Fazelina G, Feldblyum T, Ferella M, Frasch AC, Gull K, Horn D, Hou L, Huang Y, Kindlund E, Klingbeil M, Kluge S, Koo H, Lacerda D, Levin MJ, Lorenzi H, Louie T, Machado CR, McCulloch R, McKenna A, Mizuno Y, Mottram JC, Nelson S, Ochaya S, Osoegawa K, Pai G, Parsons M, Pentony M, Pettersson U, Pop M, Ramirez JL, Rinta J, Robertson L, Salzberg SL, Sanchez DO, Seyler A, Sharma R, Shetty J, Simpson AJ, Sisk E, Tammi MT, Tarleton R, Teixeira S, Van Aken S, Vogt C, Ward PN, Wickstead B, Wortman J, White O, Fraser CM, Stuart KD & Andersson B. (2005) The genome sequence of *Trypanosoma cruzi,* etiologic agent of Chagas disease. *Science.* Vol. 309, No. 5733, pp. 409-415.

Fast B, Kremp K, Boshart M & Steverding D. (1999) Iron-dependent regulation of transferrin receptor expression in *Trypanosoma brucei*. *Biochem. J.* Vol. 342, Pt 3, pp. 691–696.

Fernandes AP, Fladvad M, Berndt C, Andrésen C, Lillig CH, Neubauer P, Sunnerhagen M, Holmgren A & Vlamis-Gardikas A. (2005) A novel monothiol glutaredoxin (Grx4) from *Escherichia coli* can serve as a substrate for thioredoxin reductase. *J. Biol. Chem.* Vol. 280, No. 26, pp. 24544–24552.

Fèvre EM, Picozzi K, Jannin J, Welburn SC & Maudlin I. (2006) Human African trypanosomiasis: Epidemiology and control. *Adv. Parasitol.* Vol. 61, pp. 167–221.

Filser M, Comini MA, Molina-Navarro MM, Dirdjaja N, Herrero E & Krauth-Siegel RL. (2008) Cloning, functional analysis, and mitochondrial localization of *Trypanosoma brucei* monothiol glutaredoxin-1. *Biol. Chem.* Vol. 389, No. 1, pp. 21–32.

Ganz T. (2009) Iron in innate immunity: starve the invaders. *Curr. Opin. Immunol.* Vol. 21, No. 1, pp. 63–67.

Gerrits H, Mussmann R, Bitter W, Kieft R & Borst P. (2002). The physiological significance of transferrin receptor variations in *Trypanosoma brucei*. *Mol. Biochem. Parasitol.* Vol. 119, No. 2, pp. 237-247.

Girard M, Giraud S, Courtioux B, Jauberteau-Marchan M-O & Bouteille B.(2005) Endothelial cell activation in the presence of African trypanosomes. *Mol. Biochem. Parasitol.* Vol. 139, No. 1, pp. 41–49.

Gordeuk VR. (2002) African iron overload. *Semin. Hematol.* Vol. 39, No. 4, pp. 263–269.

Ghosh S, Goswami S & Adhya S. (2003) Role of superoxide dismutase in survival of *Leishmania* within the macrophage. *Biochem. J.* Vol. 369, Pt. 3, pp. 447–452.

Grab DJ, Wells CW, Shaw MK, Webster P & Russo DC. (1992). Endocytosed transferrin in African trypanosomes is delivered to lysosomes and may not be recycled. Eur. J. Cell Biol. Vol. 59, No. 2, pp. 398-404.

Grab DJ, Shaw MK, Wells CW, Verjee Y, Russo DC, Webster P, Naessens J, & Fish, W.R. (1993). The transferrin receptor in African trypanosomes: identification, partial characterization and subcellular localization. *Eur. J. Cell Biol.* Vol 62, No. 1, pp. 114-126.

Grant PT & Sargent JR. (1960) Properties of L-alpha-glycerophosphate oxidase and its role in the respiration of *Trypanosoma rhodesiense. Biochem. J.* Vol. 76, pp. 229–237.

Halliwel B & Gutteridge J. (1999) *Free Radical in Biology and Medicine.* Oxford University Press.ISBN 978-0198500445.

Hamilton PB, Stevens JR, Gaunt MW, Gidley J & Gibson WC. (2004). Trypanosomes are monophyletic: evidence from genes for glyceraldehyde phosphate dehydrogenase and small subunit ribosomal RNA. *Int. J. Parasitol.* Vol. 34, No. 12, pp. 1393-1404.

Hamilton PB, Gibson WC & Stevens JR (2007). Patterns of co-evolution between trypanosomes and their hosts deduced from ribosomal RNA and protein-coding gene phylogenies. *Mol. Phylogenetics Evol.* Vol. 44, No. 1, pp.15–25.

Hentze MW, Muckenthaler MU, Galy B & Camaschella C. (2010) Two to tango: regulation of Mammalian iron metabolism. *Cell.* Vol 142, No. 1, pp. 24–38.

Herrera L & Urdaneta-Morales S. (2001) Experimental transmission of *Trypanosoma cruzi* through the genitalia of albino mice. *Mem Inst Oswaldo Cruz.* Vol. 96, No. 5, pp. 713-717.

Hider RC & Kong XL. (2011) Glutathione: a key component of the cytoplasmic labile iron pool. *Biometals.* DOI: 10.1007/s10534-011-9476-8

Hofer A, Schmidt PP, Gräslund A & Thelander L. (1997) Cloning and characterization of the R1 and R2 subunits of ribonucleotide reductase from *Trypanosoma brucei. Proc. Natl. Acad. Sci. U.S.A.* Vol. 94, No. 13, pp. 6959–6964.

Hofer A, Ekanem JT & Thelander L. (1998) Allosteric regulation of *Trypanosoma brucei* ribonucleotide reductase studied *in vitro* and *in vivo. J. Biol. Chem.* Vol. 273, No. 51, pp. 34098–34104.

Horváth A, Horáková E, Dunajcíková P, Verner Z, Pravdová E, Slapetová I, Cuninková L & Lukes J. (2005) Downregulation of the nuclear-encoded subunits of the complexes III and IV disrupts their respective complexes but not complex I in procyclic *Trypanosoma brucei. Mol. Microbiol.* Vol. 58, No. 1, pp. 116-130.

Igbokwe IO, Esievo KA, Saror DI & Obagaiye OK. (1994) Increased susceptibility of erythrocytes to in vitro peroxidation in acute *Trypanosoma brucei* infection of mice. *Vet. Parasitol.* Vol. 55, No. 4, pp. 279–286.

Irigoín F, Cibils L, Comini MA, Wilkinson SR, Flohé L & Radi R.(2008) Insights into the redox biology of *Trypanosoma cruzi*: Trypanothione metabolism and oxidant detoxification. *Free Radic. Biol. Med.* Vol. 45, No. 6, pp. 733–742.

Ivens AC, Peacock CS, Worthey EA, Murphy L, Aggarwal G, Berriman M, Sisk E, Rajandream MA, Adlem E, Aert R, Anupama A, Apostolou Z, Attipoe P, Bason N, Bauser C, Beck A, Beverley SM, Bianchettin G, Borzym K, Bothe G, Bruschi CV,

Collins M, Cadag E, Ciarloni L, Clayton C, Coulson RM, Cronin A, Cruz AK, Davies RM, De Gaudenzi J, Dobson DE, Duesterhoeft A, Fazelina G, Fosker N, Frasch AC, Fraser A, Fuchs M, Gabel C, Goble A, Goffeau A, Harris D, Hertz-Fowler C, Hilbert H, Horn D, Huang Y, Klages S, Knights A, Kube M, Larke N, Litvin L, Lord A, Louie T, Marra M, Masuy D, Matthews K, Michaeli S, Mottram JC, Müller-Auer S, Munden H, Nelson S, Norbertczak H, Oliver K, O'neil S, Pentony M, Pohl TM, Price C, Purnelle B, Quail MA, Rabbinowitsch E, Reinhardt R, Rieger M, Rinta J, Robben J, Robertson L, Ruiz JC, Rutter S, Saunders D, Schäfer M, Schein J, Schwartz DC, Seeger K, Seyler A, Sharp S, Shin H, Sivam D, Squares R, Squares S, Tosato V, Vogt C, Volckaert G, Wambutt R, Warren T, Wedler H, Woodward J, Zhou S, Zimmermann W, Smith DF, Blackwell JM, Stuart KD, Barrell B &, Myler PJ. (2005) The genome of the kinetoplastid parasite, *Leishmania major*. *Science* Vol. 309, No. 5733, pp.:436-42.

Jacobs RT, Nare B & Phillips MA. (2011) State of the art in African trypanosome drug discovery. *Curr Top Med Chem*. Vol. 11, No. 10, pp. 1255–1274.

Jones MM, Singh PK, Lane JE, Rodrigues RR, Nesset A, Suarez CC, Bogitsh BJ & Carter CE. (1996) Inhibition of *Trypanosoma cruzi* epimastigotes in vitro by iron chelating agents. *Arzneimittelforschung*. Vol. 46, No. 12, pp. 1158–1162.

Kakhlon O & Cabantchik ZI. (2002) The labile iron pool: characterization, measurement, and participation in cellular processes. *Free Radic. Biol. Med.* Vol. 33, No. 8, pp. 1037–1046.

Kabiri M & Steverding D. (2000). Studies on the recycling of the transferrin receptor in *Trypanosoma brucei* using an inducible gene expression system. *Eur. J. Biochem.* Vol. 267, No. 11, pp. 3309-3314.

Kabiri M & Steverding D. (2001) Identification of a developmentally regulated iron superoxide dismutase of *Trypanosoma brucei*. *Biochem. J.* Vol. 360, Pt 1, pp. 173–177.

Kido Y, Shiba T, Inaoka DK, Sakamoto K, Nara T, Aoki T, Honma T, Tanaka A, Inoue M, Matsuoka S, Moore A, Harada S & Kita K. (2010a) Crystallization and preliminary crystallographic analysis of cyanide-insensitive alternative oxidase from *Trypanosoma brucei* brucei. *Acta Crystallogr. Sect. F Struct. Biol. Cryst. Commun.* Vol. 66, Pt 3, pp. 275–278.

Kido Y, Sakamoto K, Nakamura K, Harada M, Suzuki T, Yabu Y, Saimoto H, Yamakura F, Ohmori D, Moore A, Harada S & Kita K. (2010b) Purification and kinetic characterization of recombinant alternative oxidase from *Trypanosoma brucei* brucei. *Biochim. Biophys. Acta.* Vol. 1797, No. 4, pp. 443–450.

Kontoghiorghes GJ, Kolnagou A, Skiada A & Petrikkos G. (2010) The role of iron and chelators on infections in iron overload and non iron loaded conditions: prospects for the design of new antimicrobial therapies. *Hemoglobin.* Vol. 34, No. 3, pp. 227–239.

Koopmann E & Hahlbrock K. (1997) Differentially regulated NADPH:cytochrome P450 oxidoreductases in parsley. *Proc. Natl. Acad. Sci.* Vol. 94, pp. 14954-14959.

Korený L, Lukes, J & Oborník M. (2010) Evolution of the haem synthetic pathway in kinetoplastid flagellates: an essential pathway that is not essential after all? *International Journal for Parasitol.* Vol. 40, pp. 149-156.

Kosman DJ. (2010) Redox cycling in iron uptake, efflux, and trafficking. *J. Biol. Chem.* Vol. 285, No. 35, pp. 26729–26735.

Krauth-Siegel RL & Comini MA. (2008) Redox control in trypanosomatids, parasitic protozoa with trypanothione-based thiol metabolism. *Biochim. Biophys. Acta.* Vol. 1780, No. 11, pp. 1236–1248.

Krauth-Siegel RL & Lüdemann H. *(1996)* Reduction of dehydroascorbate by trypanothione. *Mol. Biochem. Parasitol. Vol. 80, No. 2, pp. 203-208.*

Kumánovics A, Chen OS, Li L, Bagley D, Adkins EM, Lin H, Dingra NN, Outten CE, Keller G, Winge D & Ward DM & Kaplan J. (2008) Identification of FRA1 and FRA2 as genes involved in regulating the yeast iron regulon in response to decreased mitochondrial iron-sulfur cluster synthesis. *J. Biol. Chem.* Vol. 283, No. 16, pp. 10276–10286.

Kumar C, Igbaria A, D'Autreaux B, Planson A-G, Junot C, Godat E, Bachhawat AK, Delaunay-Moisan A & Toledano MB. (2011) Glutathione revisited: a vital function in iron metabolism and ancillary role in thiol-redox control. *EMBO J.* Vol. 30, No.,10, pp-.2044–2056.

Kurz T, Eaton JW & Brunk UT. (2011) The role of lysosomes in iron metabolism and recycling. *Int. J. Biochem. Cell. Biol.,* Vol. 43, No. 12, pp. 1686-1697.

Lalonde RG & Holbein BE. (1984) Role of iron in *Trypanosoma cruzi* infection of mice. *J. Clin. Invest.* Vol. 73, No. 2, pp. 470–476.

Lara FA, Sant'Anna C, Femos D, Laranja GAT, Coelho MGP, Reis Salles I, Michael A, Oliveira PL, Cunha-e-Silva N, Salmon D & Paes MC. (2007) Heme requirement and intracellular trafficking in *Trypanosoma cruzi* epimastigotes. *Biochem. Biophys. Res. Comm.* Vol. 355, pp. 16-22.

Le Trant N, Meshnick SR, Kitchener K, Eaton JW & Cerami A. (1983) Iron-containing superoxide dismutase from *Crithidia fasciculata*. Purification, characterization, and similarity to Leishmanial and trypanosomal enzymes. *J. Biol. Chem.* Vol. 258, No. 1, pp. 125–30.

Lepesheva GI, Ott RD, Hargrove TY, Kleshchenko YY, Schuster I, Nes WD, Hill GC, Villalta F & Waterman MR. (2007) Sterol 14alpha-demethylase as a potential target for antitrypanosomal therapy: enzyme inhibition and parasite cell growth. *Chem. Biol.* Vol. 14, No. 11, pp1283-1293.

Levi S & Rovida E. (2009) The role of iron in mitochondrial function. *Biochim. Biophys. Acta.* Vol. 1790, No. 7, pp. 629–636.

Lill R & Mühlenhoff U. (2006) Iron-sulfur protein biogenesis in eukaryotes: components and mechanisms. *Annu. Rev. Cell Dev. Biol.* Vol. 22, pp. 457–486.

Lill R & Mühlenhoff U. (2008) Maturation of iron-sulfur proteins in eukaryotes: mechanisms, connected processes, and diseases. *Annu. Rev. Biochem.* Vol. 77, pp. 669–700.

Lill R. (2009) Function and biogenesis of iron-sulphur proteins. *Nature.* Vol. 460, No. 7257, pp. 831–838.

Lillig CH, Berndt C & Holmgren A. (2008) Glutaredoxin systems. *Biochim. Biophys. Acta.* Vol. 1780, No. 11, pp. 1304–1317.

Logan FJ, Taylor MC, Wilkinson SR, Kaur H & Kelly JM. (2007) The terminal step in vitamin C biosynthesis in *Trypanosoma cruzi* is mediated by a FMN-dependent galactonolactone oxidase. *Biochem. J.* Vol. 407, No. 3, pp. 419-426.

Long S, Jirku M, Ayala FJ & Lukes J. (2008a) Mitochondrial localization of human frataxin is necessary but processing is not for rescuing frataxin deficiency in *Trypanosoma brucei*. *Proc. Natl. Acad. Sci. U.S.A.* Vol. 105, No. 36, pp. 13468–13473.

Long S, Jirků M, Mach J, Ginger ML, Sutak R, Richardson D, Tachezy J & Lukes J. (2008b) Ancestral roles of eukaryotic frataxin: mitochondrial frataxin function and heterologous expression of hydrogenosomal Trichomonas homologues in trypanosomes. *Mol. Microbiol.* Vol. 69, No. 1, pp. 94–109.

Long S, Changmai P, Tsaousis AD, Skalický T, Verner Z, Wen Y-Z, Roger AJ, & Lukeš J. (2011) Stage-specific requirement for Isa1 and Isa2 proteins in the mitochondrion of *Trypanosoma brucei* and heterologous rescue by human and Blastocystis orthologues. *Mol. Microbiol.* Vol. 81, No. 6, pp. 1403–1418.

Loo VG & Lalonde RG.(1984) Role of iron in intracellular growth of *Trypanosoma cruzi*. (1984) *Infect. Immun.*Vol. 45, No. 3, pp.726–730.

Lu W, Wei G, Pan W & Tabel H. (2011) *Trypanosoma congolense* infections: induced nitric oxide inhibits parasite growth *in vivo*. *J. Parasitol. Res.*,:316067.

Lüdemann H, Dormeyer M, Sticherling C, Stallmann D, Follmann H & Krauth-Siegel RL. (1998) *Trypanosoma brucei* tryparedoxin, a thioredoxin-like protein in African trypanosomes. *FEBS Lett.* Vol. 431, No. 3, pp. 381–385.

Luckins AG & Dwinger RH. (2004). Non-tsetse-transmitted trypanosomiasis. In The Trypanosomiases, I. Maudlin, P.H. Holmes and M.A. Miles, eds. (Wallingford, UK: CA International Press), pp. 269-281.

Magez S & Caljon G. (2011) Mouse models for pathogenic African trypanosomes: unravelling the immunology of host-parasite-vector interactions. *Parasite Immunol.* Vol. 33, No. 8, pp. 423–429.

Man WC, Miyazaki M, Chu K & Ntambi JM. (2006) Membrane topology of mouse stearoyl-CoA desaturase 1. *J. Biol. Chem.* Vol. 281, No. 2, pp. 1251-1260.

Maslov DA, Lukes J, Jirku M & Simpson L. (1996). Phylogeny of trypanosomes as inferred from the small and large subunit rRNAs: implications for the evolution of parasitism in the trypanosomatid protozoa. *Mol. Biochem. Parasitol.* Vol. 75, No. 2, pp. 197-205.

Matovu E, Seebeck T, Enyaru JC & Kaminsky R. (2001) Drug resistance in *Trypanosoma brucei* spp., the causative agents of sleeping sickness in man and nagana in cattle. *Microbes Infect.* Vol. 3, No. 9, pp. 763–770.

Maudlin I. (2006) African trypanosomiasis. *Ann Trop Med Parasitol.* Vol. 100, No. 8, pp. 679–701.

Maxwell DP, Wang Y & McIntosh L. (1999) The alternative oxidase lowers mitochondrial reactive oxygen production in plant cells. *Proc. Natl. Acad. Sci. USA.* Vol. 96, No. 14, pp. 8271-8276.

Maya JD, Bollo S, Nuñez-VergaraLJ, Squella JA, Repetto Y, Morello A, Périé J & Chauvière G. (2003) *Trypanosoma cruzi*: effect and mode of action of nitroimidazole and nitrofuran derivatives. *Biochem. Pharmacol.* Vol. 65, No. 6, pp. 999-1006.

Maya JD, Cassels BK, Iturriaga-Vásquez P, Ferreira J, Faúndez M, Galanti N, Ferreira A & Morello A. (2007) Mode of action of natural and synthetic drugs against *Trypanosoma cruzi* and their interaction with the mammalian host. *Comp. Biochem. Physiol. A Mol Integr Physiol.* Vol. 146, No. 4, pp. 601–620.

McNamara L, MacPhail AP, Mandishona E, Bloom P, Paterson AC, Rouault TA & Gordeuk VR. (1999) Non-transferrin-bound iron and hepatic dysfunction in African dietary iron overload. *J. Gastroenterol. Hepatol.* Vol. 14, No. 2, pp. 126–132.

Mekata H, Konnai S, Witola WH, Inoue N, Onuma M & Ohashi K. (2009) Molecular detection of trypanosomes in cattle in South America and genetic diversity of *Trypanosoma evansi* based on expression-site-associated gene 6. *Infect. Genet. Evol.* Vol. 9, No. 6, pp. 1301–1305.

Michels PA, Bringaud F, Herman M & Hannaert V. (2006) Metabolic functions of glycosomes in trypanosomatids. *Biochim Biophys Acta.* Vol. 1763, No. 12, pp. 1463-1477.

Mochizuki N, Tanaka R, Grimm B, Masuda T, Moulin M, Smith AG, Tanaka A & Terry MJ. (2010) The cell biology of tetrapyrroles: a life and death struggle.*Trends Plant Sci.* Vol. 15, No. 9, pp. 488-498.

Moore AL & Albury MS. (2008) Further insights into the structure of the alternative oxidase: from plants to parasites. *Biochem. Soc. Trans.* Vol. 36, Pt 5, pp. 1022–1026.

Moyo VM, Mandishona E, Hasstedt SJ, Gangaidzo IT, Gomo ZA, Khumalo H, Saungweme T, Kiire CF, Paterson AC, Bloom P, MacPhail AP, Rouault T & Gordeuk VR. (1998) Evidence of genetic transmission in African iron overload. *Blood.* Vol. 91, No. 3, pp-1076–1082.

Mühlenhoff U, Molik S, Godoy JR, Uzarska MA, Richter N, Seubert A, Zhang Y, Stubbe J, Pierrel F, Herrero E, Lillig CH & Lill R. (2010) Cytosolic monothiol glutaredoxins function in intracellular iron sensing and trafficking via their bound iron-sulfur cluster. *Cell Metab.* Vol. 12, No. 4, pp. 373–385.

Murataliev MB, Feyereisen R & Walker FA. (2004) Electron transfer by diflavin reductases. *Biochim. Biophys. Acta* Vol. 1698, pp. 1-26.

Mussmann R, Janssen H, Calafat J, Engstler M, Ansorge I, Clayton C & Borst, P. (2003). The expression level determines the surface distribution of the transferrin receptor in *Trypanosoma brucei. Mol. Microbiol.* Vol. 47, No. 1, pp. 23-35.

Mussmann R, Engstler M, Gerrits H, Kieft R, Toaldo CB, Onderwater J, Koerten H, van Luenen HG & Borst, P. (2004). Factors affecting the level and localization of the transferrin receptor in *Trypanosoma brucei. J. Biol. Chem.* Vol. 279, No. 39, pp. 40690-40698.

Mwangi SM, McOdimba F & Logan-Henfrey L. (1995) The effect of *Trypanosoma brucei* brucei infection on rabbit plasma iron and zinc concentrations. *Acta Trop.* Vol. 59, No. 4, pp. 283–291.

Nakamura K, Fujioka S, Fukumoto S, Inoue N, Sakamoto K, Hirata H, Kido Y, Yabu Y, Suzuki T, Watanabe Y, Saimoto H, Akiyama H & Kita K. (2010) Trypanosome alternative oxidase, a potential therapeutic target for sleeping sickness, is conserved among *Trypanosoma brucei* subspecies. *Parasitol. Int.* Vol. 59, No. 4, pp. 560–564.

Naula C & Burchmore R. (2003) A plethora of targets, a paucity of drugs: progress towards the development of novel chemotherapies for human African trypanosomiasis. *Expert Rev. Anti Infect. Ther.* Vol 1, No. 1, pp. 157-165.

Netz DJA, Stümpfig M, Doré C, Mühlenhoff U, Pierik AJ & Lill R. (2010) Tah18 transfers electrons to Dre2 in cytosolic iron-sulfur protein biogenesis. *Nat. Chem. Biol.* Vol. 6, No. 10, pp. 758–765.

Nishimura K, Nakaya H, Nakagawa H, Matsuo S, Ohnishi Y & Yamasaki S. (2011) Effect of *Trypanosoma brucei brucei* on erythropoiesis in infected rats. *J. Parasitol.* Vol. 97, No. 1, pp. 88–93.

O'Brien TC, Mackey ZB, Fetter RD, Choe Y, O'Donoghue AJ, Zhou M, Craik CS, Caffrey CR & McKerrow JH. (2008) A parasite cysteine protease is key to host protein degradation and iron acquisition. *J. Biol Chem.* Vol. 283, No. 43, pp. 28934-28943.

Omotainse SO & Anosa VO. (1992) Erythrocyte response to *Trypanosoma brucei* in experimentally infected dogs. *Rev Elev Med Vet Pays Trop.* Vol. 45, No. 3-4, pp. 279–283.

Overath P, Czichos J & Haas C. (1986) The effect of citrate/cis-aconitate on oxidative metabolism during transformation of *Trypanosoma brucei. Eur. J. Biochem.* Vol. 160, No. 1, pp. 175–182

Paris Z, Rubio MAT, Lukes J & Alfonzo JD. (2009) Mitochondrial tRNA import in *Trypanosoma brucei* is independent of thiolation and the Rieske protein. *RNA.* Vol. 15, No. 7, pp. 1398–1406.

Paris Z, Changmai P, Rubio MAT, Zíková A, Stuart KD, Alfonzo JD & Lukes J. (2010) The Fe/S cluster assembly protein Isd11 is essential for tRNA thiolation in *Trypanosoma brucei. J. Biol. Chem.* Vol. 285, No. 29, pp. 22394–22402.

Peixoto Cupelloa M, Fernandes de Souzaa C, Buchenskyb C, Baptista Rocha Corrêa Soaresc, Augusto Travassos Laranjaa JG, Garcia Pinto Coelhoa M, Criccob JA & Paes MC. (2011) The heme uptake process in *Trypanosoma cruzi* epimastigotes is inhibited by heme analogues and by inhibitors of ABC transporters. *Acta Tropica.* Vol. 120, No. 3, pp. 211-218.

Petrini G, Altabe SG & Uttaro AD. (2004) *Trypanosoma brucei* oleate desaturase may use a cytochrome b5-like domain in another desaturase as an electron donor. *Eur. J. Biochem.* Vol. 271, pp.1079-1086.

Piacenza L, Irigoín F, Alvarez MN, Peluffo G, Taylor MC, Kelly JM, Wilkinson SR & Radi R. (2007) Mitochondrial superoxide radicals mediate programmed cell death in *Trypanosoma cruzi*: cytoprotective action of mitochondrial iron superoxide dismutase overexpression. *Biochem. J.* Vol. 403, No. 2, pp. 323–334.

Plewes KA, Barr SD, & Gedamu L. (2003) Iron superoxide dismutases targeted to the glycosomes of *Leishmania chagasi* are important for survival. *Infect. Imm.* Vol. 71, No. 1, pp. 5910–5920.

Poliak P, Van Hoewyk D, Oborník M, Zíková A, Stuart KD, Tachezy J, Pilon M & Lukes J. (2010) Functions and cellular localization of cysteine desulfurase and selenocysteine lyase in *Trypanosoma brucei. FEBS J.* Vol. 277, No. 2, pp. 383–393.

Portal P, Fernández Villamil S, Alonso GD, De Vas MG, Flawiá MM, Torres HN & Paveto C. (2008) Multiple NADPH–cytochrome P450 reductases from *Trypanosoma cruzi.* Suggested role on drug resistance. *Molec. Biochem. Parasitol.* Vol. 160, pp. 42-51

Prathalingham SR, Wilkinson SR, Horn D & Kelly JM. (2007) Deletion of the *Trypanosoma brucei* superoxide dismutase gene sodb1 increases sensitivity to nifurtimox and benznidazole. *Antimicrob. Agents Chemother.* Vol. 51, No. 2, pp. 755–758.

Priest JW & Hajduk SL. (1994) Developmental regulation of mitochondrial biogenesis in *Trypanosoma brucei. J. Bioenerg. Biomembr.* Vol. 26, No. 2, pp. 179–191.

Pujol-Carrion N, Belli G, Herrero E, Nogues A & de la Torre-Ruiz MA. (2006) Glutaredoxins Grx3 and Grx4 regulate nuclear localisation of Aft1 and the oxidative stress response in *Saccharomyces cerevisiae. J. Cell. Sci.* Vol. 119, Pt 21, pp. 4554–4564.

Py B & Barras F. (2010) Building Fe-S proteins: bacterial strategies. *Nat. Rev. Microbiol.* Vol. 8, No. 6, pp. 436–446.

Rao AU, Carta LK., Lesuisse E & Hamza I. Lack of heme synthesis in a free-living eukaryote. (2005) *Proc. Nat. Acad. Sci. USA.* Vol. 102, No. 12, pp. 4270-4275.

Ro D-K., Ehlting J & Douglas CJ. (2002) Cloning, functional expression, and subcellular localization of multiple NADPH-cytochrome P450 reductases from hybrid poplar. *Plant Physiol.* Vol. 130, pp. 1837-1851.

Roberts SA & Monfort WR. (2007) Haem proteins. In: Encyclopedia of life science. doi: 10.1002/9780470015902.a0003054

Rodríguez-Manzaneque MT, Ros J, Cabiscol E, Sorribas A & Herrero E. (1999) Grx5 glutaredoxin plays a central role in protection against protein oxidative damage in *Saccharomyces cerevisiae. Mol. Cell. Biol.* Vol. 19, No. 12, pp. 8180–8190.

Rodríguez-Manzaneque MT, Tamarit J, Bellí G, Ros J & Herrero E. (2002) Grx5 is a mitochondrial glutaredoxin required for the activity of iron/sulfur enzymes. *Mol. Biol. Cell.* Vol. 13, No. 4, pp. 1109–1121.

Roger AJ & Simpson AGB. (2009) Evolution: revisiting the root of the eukaryote tree. *Curr. Biol.* Vol. 19, No. 4, pp. 165–167.

Rouault TA & Tong W-H. (2005) Iron-sulphur cluster biogenesis and mitochondrial iron homeostasis. *Nat. Rev. Mol. Cell Biol.* Vol 6, No. 4, pp. 345–351.

Rouhier N, Couturier J, Johnson MK & Jacquot J-P. (2010) Glutaredoxins: roles in iron homeostasis. *Trends Biochem. Sci.* Vol. 35, No. 1, pp. 43–52.

Saas J, Ziegelbauer K, von Haeseler A, Fast B & Boshart M. (2000) A developmentally regulated aconitase related to iron-regulatory protein-1 is localized in the cytoplasm and in the mitochondrion of *Trypanosoma brucei*. *J. Biol. Chem.* Vol. 275, No. 4, pp. 2745–2755.

Salmon D, Geuskens M, Hanocq F, Hanocq-Quertier J, Nolan D, Ruben L & Pays E. (1994). A novel heterodimeric transferrin receptor encoded by a pair of VSG expression site-associated genes in *T. brucei*. Cell. Vol. 78, No. 1, pp. 75-86.

Salzman TA, Stella AM., Wider de Xifra EA., Del Batlle AM, Docampo R & Stoppani AOM. (1982) Porphyrin biosynthesis in parasitic hemoflagellates: functional and defective enzymes in *Trypanosoma cruzi*. *Comp. Biochem. Physiol.* Vol. 72B, No. 4, pp. 663-667.

Sauvage V, Aubert D, Escotte-Binet S & Villena I. (2009) The role of ATP-binding cassette (ABC) proteins in protozoan parasites. *Mol. Biochem. Parasitol.* Vol. 167, No. 2, pp. 81–94.

Schlecker T, Comini MA, & Krauth-Siegel RL. (2007) Chapter 11: The trypanothione system, pp. 231-252. In: Peroxiredoxin systems: Structures and functions. Eds. Leopold Flohé and Robin J. Harris. Springer-Verlag, Berlin, Germany. ISBN 9781402060502

Schultz IJ, Chen C, Paw BH & Hamza I. (2010) Iron and porphyrin trafficking in heme biogenesis. *J. Biol. Chem.* Vol. 285, No. 35, pp. 26753–26759.

Severance S & Hamza, I. Trafficking of heme and porphyrins in metazoa. (2009) *Chem. Rev.* Vol. 109, pp. 4596-4616.

Sharma AK, Pallesen LJ, Spang RJ & Walden WE. (2010) Cytosolic iron-sulfur cluster assembly (CIA) system: factors, mechanism, and relevance to cellular iron regulation. *J. Biol. Chem.* Vol. 285, No. 35, pp. 26745–26751.

Sharma RN & Pancholi SS. (2010) Oral Iron Chelators: A New Avenue for the Management of Thalassemia Major. *J. Curr. Pharm. Res.* Vol. 1, pp. 1-7.

Shi Y, Ghosh MC, Tong W-H & Rouault TA. (2009) Human ISD11 is essential for both iron-sulfur cluster assembly and maintenance of normal cellular iron homeostasis. *Hum. Mol. Genet.* Vol. 18, No. 16, pp. 3014–3025.

Simpson AG, Lukes, J & Roger, AJ (2002) The evolutionary history of kinetoplastids and their kinetoplasts. *Mol. Biol. Evol.* Vol. 19, No. 12, pp. 2071-2083.

Simpson AGB, Stevens JR & Lukes J. (2006) The evolution and diversity of kinetoplastid flagellates. *Trends Parasitol.* Vol. 22, No. 4, pp. 168–174.

Smíd O, Horáková E, Vilímová V, Hrdy I, Cammack R, Horváth A, Lukes J & Tachezy J. (2006) Knock-downs of iron-sulfur cluster assembly proteins IscS and IscU down-regulate the active mitochondrion of procyclic *Trypanosoma brucei*. *J. Biol. Chem.* Vol. 281, No. 39, pp. 28679–28686.

Stemmler TL, Lesuisse E, Pain D & Dancis A. (2010) Frataxin and mitochondrial FeS cluster biogenesis. *J. Biol. Chem.* Vol. 285, No. 35, pp. 26737–26743.

Stevens JR, Noyes H & Gibson W. (1998) The evolution of trypanosomes infecting humans and primates. *Mem. Inst. Oswaldo Cruz.* Vol. 93, No. 5, pp. 669-676.

Stevens JR, Noyes HA, Schofield CJ & Gibson W. (2001) The molecular evolution of Trypanosomatidae. *Adv. Parasitol.* Vol. 48, pp. 1-56.

Steverding D, Stierhof YD, Fuchs H, Tauber R & Overath P. (1995) Transferrin-binding protein complex is the receptor for transferrin uptake in *Trypanosoma brucei*. *J. Cell Biol.* Vol. 131, No. 5, pp. 1173-1182.

Steverding D. (1998). Bloodstream forms of *Trypanosoma brucei* require only small amounts of iron for growth. *Parasitol. Res.* Vol. 84, No. 1, pp, 59-62.

Steverding D. (2003). The significance of transferrin receptor variation in *Trypanosoma brucei*. *Trends Parasitol.* Vol. 19, No. 3, pp. 125-127.

Steverding D. (2006). On the significance of host antibody response to the *Trypanosoma brucei* transferrin receptor during chronic infection. *Microbes Infect.* Vol. 8, pp. 2777-2782.

Steverding D, Wang X & Sexton DW. (2009) The trypanocidal effect of NO-releasing agents is not due to inhibition of the major cysteine proteinase in *Trypanosoma brucei*. *Parasitol. Res.* Vol. 105, No. 5, pp. 1333–1338.

Steverding D. (2010) The development of drugs for treatment of sleeping sickness: a historical review. *Parasit. Vectors.* Vol. 3, No. 1, pp. 15.

Stijlemans B, Vankrunkelsven A, Brys L, Magez S & De Baetselier P. (2008) Role of iron homeostasis in trypanosomiasis-associated anemia. *Immunobiology.* Vol. 213, No. 9-10, pp. 823–835.

Stijlemans B, Vankrunkelsven A, Brys L, Raes G, Magez S & De Baetselier P. (2010a) Scrutinizing the mechanisms underlying the induction of anemia of inflammation through GPI-mediated modulation of macrophage activation in a model of African trypanosomiasis. Microbes Infect. Vol. 12, No. 5, pp. 389–399.

Stijlemans B, Vankrunkelsven A, Caljon G, Bockstal V, Guilliams M, Bosschaerts T, Beschin A, Raes G, Magez S & De Baetselier P. (2010b) The central role of macrophages in trypanosomiasis-associated anemia: rationale for therapeutical approaches. *Endocr. Metab. Immune Disord. Drug Targets.* Vol. 10, No. 1, pp. 71–82.

Subramanian P, Rodrigues AV, Ghimire-Rijal S & Stemmler TL. (2011) Iron chaperones for mitochondrial Fe-S cluster biosynthesis and ferritin iron storage. *Curr Opin Chem Biol.* Vol. 15, No. 2, pp. 312–318.

Sutak R, Lesuisse E, Tachezy J & Richardson DR. (2008) Crusade for iron: iron uptake in unicellular eukaryotes and its significance for virulence. *Trends Microbiol.* Vol. 16, No. 6, pp. 261–268.

Taylor MC & Kelly JM. (2010) Iron metabolism in trypanosomatids, and its crucial role in infection. *Parasitology.* Vol. 137, No. 6, pp. 899–917.

Temperton NJ, Wilkinson SR, Meyer DJ & Kelly JM. (1998) Overexpression of superoxide dismutase in *Trypanosoma cruzi* results in increased sensitivity to the trypanocidal agents gentian violet and benznidazole. *Mol. Biochem. Parasitol.* Vol. 96, No. 1-2, pp. 67–76.

Tripodi KE, Menendez Bravo SM, & Cricco JA. *(2011)* Role of heme and heme-proteins in trypanosomatid essential metabolic pathways. *Enzyme Res.* 873230.

Tsuda A, Witola WH, Ohashi K & Onuma M. (2005) Expression of alternative oxidase inhibits programmed cell death-like phenomenon in bloodstream form of *Trypanosoma brucei* rhodesiense. *Parasitol. Int.* Vol. 54, No. 4, pp. 243–251.

Tsuda A, Witola WH, Konnai S, Ohashi K & Onuma M. (2006) The effect of TAO expression on PCD-like phenomenon development and drug resistance in *Trypanosoma brucei*. *Parasitol. Int.* Vol. 55, No. 2, pp. 135–142.

Tyler KM, Matthews KR & Gull K. (1997) The bloodstream differentiation-division of *Trypanosoma brucei* studied using mitochondrial markers. *Proc. Biol. Sci.* Vol. 264, No. 1387, pp. 1481–1490.

Urban P, Mignotte C, Kazmaier MI, Delorme F & Pompon D. (1997) Cloning, yeast expression, and characterization of the coupling of two distantly related *Arabidopsis thaliana* NADPH-Cytochrome P450 reductases with P450 CYP73A5. *J. Biol. Chem. Vol.* 272, No. 31, pp. 19176-19186.

Uttaro AD (2006) Biosynthesis of polyunsaturated fatty acids in lower eukaryotes. *IUBMB Life*, Vol. 58, No. 10, pp. 563–571.

van Luenen HG, Kieft R, Mussmann R, Engstler M, ter Riet B & Borst P. (2004). Trypanosomes change their transferrin receptor expression to allow effective uptake of host transferrin. *Mol. Microbiol.* Vol. 58, No. 1, pp. 151-165.

van Weelden SWH, Fast B, Vogt A, van der Meer P, Saas J, van Hellemond JJ, Tielens AGM & Boshart M. (2003) Procyclic *Trypanosoma brucei* Do Not Use Krebs Cycle Activity for Energy Generation. *J. Biol. Chem.* Vol. 278, No. 15, pp. 12854–12863.

Vanden Bosschef H, Koymans L & Moereels H. (1995) P450 inhibitors of use in medical treatment: focus on mechanisms of action. *Pharmac. Ther.* Vol. 67, No. 1, pp. 79-100.

Vanhollebeke B, De Muylder G, Nielsen MJ, Pays A, Tebabi P, Dieu M, Raes M, Moestrup SK & Pays E. (2008) A haptoglobin-hemoglobin receptor conveys innate immunity to *Trypanosoma brucei* in humans. *Science.* Vol. 320, pp. 677-671.

Vanin AF. (2009) Dinitrosyl iron complexes with thiolate ligands: physico-chemistry, biochemistry and physiology. *Nitric Oxide.* Vol. 21, No. 1, pp. 1–13.

Vankrunkelsven A, De Ceulaer K, Hsu D, Liu F-T, De Baetselier P & Stijlemans B. (2010) Lack of galectin-3 alleviates trypanosomiasis-associated anemia of inflammation. *Immunobiology.* Vol. 215, No. 9-10, pp. 833–841.

Vincendeau P, Daulouède S, Veyret B, Darde ML, Bouteille B & Lemesre JL. (1992) Nitric oxide-mediated cytostatic activity on *Trypanosoma brucei gambiense* and *Trypanosoma brucei brucei. Exp. Parasitol.* Vol. 75, No. 3, pp. 353–360.

Welburn SC, Macleod E, Figarella K & Duzensko M. (2006) Programmed cell death in African trypanosomes. *Parasitology.* Vol. 132, Suppl: S7–18.

Wiedemann N, Urzica E, Guiard B, Müller H, Lohaus C, Meyer HE, Ryan MT, Meisinger C, Mühlenhoff U, Lill R & Pfanner N. (2006) Essential role of Isd11 in mitochondrial iron-sulfur cluster synthesis on Isu scaffold proteins. *EMBO J.* Vol. 25, No. 1, pp. 184–195.

Wilkinson SR, Obado SO, Mauricio IL & Kelly JM. (2002) *Trypanosoma cruzi* exhibits a plant-like ascorbate-dependant hemoperoxidase localized to the endoplasmic reticulum. *Proc. Nat. Acad. Sci. USA* Vol. 99, No. 21, pp. 13453-13458.

Wilkinson SR, Taylor MC, Touitha S, Mauricio IL, Meyer DJ & Kelly JM. (2002) TcGPXII, a glutathione-dependent *Trypanosoma cruzi* peroxidase with substrate specificity restricted to fatty acid and phospholipid hydroperoxides, is localized to the endoplasmic reticulum. *Biochem. J.* Vol. 364, pp. 787-794.

Wilkinson SR, Prathalingam SR, Taylor MC, Horn D & Kelly JM. (2005) Vitamin C biosynthesis in trypanosomes: A role for the glycosome. *Proc. Nat. Acad. Sci. USA* Vol. 102, No. 33, pp. 11645-11650.

Wilkinson SR, Prathalingam SR, Taylor MC, Ahmed A, Horn D & Kelly JM. (2006) Functional characterisation of the iron superoxide dismutase gene repertoire in *Trypanosoma brucei. Free Radic. Biol. Med.* Vol. 40, No. 2, pp. 198–209.

Williams S, Saha L, Singha UK, & Chaudhuri M. (2008) *Trypanosoma brucei*. Differential requirement of membrane potential for import of proteins into mitochondria in two developmental stages. *Exp Parasitol.* Vol. 118, No. 3, pp. 420–433.

Wo B, Novelli J, Foster J, Vaisvila R, Conway L, Ingram J, Ganatra M, Rao AU, Hamza I & Slatko B. (2009) The heme biosynthetic pathway of the obligate Wolbachia endosymbiont of *Brugia malayi*. *PLoS Negl. Trop. Dis.* Vol. 3, No. 7, doi:10.1371/journal.pntd.0000475.

Xu XM & Møller SG. (2011) Iron-sulfur clusters: biogenesis, molecular mechanisms, and their functional significance. *Antioxid. Redox Signal.* Vol. 15, No. 1, pp. 271–307.

Ye H & Rouault TA. (2010) Human iron-sulfur cluster assembly, cellular iron homeostasis, and disease. *Biochemistry.* Vol. 49, No. 24, pp. 4945–4956.

Ye H, Jeong SY, Ghosh MC, Kovtunovych G, Silvestri L, Ortillo D, Uchida N, Tisdale J, Camaschella C & Rouault TA. (2010) Glutaredoxin 5 deficiency causes sideroblastic anemia by specifically impairing heme biosynthesis and depleting cytosolic iron in human erythroblasts. *J. Clin. Invest.* Vol. 120, No. 5, pp. 1749–1761.

Ye H & Rouault TA. Erythropoiesis and iron sulfur cluster biogenesis. (2010) *Adv. Hematol.* 329394.

Zhang A-S & Enns CA. (2009) Iron homeostasis: recently identified proteins provide insight into novel control mechanisms. *J. Biol. Chem.* Vol. 284, No. 2, pp. 711–715.

Zhang Y, Lyver ER, Nakamaru-Ogiso E, Yoon H, Amutha B, Lee D-W, Bi E, Ohnishi T, Daldal F, Pain D & Dancis A. (2008) Dre2, a conserved eukaryotic Fe/S cluster protein, functions in cytosolic Fe/S protein biogenesis. *Mol. Cell. Biol.* Vol. 28, No. 18, pp. 5569–5582.